Medication Safety:
A Guide for Health Care Facilities

Henri R. Manasse, Jr.

Kasey K. Thompson

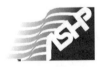

American Society of Health-System Pharmacists®
Bethesda, Maryland

For more than 60 years, ASHP has helped pharmacists who practice in hospitals and health systems improve medication use and enhance patient safety. The Society's 30,000 members include pharmacists and pharmacy technicians who practice in inpatient, outpatient, home-care, and long-term-care settings, as well as pharmacy students. For more information about the wide array of ASHP activities and the many ways in which pharmacists help people make the best use of medicines, visit ASHP's Web site, www.ashp.org, or its consumer Web site, www.SafeMedication.com.

Any correspondence regarding this publication should be sent to the publisher, American Society of Health-System Pharmacists, 7272 Wisconsin Avenue, Bethesda, MD, 20814, attn: Special Publishing.

Produced in conjunction with the ASHP Publications Production Center.

Acquisitions Editor: Cynthia M. Conner
Senior Project Editor: Bill Fogle
Design Manager: David A. Wade

ISBN: 1-58528-089-5

Table of Contents

Contributors

Editors

Henri R. Manasse, Jr., Ph.D., Sc.D.
Executive Vice President and Chief Executive Officer
American Society of Health-System Pharmacists
Bethesda, MD

Kasey K. Thompson, Pharm.D.
Director
Practice Standards and Quality Division
American Society of Health-System Pharmacists
Bethesda, MD

Contributors

C. J. Biddle, CRNA, Ph.D.
Professor and Clinical Staff Anesthetist
Department of Nurse Anesthesia
Virginia Commonwealth University
Richmond, VA

Joseph K. Bonnarens, R.Ph., Ph.D.
Assistant Professor
Social and Administrative Pharmacy Division
School of Pharmacy
University of Wisconsin-Madison

Mary E. Burkhardt, M.S., R.Ph., FASHP
Program Manager
Veterans Administration National Center for Patient Safety
Ann Arbor, MI

Daniel J. Cobaugh, Pharm.D., DABAT
Director of Research
ASHP Research and Education Foundation
American Society of Health-System Pharmacists
Bethesda, MD

Richard I. Cook, MD
Associate Professor
Department of Anesthesia and Intensive Care
Director
Cognitive Technologies Laboratory
University of Chicago

David Cousins
Head of Safe Medication Practice
National Patient Safety Agency
London, England

Vicki S. Crane, M.S., R.Ph.
Vice President, Pharmacy Services
Parkland Hospital and Health System
Dallas, TX

Richard J. Faris, B.S. Pharm., M.Sc., Ph.D.
Assistant Professor, Pharmacoeconomics and Health Policy
Department of Pharmaceutical Sciences
University of Tennessee College of Pharmacy
Memphis, TN

Roxanne J. Goeltz
Co-founder and President
Consumers Advancing Patient Safety
Professional Air Traffic Controller
Burnsville, MN

Bruce M. Gordon, Pharm.D.
Principal Consultant
Premier, Inc., Pharmacy Services
Co-coursemaster, Medication Safety in Healthcare
School of Pharmacy
University of Maryland
College Park, MD

Laura Lin Gosbee, MASc
Human Factors Engineering Consultant
Red Forest Consulting, LLC
Ann Arbor, MI

David N. Gragg, R.Ph., M.B.A.
Medication Safety Officer and Manager
Operations Development
Department of Pharmacy
The Cleveland Clinic Foundation
Cleveland, OH

William R. Hendee, Ph.D.
Senior Associate Dean and Vice President
Dean of the Graduate School of Biomedical Sciences
Professor and Vice-Chair of Radiology
Professor of Bioethics, Biophysics, and Radiation Oncology
Medical College of Wisconsin
Milwaukee, WI

Ross W. Holland, Ph.D., Ed.D.
Dean
Australian College of Pharmacy Practice
Canberra, Australia

Timothy S. Lesar, Pharm.D.
Director of Pharmacy
Patient Care Service Director
Albany Medical Center
Albany, NY

Kevin Marvin, R.Ph., M.S.
Project Manager
Information Services
Fletcher Allen Healthcare
Burlington, VT

Sondra May, Pharm.D.
Medication Safety Coordinator
University of Colorado Hospital
Aurora, CO

Gerald K. McEvoy, Pharm.D.
Assistant Vice President of Drug Information
Editor, *AHFS Drug Information*
American Society of Health-System Pharmacists
Bethesda, MD

Marsha K. Millonig, M.B.A., R.Ph.
President
Catalyst Enterprises, LLC
Eagan, MN

John F. Mitchell, Pharm.D., FASHP
Medication Safety Coordinator
Department of Pharmacy Services
University of Michigan Health System
Ann Arbor, MI

Christine M. Nimmo, Ph.D.
Director of Educational Resources
American Society of Health-System Pharmacists
Bethesda, MD

Michael F. O'Connor, MD
Associate Professor
Department of Anesthesia and Intensive Care
Head, Section of Intensive Care
University of Chicago

Jerry G. Phillips, R.Ph.
President
Drug Safety Institute
Miami, FL

Darryl S. Rich, Pharm.D., M.B.A., FASHP
Field Representative
Joint Commission on Accreditation of Healthcare Organizations
Roseville, CA

Michael D. Sanborn, M.S., R.Ph., FASHP
Director of Pharmacy Services
Baylor University Medical Center
Dallas, TX

Bruce R. Siecker, Ph.D., R.Ph.
President
Business Research Services, Inc.
Aldie, VA

Joanne E. Turnbull, Ph.D.
Executive Director
The National Patient Safety Foundation
North Adams, MA

Lee C. Vermeulen, R.Ph., M.S.
Director
Center for Drug Policy and Clinical Economics
University of Wisconsin Hospitals and Clinics
Clinical Associate Professor
University of Wisconsin School of Pharmacy
Madison, WI

Foreword

When I was a young pharmacy director, a patient at our hospital died after receiving a tenfold overdose of morphine. The overdose was caused by a miscalculation by a staff pharmacist. The incident devastated the pharmacist. She not only quit her job (without any pressure from the hospital) but left the profession of pharmacy as well.

The majority of today's pharmacists would likewise be devastated by the realization that they had committed such an error. No one wants to make an error of any kind, especially a life-threatening or fatal one. Yet many of us practice pharmacy every day without giving any thought to safety; it's as if we were on autopilot. Our clinical knowledge and skills are more commonly focused on cost-containment goals handed down by hospital administration than on patient safety. While keeping down the cost of health care serves a public good, we cannot unwittingly sacrifice patient safety in the process.

Some of us rationalize that the way we've always done things is good enough, and that "more attention to detail" is all that is needed. The scientific literature and reporting databases on medication errors prove otherwise. Medication errors are most commonly the result of systems problems. People make errors because of flaws that are inherent in the systems that they work with, not because they do not pay enough attention.

Past and current approaches to reducing medication errors, including a necessary emphasis on quality-control techniques, have clearly proved inadequate. We need creative solution—solutions that will reduce risk points and prevent errors in the medication-use system. This requires that we think beyond the routine and turn away from the status quo. And there is evidence that our profession is willing to take on the task. As I survey many organizations across the country, I am convinced that most hospital pharmacists do want to develop safer, better-performing medication systems.

It has been six years since the release of the Institute of Medicine report *To Err Is Human: Building a Safer Health System*. Despite the wide publicity and support that this landmark document received, there have been only modest gains in improving medication safety since it appeared. If a majority of hospital pharmacists do want to improve their medication systems, why haven't we have made greater progress?

I believe that it is because most pharmacists do not know how to effect the changes needed to make medication-use systems better. While pharmacists, particularly directors of pharmacy, are good at making improvements in their own domains, the fact remains that medication management is a multidisciplinary process. The medication-use system is beyond the control of the pharmacy department alone. Once they try to become change agents, pharmacists often find that things they thought were under their control are in fact not. A proposal to make even the simplest of changes, such as removing concentrated potassium chloride from all patient care units, elicits internal struggles that make the Battle of Gettysburg seem like a minor skirmish.

Why is it so difficult to make changes to improve medication safety? One reason is that health care is one of the most complex and slowest-changing systems in the United States. All organizations must deal with resistance to change, but in health care this hurdle is particularly high. The independence, or rather independent attitudes, of health care practitioners and the lack of strong clinical leadership in most hospitals make achieving a consensus very hard.

I recently attended a seminar with more than 500 health care practitioners of various professions. The speaker, a well-known former astronaut with a doctoral degree in engineering, discussed standardization and other error-reduction techniques used by the National Aeronautics and Space Administration. As I listened, I envisioned a number of ways in which the strategies he described could be applied to improving medication-management systems in hospitals. Yet during the ensuing question-and-answer period, it became obvious that people in the room felt that the presentation had no relevance to health care. Seminar participants claimed that "every patient has to be treated uniquely," and that standardization is therefore not possible. The Joint Commission on Accreditation of Healthcare Organizations gets similar feedback regarding its national patient safety goal of requiring standardization of intravenous concentrations. These examples demonstrate the strong resistance to change in health care as well as the lack of the knowledge and creativity needed to modify and apply to health care practices that have been successful in other areas.

Given such barriers, some pharmacists simply give up and try to come to terms with the status quo. Others look to organizations such as the Joint Commission to provide the "gun" that will effect change in their organizations. Usually, they find only resistance and frustration. At the Joint Commission, we have come to realize that even with all the laws, regulations, standards, goals, and other "guns" we can muster, we can achieve only modest gains unless patient safety becomes a priority in the culture of the entire organization and is supported from the top down. The organizational culture must be characterized by open-mindedness and flexibility, and by a commitment to the best interests of the patients.

How can pharmacists learn to effect necessary changes in the medication-management system that are essential for patient safety? This is where *Medication Safety: A Guide for Health Care Facilities* shines. This book is comprehensive. It recognizes medication safety as a systems problem—one that has no quick fixes. It includes topics ranging from medication safety as public policy to scientific research on patient safety to human factors engineering theory. It describes specific error-reduction and prevention strategies. Some of these strategies, such as the use of a medication-safety team and application of best practices, are broad based. Others cover specialized areas such as poison control and investigational drug use.

The book also discusses how to overcome some of the common root causes of medication errors—poor information management and ineffective communication. It gives the reader the broad background needed to effect change as well as a detailed blueprint for moving forward with an organizational medication-safety action plan. The book describes how to obtain administrative support by building a business case for patient safety. It covers reorienting the culture of the organization (and people in it) toward patient safety. It gives readers many of the tools necessary to be effective change agents for patient safety within their own organizations.

When I think of the task before us, I am reminded of a television commercial for a major national bank. In this ad, the spokesperson for the bank, which processes millions of checks daily, states that, "not one error in tens of millions is acceptable, when it is your money." Wouldn't it be wonderful if all pharmacists would voice a similar message— "Not one error in tens of millions of drugs dispensed is acceptable, when it is your life on the line"?

By applying the principles in this book, some sustained creative thinking, and a willingness to become strong leaders and advocates for medication safety, we can make this happen.

Darryl S. Rich, Pharm.D., M.B.A, FASHP
Field Representative
Joint Commission on Accreditation
of Healthcare Organizations
Roseville, California

Acknowledgements

The authors would like to acknowledge the following individuals:

First and foremost we would like to acknowledge the patients and families who have suffered as a result of preventable medication errors. Only through study of their misfortunes can we hope to gain a better understanding of how errors occur and, even more importantly, how to prevent them. Their losses inspire us to zealously seek ways to make health care safer.

We would like to thank the health care professionals who work diligently day after day to provide the safest and most effective care to their patients, often with inadequate resources and in workplace cultures that haven't made safety a priority. We applaud those who persevere despite these challenges, working to compel administrators to provide the necessary resources and engaging with other health professionals, patients, and families to ensure that the health care provided is safe and effective.

We would also like to thank all of the amazing contributors to this book, who volunteered their time, talents, and energy to writing what we believe is one of the best and most useful contributions to the patient safety literature to date. We send a personal thanks to our friend and colleague, Scott Cowan, for embracing the vision we had for this book and for working with us as a key member of the editing and writing team.

Finally, we would like to acknowledge the loving support of our families, especially our wives, Arlynn Manasse and Christina Thompson, without which none of this would have been possible.

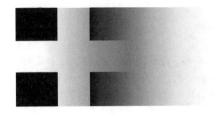

CHAPTER 1

Medication-Use Safety as a Problem in Public Policy

Henri R. Manasse, Jr., and
Kasey K. Thompson

The Nature of the Problem

In 1989, Manasse[1,2] published a series of papers entitled Medication Use in an Imperfect World: Drug Misadventuring as an Issue of Public Policy. The intent of that work was to articulate the prevalence of medication use among Americans, to discuss the risks associated with chemical therapeutics, and to communicate the significance of medication misadventuring as an issue demanding review in American public policy. In this chapter, we review some of the progress that has been achieved in the intervening years, identify some areas where conditions may have in fact deteriorated, and suggest critical issues that need to be addressed, now and in the near future, to facilitate meaningful policy discussion, planning, and action.

Americans have been conditioned and acculturated to believe that there is a "pill for every ill." Whatever the cause of our illness, injury, or discomfort—heredity, unintended exposure to pathogens, or our own behavior—there is almost always a pill, powder, or potion that promises to heal or at least help us. Trends in drug development, marketing, utilization, and spending reflect these attitudes. Direct-to-consumer advertising of prescription drugs takes advantage of these cultural views.

DRUG RESEARCH AND DEVELOPMENT

Since the U.S. Food and Drug Administration (FDA) began approving new drug products in 1939, more than 3,200 FDA-approved prescription drugs have entered the U.S. market as new chemical entities.[3] Some 18,000 drugs and their dosage forms, containing more than 4,750 active ingredients, have been approved for U.S. marketing.[4] The pharmaceutical industry estimates that more than $800 million is spent to develop a single new pharmaceutical product to market readiness. Others have suggested that that figure is inflated; nonetheless, drug development is a high-tech, expensive enterprise.[5] Since the middle of the twentieth century, advances in science and technology have driven unrelenting innovation in the biological and chemical treatment of disease. Current work in genomic and proteomic medicine promises to open new doors in the treatment of disorders once thought untreatable. Aside from the obvious social and medical benefits of this ongoing innovation, drug development and marketing continue to be exceptionally good business, garnering double-digit profit margins for pharmaceutical manufacturers and making the largest few such companies among America's most profitable businesses. In 2003, sales of prescription medicines in the United States exceeded $215 billion.[6]

DRUG UTILIZATION AND EXPENDITURES

As pharmaceutical production and innovation increase, utilization responds in kind. More than 3.4 billion prescriptions were filled in the United States in 2003, an increase of 60 percent from 1992.[6] A recent survey by the American Society of Health-System Pharmacists indicates that 46 percent of Americans regularly take one or more prescription drugs.[7] Drug therapy is increasingly relied upon to supplement, and in many cases to replace, surgical and other types of interventions. This shift is particularly prevalent in the treatment of chronic diseases, which have replaced infectious diseases as the primary causes of death in the United States and as the prime drivers of U.S. health spending. Of the 36 million persons aged 65 or older in the United States (constituting one citizen in eight), an estimated 53 percent use three or more prescription medications concurrently.[8] Census projections indicate that the elderly will make up at least 20 percent of the U.S. population by the year 2030. It is reasonable to expect a concomitant increase in medication utilization and expenditure.

National health expenditures accounted for 14.9 percent of the U.S. gross domestic product in 2002, totaling nearly $1.6 trillion.[9] Of that amount, 12.5 percent, or $194 billion, was spent on prescription drugs, making them the third-highest type of health care expenditure, after hospital costs and physician fees.[9,10] Americans spent at least an additional $17 billion on over-the-counter drugs in 2002,[11] and hospitals spent $21.3 billion to acquire prescription drugs for their patients.[6]

POTENCY AND COMPLEXITY OF CHEMICAL THERAPEUTICS

The introduction of a foreign chemical or biological agent into the human body carries with it a degree of inextricable risk. As new drug products are developed that possess not only greater therapeutic potential but also greater toxic power, the risks of undesirable and significant side effects increase. Moreover, as prescribers face an ever-wider array of drugs from which to choose, the likelihood that the same patient will use multiple drugs concurrently will increase—whether as part of a coordinated therapeutic regimen or as the accidental result of multiple, unconnected prescribers along the continuum of care. Preskorn[3] calculates that if a prescriber had access to the entire "menu" of 3,200 drugs available on the U.S. market, and the patient was prescribed five different drugs from that list during the course of treatment, there could potentially be 2.79×10^{15} drug combinations—certainly posing the threat of harmful drug-drug interactions.

As the volume and potency of drugs increase, so do the complexity and risk involved in conveying them from producer to patient. Substantial research, not only in medication safety but also in accident theory and systems science, has demonstrated the capacity of high-hazard industries for improving safety through system design. Stakeholder groups have undertaken a number of national initiatives in recent years to draw attention to the criticality of public commitment and political will to ensure that such improvements are broadly applied and, where necessary, publicly mandated and supported. Public policy has endeavored over the past century to ensure that medications are appropriately labeled, that drug products are chemically safe when used in the intended strength and setting, and that patients can obtain particularly potent drugs only through the prescription process. However, government legislation and regulation have not kept pace with the complexity of the use—the movement, management, and application—of medications.

CONTEMPORARY TERMINOLOGY USED TO DEFINE MEDICATION ERRORS

Meaningful policy must use language that articulates its scope and intent as clearly as possible. The lexicon of medication safety is not adequately standardized among health care organizations, health professionals, and policy makers. Think for a moment about the myriad terms used to describe medication errors. Terms such as *medication misadventure, adverse drug event, preventable adverse drug event, unpreventable adverse drug event,* and others are used in so many variations and permutations as to make consistent analysis or meaningful discussion seem impossible. The challenges presented by the lack of standardization in terminology hamper internal error-reporting efforts in hospitals, state-based initiatives to share data reported to voluntary reporting systems, and national efforts to develop effective public policy. Significant efforts have been made, however, to attempt to develop universally recognized terms.

The National Coordinating Council for Medication Error Reporting and Prevention (NCC MERP) has developed perhaps the most comprehensive definition of medication error.[12]

> A medication error is any preventable event that may cause or lead to inappropriate medication use or patient harm while the medication is in the control of the health care professional, patient, or consumer. Such events may be related to professional practice, health care products, procedures, and systems, including prescribing; order communication; product labeling, packaging, and nomenclature; compounding; dispensing; distribution; administration; education; monitoring; and use.

The NCC MERP has also developed a widely used taxonomy for error reporting. The taxonomy provides a logical framework for the development of internal error-reporting programs as well as a means to classify and analyze medication errors consistent with the NCC MERP or institution-specific definition.

More broadly defined terminology has been developed by the U.S. Department of Veterans Affairs to encompass the potential universe of adverse events, including medication errors.[13]

> Adverse events are untoward incidents, therapeutic misadventures, iatrogenic injuries or other adverse occurrences directly associated with care or services provided within the jurisdiction of a medical center, outpatient clinic or other facility. Adverse events may result from acts of commission or omission (e.g., administration of the wrong medication, failure to make a timely diagnosis or institute the appropriate therapeutic intervention, adverse reactions or negative outcomes of treatment, etc.).

In 1995, Bates and colleagues[14] more narrowly defined an adverse *drug* event as an injury resulting from medical intervention related to a drug.

Manasse[1] has characterized drug misadventuring as follows.

Any iatrogenic hazard or incident

1. that is an inherent risk when drug therapy is indicated;

2. that is created through either omission or commission by the administration of a drug or drugs during which a patient is harmed, with effects ranging from mild discomfort to fatality;

3. whose outcome may or may not be independent of the preexisting pathology or disease process;

4. that may be attributable to error (human or system or both), immunological response, or idiosyncratic response;

5. that is always unexpected and thus unacceptable to patient and prescriber.

Although these definitions vary in scope and intent, an integral component of each of them is patient harm. Outcomes from medication therapy are always intended to be positive. There is little disagreement on this point. However, the challenges arise when organizations seek to measure their medication-error rates in order to identify trends and to design and effect improvements. At the organizational level, in addition to having clearly defined terms, it is important that the individuals reporting errors have a general understanding of what defines an error in their organization. The level of understanding must be extremely high for individuals who are responsible for analyzing error data on the basis on narrative reports submitted by health care professionals and other staff.

Challenges deepen when attempts to gather and compare error data at the national level are considered. Many believe that a voluntary national reporting system for medication errors would facilitate learning and quality improvement. However, the challenges in comparing data from one organization to the next—challenges stemming from lack of standardization of terminology, of measurement strategies, and of individuals' understanding of the reporting system—diminish the prospect that a great deal can be learned from national error data.

Many hope that as individual hospitals continue to enhance their commitment to learning from errors, a push to standardize terminology at the local, state, and national levels will emerge and prevail. Technology used in a real-time fashion to passively and actively capture error data will likely be a prime driver toward standardization. Technologies such as computerized prescriber order entry (CPOE), bedside scanning using bar-code technology, electronic medical records, "smart" infusion devices, and automated storage and distribution devices that record information at the point of care hold great promise, especially if the data being captured are analyzed using standard terminology and translated into quality improvement at all levels.

Overview of Current Literature

For any issue to merit attention on a level of national policy, sufficient data must be available to demonstrate its relevance and urgency on a national scale. Policy makers must be educated—and convinced—by objective, balanced analysis of all facets of a problem, so that policy is not driven by political or otherwise-unbalanced purposes. In our particular case, the question becomes: Just how prevalent and how severe are medication misadventures? Do they constitute a problem that genuinely demands the attention and full weight of law and regulation?

Research and experience amassed over the past two decades tell us that the answer to this question is an emphatic yes. Medication misadventures, the data demonstrate, are common, costly, and—by and large—preventable. Additional human, economic, technological, and political resources need to be brought to bear to combat what can accurately be described as a significant threat to public health.

THREE CHARACTERISTICS OF MEDICATION MISADVENTURES

Medication misadventuring is *common*. The late 1990s, in particular, witnessed an upsurge in public and political concern over the quality and cost of health care. This increased concern was driven largely by significant year-to-year growth in health insurance premiums, a continual paring down of health benefits and services offered by employers and managed care entities, and frequent news reports making it plain that the quality and safety of health care were not what they should be. In addition to several tragic medical and medication-related accidents that appeared in news headlines during the 1990s, *To Err Is Human: Building a Safer Health System*, the much-publicized report by the Institute of Medicine (IOM) of the National Academy of Sciences, painted a grim picture of the "brokenness" of health care services in the United States.[15]

The IOM reported the findings of two large studies among hospitalized patients in New York, Colorado, and Utah that estimated that adverse medical events occur in between 2.9 percent and 3.7 percent of all hospital admissions, that more than half of those events are preventable, and that preventable adverse events kill between 44,000 and 98,000 Americans in hospitals each year—ranking them within the top 10 causes of death in the United States.[15-18] Of particular concern to health professionals involved in the medication-use process was the additional finding, in the same (and other) studies, that adverse medical events originate more frequently from errors and accidents in the processes of prescribing, ordering, dispensing, administration, and monitoring of medications than from any other source.[19] Lazarou et al.[20] determined that adverse drug reactions (a subset of adverse drug events that does not include events caused by human error but rather pertains to adverse events stemming from the proper, intended use of medications) cause 4.7 percent of hospital admissions and may kill as many as 76,000 to 137,000 hospital patients annually—a much bleaker picture than that conveyed by the IOM.

Although adverse drug events are perhaps easiest to identify and study in the adult acute-care hospital setting, they have an impact on the entire continuum of care. Significant incidences of medication misadventuring have been identified in pediatric facilities[21]; emergency departments (both as a reason for admission to trauma centers[22,23] and as a result of trauma-based care[24]); surgical intensive-care units[25,26]; outpatient settings (both hospital-based clinics and physicians' offices)[27]; community pharmacies[28,29]; nursing and long-term care facilities[30,31]; home care settings[32]; and even schools and day care centers where medications are administered to children.[33-35]

Medication misadventuring is *costly*. The statistics just cited give an idea of the considerable morbidity, mortality, and loss of quality of life and human productivity associated with adverse drug events. Other researchers have suggested that drug-related problems have cost hospitals thousands of dollars per admission,[36,37] nursing homes more than 133 percent the amount they actually spend on medications,[38] and the nation in excess of $177 billion annually since 2000.[39]

Finally, medication misadventuring is often *preventable*. The IOM report was both the product and the genesis of a growing body of research that centers on the reporting, quantification, classification, root causes, and, ultimately, the development of strategies for prevention of, adverse medical events.[15] One of its overarching conclusions was that adverse events (among them, medication misadventures) are, in the main, not the results of human incompetence or negligence, but can often be identified, then minimized or prevented, by addressing flaws in the systems engaged in the delivery of health care.

CAUSES OF SYSTEMIC FLAWS

Systemic flaws identified as frequent causes of medication misadventures include[14, 40-42]

- inadequate dissemination and application of drug knowledge to and by prescribing physicians;
- lack of availability to physicians of needed patient information;
- failure to follow organizational rules and protocols governing medication use;
- mental errors and lapses;
- failure to accurately identify drugs in the prescribing or dispensing process;
- failure to accurately interpret handwritten prescriptions;
- inaccurate transcription of dosing instructions, resulting in under- or overdoses; and
- inadequate or unsafe working conditions for the professionals engaged in managing medication use.

As it became increasingly apparent that most medication misadventures were due to system vulnerabilities, innovative researchers and practitioners began to experiment with strategies for correcting these vulnerabilities. Strategies discussed in the literature that show significant promise include

- pharmacist participation on medical rounds, on interdisciplinary health care teams, and in broader direct patient-care roles[14,43-51];
- pharmacist-conducted prospective review of prescription orders;
- CPOE;

- machine-readable coding for identifying drugs and patients and for tracking the flow of products and data throughout the continuum of care;
- electronic medical records;
- clinical decision support;
- automated pharmacy stocking and dispensing;
- interoperability between electronic data and clinical decision-support systems;
- better systems for monitoring and reporting adverse drug events by type, drug class, and severity;
- unit dose and pharmacy-based i.v. admixture systems for drug distribution;
- improved interaction between pharmacists, prescribers, and nurses to resolve discrepancies observed in medication orders; and
- failure mode and effects analysis (FMEA) to anticipate and address potential problems in medication-use systems.

SIGNS OF PROGRESS

Research on the nature, frequency, and preventability of adverse drug events has begun to bear fruit as health insurance payers and companies grow more insistent that providers demonstrate they are implementing these strategies for patients' safety. As discussed below, the Agency for Healthcare Research and Quality has received tens of millions of federal dollars to create grants for safety-related research. Finally, a number of federal and state policy initiatives have been passed in recent years, or are currently under discussion among legislative and regulatory bodies, that follow directly from the professional advocacy that stems from these discoveries.

National Initiatives: The Players and Drivers of Change

Health policy is particularly difficult to develop and enact because it involves such a diverse array of stakeholders. Simply involving health professionals, industry leaders, and politicians will not produce effective policy. Patients, payers, and the legal profession must also be vested with power and accountability.

Expanding access to health care and controlling costs are well-recognized national priorities. One out of six Americans under age 65, or some 40 million people, lacks health insurance. The lower-bound estimate of the annual national economic loss due to lack of insurance is $65 to $130 billion.[52]

Less consideration and fewer resources have been devoted to improving patient safety and overall quality of care as key elements to access and cost control. The aforementioned IOM report *To Err Is Human* shocked the public by stating that nearly 100,000 patients die each year as a result of preventable medical errors. It generated a flurry of activity among both public and private organizations.[16] Since that time, numerous initiatives, with varying degrees of coordination and purpose, have emerged to address and solve the problems associated with medical error. Indeed, the Institute of Medicine itself has orchestrated the drive to improve safety and quality in U.S. health care through publishing a series of reports on various problems associated with the health care delivery system.[15,53-58]

In 1998, the President's Advisory Commission on Consumer Protection and Quality in the Health Care Industry recommended the creation of the National Quality Forum (NQF) as part of an integrated national quality-improvement agenda. The NQF is a public-private partnership whose members represent all parts of the health care system. The NQF is charged with promoting a common approach to measuring health care quality and fostering systemwide capacity for quality improvement.

One of NQF's most successful initiatives to date is the Safe Practices for Better Healthcare project. The project produced 30 safe health care practices that should be universally used in applicable clinical care settings to reduce the risk of harm to patients. Many of the practices, including one in support of the pharmacist's role in the medication-use process, have been adopted by various stakeholder groups, including the Leapfrog Group for Patient Safety.

The Leapfrog Group was founded in 2000 by the Business Roundtable, a national association of Fortune 500 chief executive officers (CEOs). The Leapfrog Group was created to help save lives and reduce preventable medical mistakes by mobilizing employer purchasing power to initiate improvements in the safety of health care and by giving consumers information to make more-informed hospital choices. The Leapfrog Group's primary focus has been to advocate for the use of CPOE, evidence-based hospital referrals, intensivists in intensive-care units, and the most recent "leap," the NQF Safe Practices leap.

Since 2000, the Joint Commission on Accreditation of Healthcare Organizations (JCAHO) has engaged in significant efforts to redesign standards and survey processes to better reflect quality- improvement and patient-safety goals. JCAHO made medication management a top priority by increasing the stringency of these standards and aligning them with a survey process that traces patients' interaction through the process of care. JCAHO has also established a series of patient-safety goals in areas such as improving communication, eliminating dangerous abbreviations, reducing patient harm due to i.v. therapy, and ensuring that health care organizations develop a process for identifying a complete list of a patient's current medications upon admission and for communicating that information to the patient's next provider.

In the late 1990s, the U.S. Department of Veterans Affairs (VA) underwent a seemingly miraculous transformation under the leadership of then-Undersecretary for Health Kenneth Kizer. The VA devoted significant resources to implementing technologies such as bar coding, electronic medical records, and CPOE. It also established its National Center for Patient Safety to coordinate efforts to continuously learn from errors and to develop innovative approaches to improving patient safety. Today, the VA is a shining example of the transformational power of leadership and commitment in effecting culture change and of the subsequent effects of such a commitment on improving patient safety.

The Agency for Healthcare Research and Quality (AHRQ) of the U.S. Department of Health and Human Services (DHHS) has provided grants in excess of $50 million to sponsor studies aimed at learning more about how errors occur, how technology can be used most effectively, and how processes of care can be improved. AHRQ continues to be the conduit through which the Congress provides limited resources for patient-safety research.

The list of organizations involved in one way or another in patient-safety efforts continues to grow. Key challenges remain in how to finance patient safety at the local, state, and federal levels. The cost savings associated with error prevention surely outweigh the high social and financial costs of preventable patient injury, but the true cost savings associated with preventing an event is difficult to determine with current methods of research and accounting.

Continuing to link national safety efforts with state and local programs will eventually result in safer health care organizations. But until protecting patients from harm associated with the process of care becomes engrained in the health provider culture, there will likely continue to be stumbling blocks in the road to progress.

Social and Professional Questions

The complexity of medication use, combined with its social and economic implications, forces a number of critical questions to the surface of professional and political dialogue. Key questions are as follows.

ARE THE HEALTH PROFESSIONS READY TO TRADE "TURF" FOR TEAMS?

Patient care is a collective effort: Patients may require service at any time, at any location, and from any specialty along the continuum of care. Any number of uniquely trained professionals may be involved—from health professionals to health care administrators to support personnel. However, despite its collective nature, patient care can hardly be characterized as coordinated. For example, a community pharmacist may be called on to counsel a patient on a new drug but may have no access to information on that patient's medication history, allergy profile, or other concurrent prescriptions. In such a situation, a harmful reaction may occur. Or a nurse or medical resident may notice an unexpected complication in a patient but fail to suggest the appropriate intervention, for fear of "trumping" the authority of the senior attending physician.

The organizational and systemic complexity of patient care, compounded by the ever-expanding universe of scientific knowledge, demand a departure from the classical model of physician-centered care. The physician has historically been the source of all therapeutic decisions and the gatekeeper between the patient and the rest of the health care system. However, no single health profession or individual practitioner can claim an adequate grasp of all the information needed to treat and manage a patient. Science is simply moving too rapidly and in too many specialized directions. Instead, a new model must emerge—and, in some places, is emerging—where practitioners of different stripes work as a team and are jointly accountable to the patient and the patient's family.

Unfortunately, numerous barriers lurk within current public policy that limit the potential for broad application of team-based care. For example, scope-of-practice acts in 10 states prevent pharmacists from engaging in collaborative practice with physicians. Public health insurance programs fail to provide any incentive for team-based care by failing to recognize certain types of health professionals, including pharmacists, as reimbursable care providers.

Dialogue concerning team-based care is under way among key stakeholders. The IOM endorses the interdisciplinary model in practice and education.[53,55] JCAHO has convened leaders from medicine, nursing, pharmacy, and health administration in a Health Professions Education Roundtable to address these issues. It is still too early to tell when, or whether, the forces of innovation can overcome professional inertia and territorialism. Still, since IOM is specifically charged with advising national health policy, there is hope that its recommendations may someday stimulate public support for a new, team-based care model.

ARE HEALTH CARE ORGANIZATIONS READY TO EMBRACE AND EMBODY A CULTURE OF SAFETY?

The 1994 death of journalist Betsy Lehman from a massive chemotherapy overdose in a Boston hospital was followed by years of litigation, negative publicity, and organizational turmoil. But when young Ben Kolb died from a medication mix-up during routine surgery in a Florida hospital 1995, the family and the hospital quietly reached a financial settlement. The story stayed only briefly in the headlines, and the institution became a leader and model for organizational commitment to safety, transparency, and continuous quality improvement. (It should be noted that in the intervening years, the Boston hospital where Ms. Lehman died has undergone a fundamental transformation, adopting patient safety as its chief organizational priority.)

While these two stories were legally resolved in very different ways, they illustrate a common underlying issue in contemporary health care—the gulf between the "now" and the "not yet"— between a deeply entrenched organizational, even national, culture of blame and a culture of safety. Nearly 10 years have passed since these tragedies occurred, but similar stories continue to appear in the general and health care news media. Health care institutions remain slow to undertake the broad changes necessitated by the complexities and risks associated with caring for patients. They are broad changes that demand a fundamental shift from a mindset that finds and punishes the individuals most closely involved in adverse events (while stonewalling any external inquiry by the patient, family, or community) to a new organizational philosophy that shatters the time-honored model of organizational hierarchy and accountability.

The organizational elements of a safety culture are discussed in detail elsewhere in this book. More appropriate here is a discussion of the roles that public policy plays, and may play in the future, in both helping and hindering the emergence of a national commitment to safety in health care.

REPORTING OF ERRORS AND ADVERSE EVENTS

Mechanisms to facilitate and encourage the reporting of errors and adverse events by health care personnel are starting to surface as a priority in U.S. hospitals and health systems. National reporting frameworks exist in the form of the FDA's MedWatch, the United States Pharmacopeia's MEDMARX, and the recently launched Patient Safety Reporting System, developed jointly by the Department of Veterans Affairs and National Aeronautics and Space Administration. Individual hospitals and health systems are developing reporting systems as well.

While increased use of these systems reflects the growing attention to safety, these systems, with their separate databases and data parameters, do not provide the volume or breadth of data to permit a balanced analysis that would allow the development of broadly applicable solutions. For example, although more than 530,000 reports from roughly 700 hospitals have been submitted to the MEDMARX database since its deployment in 1998, these voluntarily submitted reports hardly constitute a representative sampling of error "nodes" across the U.S. health care continuum. Needed is a coordinated system that can aggregate and analyze data from hospitals, community pharmacies, ambulatory care centers, physicians' offices, long-term care facilities, and even the home care sector.

At present, no U.S. government entity is charged with the collection and analysis of patient-safety data, though other intrinsically hazardous industries are accountable to federal agencies such as the National Transportation Safety Board, the Nuclear Regulatory Commission, the Chemical Safety Board, and the Consumer Product Safety Agency. In 2003, however, the Patient Safety and Quality Improvement Act was introduced in both chambers of Congress. The act would authorize the DHHS to implement a national reporting system. The information gathered by this system would be protected from legal discovery. Patient-safety advocates hoped that this protection would make practitioners more willing to report errors and near misses because the threat of legal and professional reprisal would have been lifted. The House and Senate versions of this legislation passed with great support; however, Congress was not able to work out minor differences between the bills in time to pass the final legislation. This legislation remains a priority, and in late 2004, the incoming chair of the Senate Health, Education, Labor and Pensions Committee vowed to address this issue early in the next session of the Congress.

Another significant piece of legislation introduced to both chambers in 2003 would direct the DHHS to establish a national health information infrastructure, with the aim of electronifying patient medical records, reducing paperwork, ensuring access to patient data across the spectrum of care, and thereby reducing the risk of medical errors and suboptimal treatment. Although this legislation was not enacted, it, too, remains a priority.

PERVERSE FINANCIAL INCENTIVES

A 2003 survey by the American College of Healthcare Executives found that among the top 12 concerns of CEOs of health organizations, patient safety ranked tenth. Only 9 percent of

CEOs placed patient safety first on their lists (a drop of 5 percent from the same survey in 2002). With all the clamor about systemic and culture change, why does safety remain such a low priority among executives?

Not surprisingly, CEOs' chief concern, as revealed by the survey, is securing adequate reimbursement and financing for services. Why should they, or rather how can they, invest millions in the technical resources to improve safety when there is barely enough cash in the coffers to maintain the status quo and little or no prospect exists that those millions will be recouped under current reimbursement mechanisms?

It is not the government's duty to bankroll all health care services in a country without national health insurance. However, in the United States, public funds do account for more than half of health care expenditures. Consequently, public policy decisions can in fact influence how health care is incentivized and reimbursed. When Medicare or Medicaid adopts a certain reimbursement scheme, private insurers normally follow suit. But are we getting what we're paying for? Are we as a nation (or, more to the point, are our employers, who fund most of our health insurance) reimbursing our health providers in a way that rewards them for providing high-quality care? And is there a causal relationship between what we spend and the quality of outcomes?

The answers on both counts appear to be no. The World Health Organization in 2000 ranked the United States 37th (and last among the Group of 7 [G-7] nations) in overall health system performance among more than 190 countries tabulated. This country spends more per capita on health care than does any other country, yet a 2002 study by the Centers for Medicare & Medicaid Services (CMS) indicated that more than 25 percent of Medicare beneficiaries do not receive appropriate care for their particular conditions. It seems clear that the time has come to discard the old model of reimbursing the sheer volume of visits, procedures, and prescriptions provided and to begin to design rewards that recognize the prevention or reversal of illness, the application of current scientific evidence to clinical decisions, and the reduction of harm caused patients by the health system. CMS and some private insurers have recently introduced pay-for-quality incentives. Medicare reform legislation of 2003 cuts reimbursement by 0.4 percent to hospitals that fail to report data on a list of 10 quality measurers developed by CMS and endorsed by the NQF. In 2003, the Blue Cross of California Quality ScoreCard program paid out $28 million in bonuses to participating providers who performed well on an array of quality standards. Several states are reaping improved outcomes and decreased costs by using a disease-management approach, often by means of pharmacist-run clinics. As these and other payment schemes become more prevalent, it seems reasonable to hope that the business case for patient safety will become clearer and that CEOs and chief financial officers will adopt safety not only as a philosophical construct but as a material reality, borne out in daily practice and financial stewardship.

Conceptual Framework and Recommendations for the Design of a New Medication-Use System

We commonly speak of the "health care system" or the "medication-use system." In fact, these terms are misnomers. In *To Err Is Human*, the IOM defines a system as a "set of interdependent elements interacting to achieve a common aim."[15] If this definition is accurate, then one cannot describe health care delivery in the United States as a "system." Rather, it is better described as a hodgepodge of independent processes and silos with very few systematic connections to facilitate communication, teamwork, or safety.

We should not attempt to repair the current medication-use process. Instead, it is time for all health care stakeholders, including patients, to take a blank sheet of paper and begin to conceptualize a new model for a safe, effective, patient-centered, timely, efficient, and equitable medication-use system. The aforementioned elements make up the "six aims for improvement" in health care urged by the Institute of Medicine in its 2001 report *Crossing the Quality Chasm, A New Health System for the 21st Century* (see **Table 1-1**).[53] They should be applied as well in our focused efforts to redesign medication use, so that it takes on the true nature of a system.

Table 1-1. Institute of Medicine's Six Aims for Quality Improvement[53]

Safe	Avoiding injuries to patients from the care that is intended to help them.
Effective	Providing services based on scientific knowledge to all who could benefit and refraining from providing services to those not likely to benefit (avoiding underuse or overuse).
Patient-Centered	Providing care that is respectful of and responsive to individual patient preferences, needs, and values, and ensuring that patient values guide all clinical decisions.
Timely	Reducing waits and sometimes harmful delays for both those who receive and those who give care.
Efficient	Avoiding waste, in particular, waste of equipment, supplies, ideas, and energy.
Equitable	Providing care that does not vary in quality because of personal characteristics such as gender, ethnicity, geographic location, and socioeconomic status.

Safety is the foundation on which the new system should be built. A system cannot meet any of the aims for improvement if it injures the people it is designed to help. The first step, then, will be to understand how people and technology can work in concert to ensure that the system is fundamentally safe. This will demand that stakeholders clear their minds of all preconceived notions about how things have traditionally been done and that they think creatively about what makes sense in terms of using technology in a safe and effective manner, while recognizing its limitations. It will also require that the skill sets of health professionals be scrutinized to ensure that the right people are doing the right jobs in order to meet the needs of patients consistent with the six aims of the IOM.

In recent years, considerable effort has been devoted to describing the ideal design features of the 21st-century health care system, as published in reports by the IOM, patient-safety research, and the work of numerous health care professional organizations, accrediting bodies, and patient-advocacy groups. In most cases, an incrementalist model for change has been applied. Small steps and successes may be the most practical way to improve patient safety, but they certainly will not address the monumental problems we currently face in a timely manner to assure patients that the system designed to help will not cause undue harm. Further, it must be recognized that patient safety is a continuum, which means that we will not suddenly find the perfect solution that "fixes" the system. A reliable mechanism will evolve only if meaningful and ongoing commitments to continuous improvement are agreed on and followed through.

The practical approaches and concepts described by authors throughout this book provide a strong basis for a discussion on building a new medication-use system that meets the six aims for improvement described by the IOM. Underlying the various improvements organizations can implement to make the system safer is the fact that many of the problems that plague our system reside in the belief systems and perceptions of the people that work in that system. Therefore, discussions on how to redesign processes and nonhuman components of systems will have to begin with a discussion on how we, as practitioners and patients, currently perceive the system. If our work is truly about helping people, then our minds must be open to hearing challenges and criticisms of many of the things we have accepted as tried and true.

Many efforts are under way at the national level to support these aims with a policy framework—to protect the data and reporters involved in voluntary error-reporting systems, enhance research, increase the utility and accessibility of electronic information, and attain other laudable goals. These initiatives will likely continue, but discussions on system redesign and culture change must be going on simultaneously at the local level to ensure that innovative approaches and policies are adopted in a timely fashion by individual health care providers and organizations.

Medication errors are no longer a guarded, guilty professional secret. They are a public concern. This is a good thing. It will take passionate voices, political will, and common action to move closer to a true health care system, where every patient can count on care that is safe, effective, patient-centered, timely, efficient, and equitable.

References

1. Manasse HR. Medication use in an imperfect world: drug misadventuring as an issue of public policy, part 1. *Am J Hosp Pharm.*1989;46:929-944.

2. Manasse HR. Medication use in an imperfect world: drug misadventuring as an issue of public policy, part 2. *Am J Hosp Pharm.* 1989;46:1141-1152.

3. Preskorn SH. Drug approvals and withdrawals over the last 60 years. *J Psychiatric Pract.* 2002;8:41-50.

4. Wilson J. Epidemiology and public health impact of drug-induced diseases. In: Miller J, Tisdale D, eds. *Drug-Induced Diseases: Prevention, Detection, and Management.* Bethesda, MD: American Society of Health-System Pharmacists; 2005.

5. Relman AS, Angell M. How the drug industry distorts medicines and politics: America's other drug problem. *New Republic.* 2002(Dec 16);27-41.

6. IMS Health. U.S. purchase activity by channel, 2003. Available at: www.imshealth.org/ims/portal/frontarticleC/0,2777,6599_42720942_44800060,00.html. Accessed July 21, 2004.

7. American Society of Health-System Pharmacists. Snapshot of medication use in the United States. Available at: http://www.ashp.org/pr/snapshot.pdf. Accessed July 21, 2004.

8. American Society of Health-System Pharmacists. Medication use among older Americans. Available at: www.ashp.org/pr/over65.pdf. Accessed July 21, 2004.

9. Levit K, Smith C, Cowan C, et al. Health spending rebound continues in 2002. *Health Affairs.* 2004;23(1):147-59.

10. Hoffman JM, Shah ND, Vermeulen LC, et al. Projecting future drug expenditures–2004. *Am J Health-Syst Pharm.* 2004;61:145-158.

11. Consumer Healthcare Products Association. OTC retail sales—1964–2002. Available at: www.chpa-info.org/web/press_room/statistics/otc_retail_sales.aspx. Accessed July 21, 2004.

12. National Coordinating Council for Medication Error Reporting and Prevention. What Is a Medication Error? Available at: www.nccmerp.org/aboutMedErrors.html. Accessed July 21, 2004.

13. Veterans Administration National Center for Patient Safety. Adverse Events. Available at: www.patientsafety.gov/ae.html. Accessed July 21, 2004.

14. Bates DW, Boyle DL, Vander Vliet MB, et al. Relationship between medication errors and adverse drug events. *J Gen Intern Med.* 1995:10:199-205.

15. Kohn LT, Corrigan JM, Donaldson MD, eds. Committee on Quality of Health in America, Institute of Medicine. *To Err Is Human: Building a Safer Health System.* Washington, DC: National Academy Press; 1999.

16. Brennan TA, Leape LL, Laird NM, et al. Incidence of adverse events and negligence in hospitalized patients: results of the Harvard Medical Practice Study I. *N Engl J Med.* 1991;324:370-376.

17. Brennan TA, Leape LL, Laird NM, et al. The nature of adverse events in hospitalized patients: results of the Harvard Medical Practice Study II. *N Engl J Med.* 1991;324:377-384.

18. Thomas EJ, Studdert DM, Burstin HR, et al. Incidence and types of adverse events and negligent care in Utah and Colorado. *Med Care.* 2000;38:261-271.

19. Bates DW, Cullen DJ, Laird N, et al. Incidence of adverse drug events and potential adverse drug events: implications for prevention. *JAMA.* 1995;274:29-34.

20. Lazarou J, Pomeranz BH, Corey PN. Incidence of adverse drug reactions in hospitalized patients: a meta-analysis of prospective studies. *JAMA.* 1998;279:1200-1205.

21. Fortescue EB, Kaushal R, Landrigan CP, et al. Prioritizing strategies for preventing medication errors and adverse drug events in pediatric inpatients. *Pediatrics.* 2003; 111:722-729.

22. Tafreshi MJ, Melby MJ, Kabck KR, et al. Medication-related visits to the emergency department: a prospective study. *Ann Pharmacother.* 1999;33:1252-1257.

23. Aparasu RR. Drug-related-injury visits to hospital emergency departments. *Am J Health-Syst Pharm.* 1998;55:1158-1161.

24. Lazarus HM, Fox J, Evans RS. Adverse drug events in trauma patients. *J Trauma.* 2003;54:337-343.

25. Herout PM, Erstad BL. Medication errors involving continuously infused medications in a surgical intensive care unit. *Crit Care Med.* 2004;32:428-432.

26. Calabrese AD, Erstad BL, Brandle K, et al.

Medication administration errors in adult patients in the ICU. *Intensive Care Med.* 2001;27:1592-1598.

27. Gandhi TK, Weingart SN, Borus J, et al. Adverse drug events in ambulatory care. *N Engl J Med.* 2003;348:1556-1564.

28. Camp SC, Hallemeskel B, Rogers TL. Telephone prescription errors in two community pharmacies. *Am J Health-Syst Pharm.* 2003;60:13-14.

29. Currie JD, Chrischilles EA, Kuehl AK, et al. Effect of a training program on community pharmacists' detection of and intervention in drug-related problems. *J Am Pharm Assoc.* 1997;NS37:182-191.

30. Monette J, Gurwitz JH, Avorn J. Epidemiology of adverse drug events in the nursing home setting. *Drugs Aging.* 1995;7:203-211.

31. Field TS, Gurwitz JH, Avorn J, et al. Risk factors for adverse drug events among nursing home residents. *Arch Intern Med.* 2001;161:1629-1634.

32. Meredith S, Feldman P, Frey D, et al. Possible medication errors in home healthcare patients. *J Am Geriatr Soc.* 2001;49:719-724.

33. McCarthy AM, Kelly MW, Reed D. Medication administration practices of school nurses. *J School Health.* 2000;70:371-376.

34. Reutzel TJ, Rinku P. Medication management problems reported by subscribers to a school nurse listserv. *J School Nursing.* 2001;17:131-139.

35. Sinkovits HS, Kelly MW, Ernst ME. Medication administration in day care centers for children. *J Am Pharm Assoc.* 2003;43:379-382.

36. Classen DC, Pestonik SL, Evans RS, et al. Adverse drug events in hospitalized patients: excess length of stay, extra costs, and attributable mortality. *JAMA.* 1997;277:301-306.

37. Bates DW, Spell N, Cullen DJ, et al. The costs of adverse drug events in hospitalized patients. *JAMA.* 1997;277:307-311.

38. Bootman JL, Harrison DL, Cox E. The health care cost of drug-related morbidity and mortality in nursing facilities. *Arch Intern Med.* 1997;157:2089-2096.

39. Ernst FR, Grizzle AJ. Drug-related morbidity and mortality: updating the cost-of-illness model. *J Am Pharm Assoc.* 2001;41:192-199.

40. Leape LL, Bates DW, Cullen DJ, et al. Systems analysis of adverse drug events. *JAMA.* 1995;274:35-43.

41. Lesar TS, Briceland L, Stein DS. Factors related to errors in medication prescribing. *JAMA.* 1997;277:312-317.

42. Lesar TS, Lomaestro BM, Pohl H. Medication-prescribing errors in a teaching hospital: a 9-year experience. *Arch Intern Med.* 1997;157:1569-1576.

43. Leape LL, Cullen DJ, Clapp MD, et al. Pharmacist participation on physician rounds and adverse drug events in the intensive care unit. *JAMA.* 1999;282:267-270.

44. Bond CA, Raehl CL, Franke T. Medication errors in United States hospitals. *Pharmacotherapy.* 2001;21:1023-1036.

45. Kucukarslan SN, Peters M, Mlynarek M, et al. Pharmacists on rounding teams reduce preventable adverse drug events in hospital general medicine units. *Arch Intern Med.* 2003;163:2014-2018.

46. American Society of Health-System Pharmacists. Top-priority actions for preventing adverse drug events in hospitals: recommendations of an expert panel. *Am J Health-Syst Pharm.* 1996;53:747-751.

47. Bates DW, Leape LL, Cullen DJ, et al. Effect of computerized physician order entry and a team intervention on prevention of serious medication errors. *JAMA.* 1998;280:1311-1316.

48. Bates DW. Using information technology to reduce rates of medication errors in hospitals. *Br Med J.* 2000;320:778-791.

49. Bates DW, Gawande AA. Improving safety with information technology. *N Engl J Med.* 2003;348:2526-2534.

50. Cohen MR, Senders J, Davis NM. Failure mode and effects analysis: a novel approach to avoiding dangerous medication errors and accidents. *Hosp Pharm.* 1994;29:319-330.

51. Schneider PJ, Hartwig SC. Use of severity-indexed medication error reports to improve quality. *Hosp Pharm.* 1994;29:205-211.

52. Miller W, Vigdor ER, Manning WG. Covering the uninsured: what is it worth? Health Affairs Web exclusive. Available at: http://content.healthaffairs.org/cgi/content/full/hlthaff.w4.157v1/DC1. Accessed July 21, 2004.

53. Committee on Quality of Health Care in America, Institute of Medicine. *Crossing the Quality Chasm: A New Health System for the 21st Century.* Washington, DC: National Academy Press; 2001.

54. Corrigan JM, Adams K, eds. *Priority Areas for*

National Action: Transforming Healthcare Quality. Washington, DC: National Academy Press; 2003.

55. Greiner AC, Knebel E, eds. *Health Professions Education: A Bridge to Quality.* Washington, DC: National Academy Press; 2003.

56. Aspden P, Corrigan JM, Wolcott J, et al, eds. *Patient Safety: Achieving a New Standard for Care.* Washington, DC: National Academy Press; 2004.

57. Corrigan JM, Eden J, Smith BM, eds. *Leadership by Example: Coordinating Government Roles in Improving Health Care Quality.* Washington, DC: National Academy Press; 2003.

58. Page A, ed. *Keeping Patients Safe: Transforming the Work Environment of Nurses.* Washington, DC: National Academy Press; 2004.

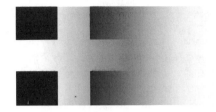

CHAPTER 2

The Role of the Leader in Advancing Patient Safety

Vicki Crane

Introduction

Leadership is a prerequisite of patient safety. Leaders transform themselves and their organizations by conducting honest assessments of patient safety in their practice environments, being willing to adopt new leadership behaviors to enhance patient safety, and having the tenacity to embed the needed changes into their health care cultures.

Patient safety has traditionally been viewed as the responsibility of a select few at the top of the organizational pyramid. Although members of the organization's quality-management department or team generally had roles in patient safety, the rest of the staff were merely spectators. That approach is no longer safe, if indeed it ever was. Everyone must participate in patient safety.

The health care culture has several other traps that leaders must overcome in order to enhance patient safety. These traps erroneously assume that

- Leaders have to react defensively, rather than proactively, to patient-safety issues because they are burdened by production pressures, regulatory issues, time constraints, and financial limitations.
- Health care providers should be able to deliver errorfree care if they work hard and pay attention; thus, if a safety issue does arise, the providers should be blamed.
- Conventional behaviors, levels of thinking, and technical excellence will produce patient-safety results that are different from those they have produced in the past.
- Employee safety is not a precondition to patient safety.
- Withholding the truth about patient-safety problems protects everyone.

Overcoming these erroneous assumptions problems will require a leadership approach that balances individual accountability with systems enhancements in order to provide reliable, safe care to each patient. Only leaders can rise above the daily production pressures, recognize dynamic couplings between process improvements and personnel, and identify, execute, and sustain maximum points for maximum patient safety. It is not easy work; it requires leaders to think in transformational ways about what they are doing and how to do it better. This chapter discusses transformational changes in the way leaders can think about and approach work in patient safety and reduce medication errors and adverse events. It is based on five leadership behaviors that have been adopted from the work of Greg Hicks.[1]

Leadership Behavior #1: Activate Intentions for Patient Safety[1]

Most leaders feel constantly overwhelmed. In such a situation, the natural tendency is react to each circumstance with a rigid, one-outcome solution rather than to consider other alternatives that might yield better outcomes. Some leaders feel as if they are victims of their circumstances, even though setting and declaring their intentions is actually 100 percent under their control. How can setting and declaring clear intentions contribute to patient safety?

Numerous studies have documented that the existing health care culture is likely the greatest barrier to improving patient safety.[2-4] This barrier may be largely removed by embedding change within the culture so that culture is working for, rather than against, patient safety. Culture can work for patient safety in many ways. Culture gets the employees' attention, influences their thinking, wins their affections, redirects their focus, dominates their conversation, influences their behaviors, and alters how they spend their time.[5] Culture will win out over policies and procedures every time. Thus, the primary intention of the patient-safety leader should be to embed patient safety into the culture such that the culture supports patient safety as "job 1."

Schein[6] has defined the word *culture* as a set of values, guiding beliefs, and understanding that is shared by members of an organization. Culture defines the way in which an organization communicates its values to new members. This, in turn, helps newcomers understand how to think and act and how things ought to be done. The culture of an organization has an impact on patient-safety intentions because it influences an organization's goals and strategies as well as employee attitudes and performance. Three levels of culture exist: (1) artifacts, or the visible organizational structures and processes; (2) values, strategies, goals, and philosophies; and (3) assumptions, which include beliefs, perceptions, thoughts, and feelings.[6]

Leaders can use a variety of mechanisms for embedding patient-safety culture change within their organizations. Craig[7] has described seven such mechanisms. They are introduced here in philosophical terms; the section entitled Seven Components of Cultural Change (see below) discusses their practical application.

1. Setting criteria for selection of employees. The criteria used to select leaders and employees have a powerful influence on organizational culture. An organization's culture is maintained through the hiring of personnel who fit into the existing culture. Conversely, cultural change can be made by hiring employees who do not fit into the existing culture. The kinds of employees recruited and how they are oriented to the organization send strong messages about the organization's culture. As patient safety is embedded into an organization's culture, selection of personnel who fit the new culture becomes increasingly important.

2. Providing employee training. Organizational culture is the result of a complex learning process. Well-planned education and training initiatives not only enhance an employee's knowledge and skills but also convey messages about the organization's goals and priorities. What is taught during such sessions provides important clues about an organization's culture. Thus, if the organization values patient safety, safety must figure prominently in training sessions.

3. Changing an organizational structure. The strategy, structure, and culture of an organization are interwoven. Culture change usually cannot happen without structural change. Both the moment at which an organization is formed and the periodic reorganizations that it goes through provide opportunities for leaders to lay the groundwork for culture change. Considerations to be borne in mind include existing as-

sumptions about the task, the means to accomplish the task, the nature of people, and the kinds of relationships that should be fostered. In preparation for a new emphasis on patient safety, leaders must identify and implement structural changes within the organizations.

4. Using specific reward systems. Leaders can communicate their priorities and values by linking rewards to behaviors. Employees will direct their energy toward rewards that they value. Using rewards for patient safety (if valued by the employee) will strengthen positive behaviors and diminish negative ones.

5. Socializing. Socialization is the process by which new members adapt to a new culture or existing members adapt to a changed culture. It is an active process by which the organization teaches its rules of behavior and the assumptions that lie behind them. Leaders must use the other six components presented here, as well as leadership skills, to make sure socialization occur.

6. Changing an organization's systems and procedures. The systems and processes of an organization formalize what its leaders value. They reinforce that leaders care about certain things. If an organization's leaders pay attention to patient safety, its systems and procedures will be designed as reinforcement mechanisms to strengthen the culture of patient safety.

7. Designing physical spaces. An organization's physical design conveys messages about its culture to employees, customers or patients, vendors, and visitors. Design demonstrates the value that the organization places on quality, ease of communication, and relationships. What patients and employees see throughout the facility is the picture of the organization's most deeply held assumptions.

In summary, leaders embed organizational culture in different ways. They do it by what they pay attention to, how they react to critical incidents and accidents, and how they set and state intentions, model roles, and coach their subordinates. Leaders can plan for management interventions that can change the form and the content of an organization's culture. As patient-safety initiatives are implemented, leaders set intentions and model behaviors for their subordinates.

Simply stated, when culture doesn't change, it's often because leadership behaviors don't change. New outcomes cannot come from old methods. Leaders must set, and then clearly articulate, patient-safety intentions.

Leadership Behavior #2: Own Accountability for All of Patient Safety[1]

Once a leader has set and articulated organizational patient-safety intentions, he or she becomes accountable for patient safety. Responsibility for errors and adverse events cannot be shunted elsewhere. The productive patient-safety leader asks, "What did I do to contribute to the problem?" and "What can I do to make things better?" As accountability spreads throughout the organization, these questions become everyone's questions.

The leader must integrate patient safety into the cultural fabric. This entails developing a conceptual model of a culture of safety. The old saying, "What you focus on is what you become" is true in patient safety.

Marx's[8] "just culture" model provides an excellent conceptual model for patient safety. The just culture acknowledges that providers may make errors.[8,9] It emphasizes learning rather than disciplinary action; its focus is not retaliatory.[8,9] The just culture offers a process for the reporting, investigating, tracking, and determining the cause of errors so that improvements can be made.[8,9]

THREE TYPES OF BEHAVIORS

The just culture model recognizes that errors can be caused by any of three types of behaviors: imperfect behavior, at-risk behavior, or reckless behavior (see **Figure** 2-1). These three behaviors must be managed in order to enhance patient safety.

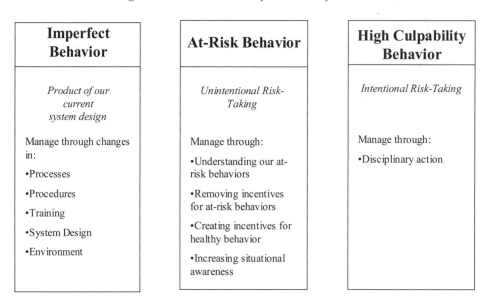

Figure 2-1. *Three Manageable Behaviors (Marx, reference #8)*

Imperfect Behavior

Humans cannot perform with 100 percent reliability all the time, but systems can be designed to enhance human reliability. The custom of having physicians write prescriptions by hand is a classic example of a system designed to produce errors and decrease patient safety. Illegible or incomplete physician handwriting leads to many types of interpretation errors (e.g., wrong drug, wrong dose).

The solution to imperfect behavior is to analyze and design systems that increase human reliability. One systems solution for illegible handwritten prescriptions, for example, is to switch to a computerized physician order entry system. Systems design includes such things as processes, procedures, environmental factors, and staff training and development. Reducing errors requires systems improvements, not disciplinary actions. If systems changes are not made, the problems will recur.

At-Risk Behavior

At-risk behavior is intentional conduct that unintentionally creates a risk that may produce an undesirable outcome. The health care provider is typically under the twin stress of providing patient care quickly and accurately. In such a situation, trade-offs may have to be made between completeness and getting the job done, and the outcome of such trade-offs may sometimes be negative. As providers gain experience, they drift away from what they were taught in order to save time or other resources. Over time, and at first with no adverse consequences, they deviate from norms of practice, just as a driver over time drifts away from keeping both hands positioned on the steering wheel of a car. If a driver finds that he or she can steer with just one hand, he or she has created a new, and at least temporarily acceptable, norm. In both cases—that of the health care provider and the driver—the conduct is intentional but its potential effect is unintentional. Neither recognizes that the conduct increases the risk of a negative consequence or that they have placed themselves in a situation where their human reliability or performance is shaped by expediency rather than by tested, safe practices. The ill effects of the trade-off cannot be foreseen; they become obvious only after the negative outcome. This phenomenon is called hindsight bias.[10,11]

The correct solution to at-risk behaviors is not disciplinary action. The solution is to change the incentives so that people choose safe behaviors over at-risk behaviors. It includes such things as improved communications between managers and workers, direction regarding workload and other key factors, increased health care team training, increased risk awareness, and removal of the incentives for at-risk behavior. In many health care organizations, changing at-risk behaviors represents the largest opportunity to prevent errors.

Reckless Behavior

Reckless behavior is intentional risk taking that blatantly disregards safe practices and jeopardizes the life or welfare of another individual. The approach to decreasing reckless behavior is disciplinary because the behavior must be changed or the person cannot continue to function as a health care provider. This is the only behavior where punitive sanctions should be the solution. Punitive sanctions include progressive disciplinary actions, time off, or even termination.

SEVEN COMPONENTS OF CULTURAL CHANGE

Once the culture of safety is defined and described, integrative action steps under the seven components of culture change described earlier in this chapter can be taken. These steps are as follows:

Set Criteria for Selection of Employees[7]

Behavioral position descriptions or behavior-based interviewing can be used to articulate the prerequisites for success for a given job. Behavior-description interviewing can predict for the applicant, the line manager, and the human resource specialist the candidate that possesses the attributes critical to success in a given job.[12] Managers and human-resource specialists should be trained in how to conduct a defined, consistent, behavior-based patient-safety assessment with potential employees. Expected patient-safety behaviors should be included in organizational and departmental recruitment materials. Candidates for employment should be aware of the organization's commitment to shared responsibility for patient safety of what specific patient-safety behaviors will be required of them.

Provide Training for Employees[7]

When an organization moves from a punitive to a just-culture system, it is especially important to provide appropriate training so that the employees, especially managers, know how to perform their responsibilities in the new system as the old system is phased out.

Employee and medical staff orientations at the organizational, departmental, and work-unit levels should include presentations on patient-safety standards. Management buy-in is essential to the creation of an environment in which patient safety is everyone's business. Opportunities for training in patient safety must be included in such courses as management development, behavior-description interviewing, and coaching and counseling. For example, the coaching and counseling course should include concepts relating to a just culture and to patient safety, as well as to differentiating between imperfect, at-risk, and reckless behaviors. All employees and medical staff should undergo mandatory training on patient safety annually. Standards of performance should include putting patient safety first. The patient-safety monitoring system (e.g., for iatrogenic incidents and sentinel events) should provide feedback and goal setting for continuous safety communication, training, and development.

Change the Organizational Structure to Support Patient Safety[7]

There is no single or universal design for a patient-safety infrastructure; there are, however, patient-safety building blocks. Typical building blocks include

- a system for coordinating responsibility for patient safety (e.g., creating a patient-safety department or appointing a patient-safety officer from senior management) for patient-safety goals and initiatives, such as implementation of Joint Commission on Accreditation of Healthcare Organization patient-safety standards;

- a reporting system;

- communication and awareness campaigns (e.g., patient-safety hotline, patient-safety fair);

- patient-safety rounds and briefings by executives and supervisors;

- employee training and development in patient safety; and

- employee-safety questionnaires and checklists.

Use Specific Reward Systems[7]

If a certain activity is recognized and rewarded, chances are it will get done. Reward systems for patient safety usually involve a combination of "push" and "pull" tools. Push tools include the employee's annual evaluation (with patient safety recognized as a core competency), bonus plans, budgets, awards, and mandatory training that focuses on or includes patient safety. Pull tools include painting a picture of how to optimize patient safety and telling stories of patient-safety heroes. The choice of tools depends on the organization's ability to employ them effectively (e.g., not all organizations may have a bonus plan) and whether the rewards need to be based on individual performance, team performance, or a combination of the two.

Provide Opportunities for Socialization[7]

Socialization is the process by which the norms and standards embedded in the culture are passed on to members joining the culture. Success at transitioning to a new culture depends on the organization's ability to transform current members to its new ways and to hire new staff that have bought into that culture. This process does not occur overnight; for that reason, it is essential that leadership start the process as early as possible by altering the parts of the culture that are most out of alignment with regard to a new cultural norm. Only about 5 percent of a culture's norms and standards significantly affect the mission-critical aspects of patient safety.[13] Leaders must discern between the "vital few" and the "trivial many" norms and standards with regard to culture change. For example, one of the vital few would be to stop responding to medication-error reports in a punitive fashion and to begin using them as a basis for systems improvement.[14]

Change the Organization's Systems and Procedures

Each organization must design and sustain patient-safety considerations around its key activities. Guidelines to follow during this process include the following:

- Do not expect different results or outcomes from the same systems and procedures.

- Conduct integrated process redesign in both patient care and support areas. Redesigned care management cannot be effective, safe, and efficient unless support area redesign is included in the process.

- Integrate process redesign with information technology upgrades to sustain quality and safety gains. Gains achieved through process redesign are generally sustained by information technology.

- Base redesign processes on best practices, evidence-based medicine, regulatory mandates, and internal quality and safety data, as well as input from colleagues[15,16] on initiatives rather than on analyzing the reasons for the gap.

- Perform ongoing assessments of systems and procedures (e.g., medication-use cycle safety plan) and develop ways of enhancing them.

Pay Attention to the Design of Physical Spaces[7]

The design of physical space has both material and social implications. Rarely does a health care organization have the luxury of building a totally new facility. Health care organizations are, however, constantly renovating work areas and redesigning patient-flow procedures and systems to accommodate new demands. Physical design has an impact on patient safety, and the process of redesign can be used to influence the change to a culture of safety.

Reiling[17] has suggested 10 principles for redesigning hospital space for patient safety:

1. Ensure that design processes for physical space are data driven and use tools such as failure mode and effects analysis.

2. Include stakeholders at every step in the design process.

3. Make sure that leaders support the design process.

4. Use design mock-ups, and test equipment at every major step of the redesign process.

5. Pay attention to the environmental and human factors that will affect the safety of staff, patients, and families.

6. Design the space to safely accommodate the most vulnerable patient populations (e.g., newborns, elderly persons).

7. Ensure that the design is sufficiently adaptable to enable the organization to respond to future changes in patient populations, technology, and processes.

8. Standardize design whenever possible (e.g., medical records organization and forms storage in patient care areas).

9. Provide user-friendly access to information systems.

10. Address all safety issues identified through the literature, internal data, or regulatory standards.

In summary, accountability for the transition to a culture of safety lies with patient-safety leadership. The culture of safety and patient-safety leadership are two sides of the same coin. Leaders create a culture when they create the organization's mission, goals, and objectives and hire the appropriate personnel to achieve those goals. The most important function of the leader is to ensure that patient safety is "job 1" of the organization.[18]

Leadership Behavior #3: Recast Stress and Conformity into Strengths and Possibilities[18]

A just culture is a learning culture. Creating a learning culture requires that leaders recast four traditional and counterproductive approaches into patient-safety strategies that enable an organization to create a learning culture. More specifically, an organization must move

- from a culture of reporting incidents and accidents to one of *learning* from incidents and accidents;

- from an accounting approach, which tabulates events, to a synthetic approach that searches for positive and negative *patterns;*

- from looking backward to looking forward in *anticipation* of future risks; and

- from a focus on error and blame to a focus on *complexity.*[18]

The following paragraphs explore each of these four areas of transformation in greater detail.

LEARNING

Figure 2-2 pictures the traditional cycle of patient safety.[19] In such a system, the investigative procedure ends by assigning blame to an individual and by creating additional procedures

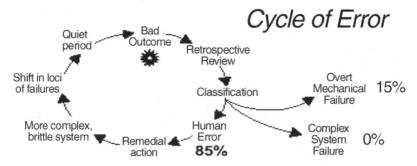

Cycle of Error

Organizational *reactions to failure* focus on human error.
The reactions to failure are: blame & train, sanctions, new
regulations, rules, and technology. These interventions
increase complexity and introduce new forms of failure.

Figure 2-2. Cycle of Error (Cook, reference #19)

that only make the system more complex and rigid. This approach overlooks the fact that success comes from the same sources as failure does. If the focus is only on errors or failures, much time is spent chasing after discrete events that change as the system changes. This approach does not optimize learning and is not conducive to patient safety.

The cycle of error is usually set off on its predetermined course by "first stories"—stories that break when an incident with a negative outcome occurs. Such stories are biased by the foreknowledge of the negative outcome and inevitably provide a simplistic view of the causal factors associated with that outcome. This bias causes investigators to limit their exploration of what happened to the proximal cause, which is usually human error.

To make patients safe and to learn from errors, an organization must examine the "second stories" behind a human error. The "third stories" must likewise be examined from an objective viewpoint. That examination must take place in the broad context of the system. Second and third stories often reveal how providers work to make care safe in spite of production pressures, at-risk behavior, and other barriers. A culture of safety develops only when those involved understand how it is created and maintained in the face of challenges.

To escape hindsight bias and to make progress in patient safety, three leverage points must be simultaneously in place: an understanding of how events happen, what events occur, and what is possible to do to prevent those events in the future.[18] A simple example illustrates this point. Suppose two different, look-alike medication vials are placed in adjoining compartments in an anesthesia box. The anesthesiologist unintentionally switches the vials, and the patient is harmed. After investigation, the health care team decides that the solution is to place the vials on opposite sides of the box. The team is surprised when, after a period of time, a similar accident happens.

Why did the error recur? The team looked only at the assumed, or immediate, cause of the first event (i.e., look-alike packaging) rather than at other possibilities (e.g., a pharmacy technician filled the compartments incorrectly), other similar events that may have occurred (e.g., the pharmacy stored the vials in the wrong places and created errors elsewhere), and the range of possible responses (e.g., the hospital could buy the products from different manufacturers so that vials do not look alike or determine whether both vials are routinely needed in the anesthesia box). The solution chosen was not the best one for other reasons as well. For example, the anesthesiologist might have left the syringes unlabeled and switched them at a later point. Also, the team did not look at solutions generally known to make medication systems safer (e.g., having a pharmacist fill and label the syringes). Although the team intended to make things safer, it did not consider the many possible reasons behind the error. It focused on a single solution of human error (hindsight bias), failed to consider that the solution might have its own set of negative consequences, and thought the event to be unique rather than part of a complex system.

In sum, to make progress in patient safety, leaders must ensure that middle managers are trained in investigative procedures that include the three leverage points, that the reporting system supports the right investigative procedures and incentives, and that employees feel welcome to raise their hands and discuss errors.

PATTERNS

If care is to become safer, reporting systems must stop categorizing errors and begin looking for underlying patterns and overarching trends. A "who, what, when, and where" approach describes the reasons for failure but does not explore the underlying patterns of systems errors. Investigations of patterns look at how health care providers, teams of providers, communication and coordination handoffs, human-computer cooperation, and other factors form overlapping interdependencies with the care-delivery system.

For example, in looking beyond categories with respect to medication- and blood-administration errors, one might find that their source is a lack of patient identification or patient-product mismatches. Absent this understanding, unneeded checking steps might be added to the medication- and blood-administration cycles. This would merely make each system more complex and error-prone while not resolving the problems leading to the continued patient-product mismatches for blood products, medications, and other products.

As leaders examine technical work, they must look for patterns in both successful and unsuccessful work and find ways to close the loop and prevent future fail points.

ANTICIPATION

The third change is a shift from analyzing past events to anticipating ways to prevent future risks. Leaders must develop predictive risk assessments and models. Vigilance is essential; even the best system, left unattended, drifts toward dysfunctionality and a lower safety margin. Complex systems are in constant flux. Changes made to the system in the name of patient safety may inadvertently introduce new failure points into that system. Shortcuts introduced in response to production pressures may cause safety margins to erode. Thus, leaders must shift organizational learning to predictive risk modeling.

The following example, based on patient flows between the emergency room (ER) and the inpatient units, illustrates this point. Each of these areas has its own staff and its own processes for providing patient care. A quality-management study notes that ER is often overflowing with patients, resulting in long waits and an increase in errors. The ER is redesigned to be more efficient and errorproof. Despite these changes, six months later, the situation is even worse. Why? Predictive risk modeling of the hospital's capacity management would have shown that while inefficiencies did exist within the ER, the primary bottleneck was delays in getting patients admitted from the ER to inpatient beds. Thus, increasing efficiencies in ER patient flow had a counterproductive effect: It brought patients more quickly to the bottleneck of admission. A capacity-management predictive-risk model would also have shown the reason for the bottlenecks in the inpatient service (i.e., time needed to clean the discharged patients' rooms).

To predict situations that contribute to errors, leaders must understand how work is performed, how safety is created, and how system-failure points arise, and then target opportunities for improvement. To make their systems safer, leaders must take the safety experiments they are performing every day and start analyzing them with predictive risk modeling. Basic tools such as total quality improvement, benchmarking, quality circles, balanced scorecards, and rapid-cycle testing can be helpful.[20] More-advanced tools, including probabilistic risk assessment[8] and six sigma,[20] can be used for comprehensive predictive-risk modeling as the organization moves forward in its efforts to create a safer medication system.

COMPLEXITY

As the shift to a learning culture continues, the organization will move from a focus on error and blame to a focus on complexity. A focus on errors assumes that the error is unique and that the cause is human unreliability. The response is to move things around (e.g., fire the provider). This technique merely squeezes the balloon at a different point; accidents will soon pop out at other points in the complex system.

A focus on complexity assumes that as systems become more complicated, dynamic couplings occur, creating overlapping interdependencies. As the system becomes more complex, it also becomes more rigid and brittle. In such a system, a small change can have a dramatic effect. Production pressures and limited resources push providers to operate at a lower and lower safety margin until an accident occurs.

The ER case study presented in the previous section illustrates how brittle many complex systems are and how quickly patient safety can erode even if one minor piece is out of place. Suppose, under that scenario, that three patients who had been in the surgery intensive-care unit (ICU) were medically ready to be discharged, but none could be discharged. One patient did not know he was ready for discharge and had not made arrangements to be picked up; the second knew but was allowed to wait until evening when a friend could pick him up; and the third wanted to eat before he left. This backed up the surgical ICU, which could not send three new patients to the general surgery unit. This backed up the operating room, which could not send three patients in recovery to the surgical ICU. Finally, this exacerbated the delay in the ER, which could not send three new patients to the operating room. The failure to communicate clear expectations about discharge to the general surgery patients ultimately produced a systemwide backup.

Complexity is the enemy of patient safety. Simplicity is the ally of patient safety. As complexity grows, human reliability decreases and safety problems increase. New technologies such as medications, medical devices, computers, and automation can either increase or decrease human reliability by removing the possibility of some failure points and introducing new ones. Leaders must learn, through understanding patterns and use of predictive risk modeling, how best to use technology and the human-technology interface to simplify the complex health care system and increase human reliability.

In summary, responsibility for recasting stress and conformity into strength and possibilities lies with patient-safety leaders. Only leaders can transform production pressures, recognize dynamic couplings between process improvements and personnel, and identify, implement, and sustain leverage points for patient safety.

Leadership Behavior #4: Put Employees First So that Employees Can Put Patients First[1]

The most crucial conversations leaders have are those they undertake with their employees. Leaders cannot make health care safe for patients if they do not first make it safe for employees. Leaders accomplish this through three key dialogues.

SHIFT THE EMPHASIS FROM FAULT FINDING TO CONTRIBUTION[21]

Finding fault with employees does little for patient safety because it inhibits those involved from investigating what really caused the problem and how to fix it. Blaming focuses on the past and punitive actions. When a medication error occurs, is it the fault of the physician who wrote an illegible order? The pharmacy technician who filled the order incorrectly? The pharmacist who didn't do a careful check against the original order? The nurse who administered the drug? When the goal is patient safety, focusing on blame is a waste of time.

Contribution, by contrast, focuses on understanding the many factors that contributed to the problem and on how to change the system so that the problem does not recur. Focusing on contribution makes investigations easier and more productive. The emphasis is on learning and enhancement. The responsibility of the patient-safety leader is to stop blaming employees and to adapt a contribution-and-learning mindset that sparks crucial conversations about enhancements and provides alternative, safe models under which employees work together to preserve the safety margin for the patient.

EMPHASIZE THE VALUE OF APPRECIATIVE INQUIRY[22]

Appreciative inquiry recognizes that many things work right in patient safety within the organization and seeks to inculcate those right things so that employees know how to repeat those patient-safety successes.[22] Appreciative inquiry sets up a series of dialogues that define where an organization wants to be with patient safety on the basis of stories and the history of the organization's patient-safety initiatives. Because the definitions are based on the organization's experience, employees begin to understand how to consistently repeat safety successes.

The assumptions of appreciative inquiry are as follows[22]:

- Every organization, group, or team has successes.
- What the organization, group, or team focuses on becomes its reality.
- Multiple realities are created at each moment.
- Asking questions has an impact on the organization, group, or team.
- The organization, group, or team will have confidence about the future if it can carry forward parts of the certainties of the past.
- If the organization, group, or team carries parts of its history with it, they should be the best parts.
- Diversity must be valued.
- The vocabulary the organization, group, or team uses creates or limits its reality.

Most health care organizations have had little practice or success at working with their frontline employees to identify what works in patient safety and at focusing on doing more of what is already successful. Instead, they fixate on errors and problems. Why don't leaders allow the frontline staff to tell them how they have kept patients safe and allow those patient-safety success stories and behaviors to multiply?

Appreciative-inquiry techniques can be carried out in a focus group/workshop setting where frontline employees share stories of patient-safety successes. The employees emerge from the process with a heightened sense of commitment and a validation that they have been successful in patient safety. They know how to make those high points of patient safety happen much more often. The positive and synergistic energy that comes from the process of appreciative inquiry is infinite.

The patient-safety leader's responsibility is to turn an appreciative eye toward patient safety (see **Figure 2-3**). This is not to say that leaders should adopt a "dumb but happy" approach to patient safety. What happens when the monthly incident report is received? The leader automatically focuses on those areas that have the most medication errors or sentinel events. Why not focus on those areas where there are fewer medication errors and no sentinel events? What are those areas doing differently to prevent medication errors and sentinel events, and how can this success be spread to other patient care areas?

The only way to discover whether positive approaches work is to try them. Leaders do not have to do a large and risky project to initiate appreciative inquiry. They can start with something simple, such as appreciative-inquiry dialogues in patient-safety meetings. The only way the leader can fail is to do nothing.

Problem Solving	**Appreciative Inquiry**
BASIC ASSUMPTION:	BASIC ASSUMPTION:
AN ORGANIZATION IS A PROBLEM TO BE SOLVED	AN ORGANIZATION IS A MYSTERY TO BE EMBRACED
Identification of Problem	Appreciating and Valuing the Best of What Is
▼	▼
Analysis of Causes	Envisioning What Might Be
▼	▼
Analysis of Possible Solutions	Dialoging What Should Be
▼	▼
Action Planning (Treatment)	Innovating What Will Be

Adapted from Cooperrider and Srivasha (1987) "Appreciative Inquiry into Organizational Life" in *Research in Organizational Change and Development*. Pasmore and Woodman (eds) Vol 1, JAI Press.

Figure 2-3. *Appreciative Inquiry into Organizational Life (Hammond, reference #22)*

HAVE THE CONSISTENT INTENTION TO GIVE TO, NOT TAKE FROM, EMPLOYEES[1]

Trust is a precondition to patient safety, and the starting point of trust is giving. Giving, in other words, is a precondition to trust. As the patient-safety leader stops blaming and starts appreciative inquiry, trust will start to develop. Giving to employees at every contact—through respect, communication, positive and negative feedback, and use of patient-safety strategies that enhance rather than restrict employee performance—inculcates trust. The minimal expectations of good leadership (e.g., training and development, competitive wages, fairness, and fulfilling job content) accomplish little if giving is not consistently present.

Leaders should give feedback, information, and compliments to employees every time they have contact with them. The consistent questions of the leader to employees should be

- What do you need to make things safe for you and for your patients?
- What motivates you to make things safe for you and for your patients?
- How can I demonstrate to you that I care about you and your patients' safety?

Answering these questions requires that the leader spend time with employees. The time should be scheduled routinely and treated as any other crucial meeting. By spending consistent time listening to employees, leaders gain more insight into patient safety than they can through any other channel. Once the leaders gain the patient-safety information and employee trust, they must translate knowledge into action on behalf of the employees and the patients, as discussed in other chapters of this book.

Motivation for patient safety comes when employees know that they can make significant and unique contributions to it. Leaders need to search for clues with employees as to what they value and to relate these values to patient-safety goals. When the leader treats employees as if they were doing all they can for patient safety, safety becomes a self-fulfilling prophecy. Being attentive to peoples' need for respect-and development motivates them to be attentive to patient safety.

In summary, when the leader empowers and validates employees through appreciative inquiry and giving techniques, employees respond by enlarging the patient-safety margin in all they do. The biblical proverb that states, "The generous soul will be made rich, and he who waters will also be watered himself"[23] is true of leadership of patient-safety endeavors.

Leaders who surround themselves with appreciative, competent, caring followers will reap infinite patient-safety dividends.

Leadership Behavior #5: Communicate the Truth About Patient Safety So that Employees Are Free to Hear and Tell the Truth About Patient Safety[1]

Feedback is a key aspect of a culture of safety. Feedback, education, and goal setting are powerful tools for advancing patient safety and for gaining support for continued safety improvements. Feedback affects performance in important ways. Objective, specific, and immediate feedback serves as a reminder to allow for individual and team corrections and adjustments. Feedback promotes goal-setting behavior and stimulates motivation. The goal-setting and achievement process for patient safety is initiated and then maintained through feedback.[24] The feedback cycle builds trust, and trust is an essential element of every successful patient-safety team.[1]

To initiate a successful cycle of feedback, the patient-safety leader must require the truth as a precondition of patient safety. Requiring truth has three components: being willing to hear, tell, and advocate the truth.[21]

- **Hear the truth.** The patient-safety leader must regard feedback as information that can be used to educate and set goals, not as criticism or any kind of attack. Some part of feedback will always be useful. The leader believes that feedback is a gift of trust. Patient-safety leaders must search for feedback about their individual performance as well as patient-safety initiatives.

- **Tell the truth.** Patient-safety leaders must tell the truth in a gracious manner. They must be able to deliver both good and bad news. The intent of feedback is not to put down someone but to build up the employee or the team and, in doing so, to advance patient safety.

- **Advocate the truth.** Each employee sees the same patient-safety story in a different way. Each individual's culture, profession, experiences, gender, hindsight bias, and perceptions, as well as many other factors, cause him or her to view a story from a unique perspective. The patient-safety leader must act as a mediator or facilitator to uncover the true (or third) story. The leader must integrate the stories into a comprehensive story as to what happened and how to enhance patient safety. If this is done, all stakeholders perceive that they are legitimate owners in the eventual enhancement.

In summary, effective patient-safety leaders lead by example, not command. To advance patient safety, leaders must have the courage to seek the truth, tell the truth, and act upon the truth.

Putting It All Together[25]

The purpose of this chapter has been to demonstrate that leadership in patient safety and culture evolution are closely connected. All patient-safety leadership behaviors interact with and reinforce one another (**Figure 2-4**). Patient-safety leaders must create, embed, and sustain patient safety within the organizational culture. If they succeed, that culture will evolve in controversial and difficult ways. Thus, it is important for the patient-safety leader not only to adapt the leadership behaviors but also know how to lead through the necessary transitions.

Several authors have developed comprehensive models for culture transition and change.[6,25,26] The following discussion introduces key ideas that may assist patient-safety leaders in transitioning a health care organization's culture to a culture or community of safety.

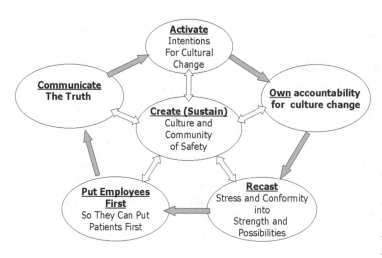

First, promote yourself. Patient-safety leaders must promote themselves in their patient-safety leadership roles. They cannot assume that behaviors that have made them successful in previous assignments, even in quality control, will make them successful in patient safety. Patient safety requires a new approach that balances individual accountability with systems enhancements.

Figure 2-4. Principles of Transformational Leadership in Patient Safety (adapted from reference #1)

The visible behaviors of the leader communicate and leverage the culture change needed to create a community where safety is everyone's business.

Second, accelerate your learning. The job of the patient-safety leader is to learn and then to manage the health care organization's culture in a way that enhances patient safety. The learning must be focused and systematic so that the key aspects of the organization's culture that are critical to patient safety can be identified and then changed as necessary. Culture's overarching goal is to preserve itself and the status quo. Too often, equilibrium is a degenerating, rather than a generating, culture, or a culture repeating the same strategies but expecting different results. Patient-safety leaders must learn which components of the culture are critical to patient safety and then manage those components to improve patient safety.

Third, match strategy to situation. Patient-safety leaders must first diagnose where current patient-safety strategies are on the evolutionary scale. They must determine where the health care organization is in order to clearly define its opportunities and challenges. The evolution may be a start-up, a turnaround, a realignment, or a sustaining of a culture of patient safety.

Fourth, create an oversight team. Leadership is about leverage. Leaders must create a leadership team that achieves organizational alignment with the vision, strategy, communication, and actions of patient safety.

Fifth, design quick wins. Transforming a culture is a long-term process, yet it also can produce some immediate results. Quick wins can create credibility and momentum for patient safety. They provide early evidence that the investment in patient safety is a worthy one, that employees will be rewarded and recognized for patient-safety endeavors, and that both senior leaders and "fence sitters" should continue their support of the patient-safety initiatives.

Sixth, consolidate gains through culture change. The work of leaders is to leverage a patient-safety culture in their organizations. Patient-safety leaders can embed changes in the culture through the integrated use of the principles discussed in the chapter. However, culture by its very nature resists change, and changing to a culture of safety often becomes the difficult process of creative destruction. The successful patient-safety leader must be willing to take the calculated risk of failure to build a culture that enhances patient safety.

Conclusion

Patient-safety leadership and a patient-safety culture are intertwined. Leaders create the patient-safety culture and then become embedded in it. The role of the patient-safety leader is to identify when components of the culture are not supporting patient safety and to lead cultural evolution to continue enhancing patient safety.

Acknowledgements

The author would like to acknowledge the contributions of cultural change leaders David Marx, Richard Cook, Greg Hicks, and Edgar Schein. An even greater debt is owed to the American Hospital Association/Health Forum Patient Safety Leadership Fellowship, 2002–2003 and the patient-safety leaders and employees of Parkland Health & Hospital System, Dallas, Texas, who made the preparation of this chapter possible.

References

1. Hicks G. *LeaderShock—And How to Triumph over It*. New York: McGraw-Hill; 2003.

2. Cohen MM, Eustis MA, Gribbins RE. Changing the culture of patient safety: leadership's role in health care quality improvement. *Jt Comm J Qual Safety*. 2003;29:329-335.

3. Leape LL. Creating a culture of safety. Paper presented at: Enhancing Patient Safety and Reducing Errors in Health Care; November 8, 1998; Rancho Mirage, CA.

4. O'Leary DS. Organization, evaluation, and a culture of safety. Paper presented at: Enhancing Patient Safety and Reducing Errors in Health Care. November 8, 1998; Rancho Mirage, CA.

5. Stanley C. Surviving Our Current Culture [audiotape]. Atlanta: In Touch Ministries; 2003.

6. Schein E. *Organizational Culture and Leadership*. 2nd ed. San Francisco: Jossey-Bass;1992.

7. Craig S. Clinical Safety Steering Committee Retreat. Parkland Health & Hospital System, Dallas, January 2002. Unpublished.

8. Marx D. Patient safety and the "just culture": A primer for health care executives. Paper prepared for Columbia University under a grant from the National Heart, Lung, and Blood Institute, U.S. Department of Health and Human Services. April 2001. Unpublished.

9. Crane VS. Medication error and adverse drug event prevention. In: Di Piro JT, ed. *Encyclopedia of Clinical Pharmacy*. New York: Marcel Dekker; 2003:533-544.

10. Baron J, Hersey J. Outcome bias in decision evaluation. *J Personality Soc Psychol*. 1988;54:569-579.

11. Caplan RA, Posner KL, Cheney FR. Effect of outcome on physician judgments of the appropriateness of care. *JAMA*. 1991; 265:1957-1960.

12. Janz T, Hellervik L, Gilmore DC. *Behavior Description Interviewing*. Englewood Cliffs, NJ: Prentice-Hall; 1986.

13. Pritchett P. *Shaping Corporate Culture*. Plano, TX: Pritchett LLC; 2002.

14. Crane VS. New perspectives on preventing medication errors and adverse drug events. *Am J Health-Syst Pharm*. 2000;57:690-697.

15. Agency for Healthcare Research and Quality. Making Health Care Safer: A Critical Analysis of Patient Safety Practices. Rockville, MD: AHRQ; 2001. Available at: www.ahrq.gov. Accessed January 11, 2005.

16. Joint Commission on Accreditation of Healthcare Organizations. JCAHO Accreditation Manual. Oak Brook Terrace, IL: JCAHO; 2003.

17. Reiling J. Healing design: redesigning hospitals to improve safety. Paper presented at: Fifth Annual National Patient Safety Foundation Patient Congress. March 14, 2003; Washington, DC.

18. Cook R. Learning to learn about patient safety. Paper presented at: AHA/Health Forum Patient Safety Leadership Fellowship. November 11, 2003; Tucson, AZ

19. Cook R. A brief look at the new look in complex system failure, error, and safety. Available at: www.ctlab.org. Accessed December 28, 2003.

20. Vonderheide-Liem D, Pate B. Applying Quality Methodologies to Improve Healthcare. Marblehead, MA: HCPro Inc; 2004.

21. Stone D, Patton B, Heen S. *Difficult Conversations*. New York: Penguin Putnam; 1999.

22. Hammond SA. *The Thin Book of Appreciative Inquiry*. 2nd ed. Plano, TX: Thin Book Publishing; 1998.

23. Proverbs 11:25. New King James Version, the Nelson Study Bible, 1997.

24. Crane VS. *Continuous Quality Improvement as an Ideal in Hospital Pharmacy Practice*. Durham, NC: Clean Data, Inc; 1990.

25. Watkins M. *The First 90 Days*. Boston: Harvard Business School Press; 2003.

26. Kotter JP. *Leading Change*. Boston: Harvard Business School Press; 1996.

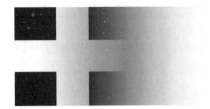

CHAPTER 3

A Business Case for Patient Safety?

Joseph K. Bonnarens and
Lee C. Vermeulen

Introduction

Patient safety is one of the most important policy issues currently facing our health care system. The Institute of Medicine's report *To Err Is Human*, published in 1999, clearly articulated the need for improvement in the systems used to deliver care safely.[1] All constituent groups—patients, funders, insurers, providers, and regulators—agree that financial investment is needed to support interventions that improve safety.[2] However, national health care expenditures exceeded $1.6 trillion in 2003 and are expected to top $3 trillion annually by 2012, even without these additional investments.[3] Although our national appetite for health care seems insatiable, investment in safety interventions must be considered in the context of increasing scrutiny that will certainly be applied to future resource-consumption patterns.

In an era where health care resources are finite, those responsible for deciding the size of investments in patient safety, as well as when, where, and how those investments will be made, need an analytic framework that considers both the cost and consequences of those investments. The term *business case* has been used to define this framework. A business case is a structured proposal for business improvement that functions as a decision package for decision makers.[4] Developing a business case entails ranking in order of priority various strategies to accomplish particular goals, taking into consideration financial and other relevant factors. Those creating a business case for improved safety must first determine the need for improvement and then assess various safety-improving interventions that meet that objective. This chapter explores the question of whether a business case for safety improvement has been made and discusses several issues to be borne in mind in making a business case for safety in health care delivery organizations.

Has a Business Case for Safety Been Made?

The literature offers limited empirical evidence to support the development of a business case for quality and safety initiatives.[5-7] In fall 2002, the Agency for Healthcare Research and Quality (AHRQ), the Centers for Medicare & Medicaid Services (CMS), the Joint Commission on Accreditation of Healthcare Organizations (JCAHO), the Department of Defense, and the American Hospital Association brought together hospital chief executives to discuss the business case for patient safety. The sponsors of this seminar believed that if a return on investment (ROI) in patient safety could be quantified, these executives would reprioritize the importance of safety initiatives in their institutions.[8] At the conclusion of the event, participants concluded that a business case has not yet been made; however, they did reach a consensus on the importance of patient safety and the need to pursue it.[9]

Several difficulties exist in making a business case for safety. According to JCAHO President Dennis O'Leary, most of these barriers are financial.[8] In testimony before the U.S. Senate Committee on Government Affairs, O'Leary noted that key barriers include insufficient capital to support major patient safety improvements and reimbursement policies that do not distinguish safe from unsafe practices and that reward systems that place too little value on investments in patient safety.[8]

Oetgen and Oetgen[5] suggest that the business case for patient safety must include not only financial considerations but also ethical, sociopolitical, and medicolegal factors. These authors emphasize that while all these components contribute to business case development, empirical evidence for the effectiveness of safety enhancements is a necessary prerequisite that many interventions do not currently meet.

One organization that has tried to develop such evidence is the AHRQ, which in 2001 provided an initial review of patient-safety practices. It identified 79 safety-enhancing interventions reported in the medical literature that have the potential to improve patient safety.[10] Interventions specified as having strong empirical support, suggesting widespread implementation, were all clinical in nature and included such practices as thromboprophylaxis to prevent perioperative clots and the use of pressure-relief devices to prevent bedsores. The effectiveness of operational and process-of-care interventions, such as computerized prescriber order entry (CPOE) and creating a "culture of safety," were less well supported by objective evidence.

Oetgen and Oetgen[5] suggest that organizations that make improvements in safety may secure a market advantage that would allow them to become more competitive and successful. However, Rosenthal and colleagues[11] argue that the market currently does not provide incentives improvement but rather "pays for performance." Organizations with strength in their structures and processes (e.g., in their ability to ensure that beta-blockers are given to patients with acute myocardial infarction) receive modest financial rewards, while those without such structures and processes do not. Organizations that make strides in their performance receive no incentive to improve their performance unless their improvements achieve a minimum standard. This makes it difficult for a poorer-performing organization to justify added investments in safety. As a result, the successful get more successful and the less successful slip further into the "quality chasm." It is unclear that any market response to safety improvement will offset the investment necessary to alter outcomes in a measurable fashion. Insofar as markets are increasingly limiting choice as a successful method of cost containment, it is doubtful that any organization can leverage its safety performance to capture a greater market share.

Making a business case for safety ultimately requires that the financial value of various interventions be proved and that a positive ROI be demonstrated. The challenge in establishing value lies in reconciling the financial fragmentation that exists among various constituent groups who participate in decisions about resource allocation.

Five Perspectives on Care

In order to build a business case for any sort of investment in health care, one must first identify the perspective from which the analysis is to be made. Perspective defines the viewpoint from which the business case is assessed and identifies what costs and resulting consequences are relevant. Subsequent financial analysis must take into account these costs and their consequences in calculating cost-effectiveness or ROI.

Investment in particular interventions may provide return to only one constituent group. For example, investments in medications that improve quality of life, while potentially valuable from patient and societal perspectives, may provide little direct return to funders and health care providers. It is this perverse lack of alignment, wherein providers are expected to invest in safety enhancements that provide a ROI only to patients and insurers, that has prevented the development of a business case for safety to date.

The choice of perspective—that is, of which constituency's interest is being measured—therefore becomes of paramount importance. In this particular case, five constituencies are particularly relevant: society, patient, funder, insurer and provider. As shown in **Table 3-1,** each constituency has a different perspective with respect to investment and return.

Table 3-1. Alignment of Investment and Return by Perspective

Perspective	Expected to Invest?	Realizes Return?
Society	Investments not made at societal level in multipayer system.	Ultimately yes, but not measured in aggregate.
Patient	No (except for self-pay patients, who are rare).	Yes, directly measurable.
Funder	No, but currently driving demand through unfunded mandates.	High return if total cost is reduced.
Insurer	No.	Increased profit margin possible if resulting savings are not passed on to funders.
Provider	Yes, mandated.	Little, unless operational efficiency accompanies safety improvement.

SOCIETAL PERSPECTIVE

In 1993, the U.S. Public Health Services' Panel on Cost-Effectiveness in Health and Medicine recommended that analyses measuring the value of health care interventions be considered from the societal perspective, taking into account all health consequences and costs associated with a particular intervention.[12] This recommendation was necessary to promote comparisons across and among various alternative investment opportunities. However, a single constituent group positioned to make such global decisions regarding resource consumption does not exist in the United States. In the United States, unlike certain other countries such as Australia and the United Kingdom, we do not choose at the societal level between spending health care resources on organ transplantation or on vaccination. While decisions regarding investment in safety interventions would ideally include the consideration of all costs and consequences, the fragmented financial structure of the U.S. health care system makes this societal perspective fundamentally irrelevant.

PATIENT PERSPECTIVE

Patients are clearly the primary benefactors of any investment made to improve the safety of the health care system. If care is safer, patient outcomes should improve. Since patients receive the greatest benefit, the ideal opportunity to demonstrate ROI for safety interventions would be from the patient perspective. However, patients are responsible for the smallest portion of the investment, since their out-of-pocket expenses for health care are minimal. Most patients today are insured through employer-based or federal and state entitlement programs. Another substantial number of Americans does not have health insurance and cannot afford to pay for care; these individuals make little to no financial contribution to the health care system, even though they consume health care at various levels. The fiscal fragmentation of the U.S. health care system prevents the measurement of a direct ROI for those patients who realize a benefit from improved safety, as they are the constituent group that is by and large making the least financial investment in that system.

FUNDER PERSPECTIVE

For purposes of this discussion, health care funders may be divided into two main categories: public and private.

Public funders include federal, state, and local governments that support various entitlement programs, primarily for the elderly and poor. Private funders are employers responsible for purchasing health care services for their employees and retirees as an employment benefit. Including tax incentives provided to employers for their payment of health care insurance premiums, public funders pay for nearly 60 percent of total U.S. health care expenditures.[13]

The largest publicly funded health care program, Medicare, drives patient safety initiatives through JCAHO accreditation surveys. Interventions such as improving patient-identification procedures and prohibiting the use of ambiguous abbreviations are critical in securing and maintaining JCAHO accreditation, which is a requirement for participation in the Medicare program. While the public payer's financial return associated with improved safety is limited by capitated prospective-reimbursement structures, public funders still realize cost advantages as a result of lower hospital readmission rates and other benefits associated with increased patient safety.

On the private side, the Leapfrog Group was founded in 2000 by the Business Roundtable, a national association of Fortune 500 chief executive officers, in an attempt to leverage the influence of 150 large employers to advance safety improvements.[14] The group advocates a variety of quality-improvement standards, including CPOE, evidence-based hospital referral, and intensive care unit physician staffing.[15] Providers meeting the Leapfrog standards receive full reimbursement for services provided to the individual funder's patients, while providers who do not meet the standards run the risk of financial disincentives.[16]

Whether public or private, whether operating in response to regulation or to market pressures, funders are mandating the adoption of safety interventions but not directly bearing the cost of those interventions. Providers, health systems, and hospitals have the full administrative and financial burden of development and implementation.

INSURER PERSPECTIVE

The two basic funder groups just described do not include insurance and managed care companies that serve as fiscal intermediaries and that, other than for their own employees, do not provide funds directly into the health care system. While their role in transferring funds and providing administrative services (e.g., claims processing, rate setting, underwriting) is important, these companies have no stake in patient safety other than their desire to secure a larger margin between what money is raised through premiums and what is paid to providers.

PROVIDER PERSPECTIVE

The word *provider* refers to various entities, including health care practitioners, hospitals, health systems, and others, that offer health care services directly to patients. Today, funders and insurers expect providers to bear a disproportionate share of the cost of safety interventions. For example, it has been estimated that the initial cost of implementing CPOE in an average 500-bed hospital is approximately $8 million, with subsequent annual costs of $1.35 million.[17] Health systems and hospitals are under increasing regulatory and financial pressures to implement such systems (indeed, the Leapfrog Group has mandated implementation), yet funders and insurers have offered little to no financial support to offset their implementation and maintenance costs. Providers remain challenged to demonstrate a positive ROI for most safety initiatives.

Is a Business Case for Patient Safety Possible?

As demonstrated in the preceding section and in Table 3-1, each perspective considered in making a business case for investment in patient safety differs in terms of expected investment and return. A review of these perspectives reveals that providers appear to face the greatest challenge with respect to demonstrating ROI and establishing a business case for the value of various safety-enhancing interventions.

Providers are expected to underwrite investments in safety-enhancing interventions with little or no additional offsetting revenue from funders and payers. Providers must meet regulatory mandates for many care-delivery processes (e.g., core measures used by CMS and JCAHO), must achieve and demonstrate positive patient outcomes, and are mandated to implement safety-improvement technologies such as CPOE, all with increasingly fewer resources. They must decide how to allocate fixed reimbursement in a way that will best serve their patients and improve safety yet enable them to maintain fiscal viability.

In a fully capitated market, where a provider accepts financial risk for all care necessary for a defined cohort of patients, improved safety may provide ROI by eliminating readmissions and their associated costs. However, in a less competitive market, where providers generally bill on a fee-for-service basis, readmissions are uniquely billable encounters, and improved safety does not provide as great a return. While the suggestion that lower-quality care is favorable for providers may seem perverse, decisions regarding how best to invest finite resources must consider the realities of our current reimbursement system.

In markets where providing more care is associated with higher reimbursement and improved financial performance, other justifications for investing in patient safety must be identified. Safety initiatives may simultaneously improve the operational efficiency of provider organizations and lower the cost of providing care. For example, robotics has been shown to reduce workforce needs for medication cart–filling functions in hospitals and reduce medication errors.[18] To the extent that provider organizations have limited capacity to care for patients, improved efficiency can produce actual revenue growth.

Lower rates of error would presumably have a positive impact on the total cost of care (e.g., by reducing the spending necessary to manage negative consequences of an error and the cost of potential malpractice awards). However, the financial value of a medication error avoided can at present be based only on speculative data.[19] It is a challenge both to measure the financial impact of something that has not happened and to attribute something that has not happened to a specific intervention. As reasonable as it might be to assume a financial benefit associated with improved safety, that benefit must be accurately quantified to establish a compelling business case.

Safety-improvement technologies that also improve documentation, such as bar code–based medication-administration systems, may increase billing compliance, given the substantial fines levied against organizations that bill for services (including provision of medications) that are not documented. Bar coding has also exhibited additional efficiencies in the administrative process by eliminating inaccuracies and delays and collecting data for future analysis.[20,21]

In markets where patients have many choices regarding providers, organizations seen in a community as being a "safe place" to receive care may also improve their financial performance. However, metrics that measure safety are simple to manipulate, data are not available, and the value of such data to consumers, even if they did exist, is unknown.

CPOE is one of the most widely promoted safety interventions, and it comes a very high price tag. Making a business case for CPOE is exceptionally difficult. Unless tied to decision-support tools that encourage cost-efficient prescribing behaviors, the benefit of CPOE is limited to a reduction in errors caused by illegible handwriting. Berger and Kishak[22] note that little data support the benefit of CPOE and even suggest that the process of implementing CPOE may temporarily cause more errors and increase the cost of care. These concerns may explain the limited diffusion of CPOE technology. In 2004, Ash and colleagues[23] reported the results of two definitive surveys regarding CPOE in U.S. hospitals over a period of seven years. They found that only 9.6 percent of hospitals currently had CPOE completely available. Devers and Liu[24] supported the findings of Ash and colleagues and identified additional barriers to CPOE, including the lack of incentives and the organizational and technological challenges surrounding the implementation of such a system.

Conclusion

A business case for investment in safety-enhancing interventions should be based on the same sort of systematic evaluation process used to make other decisions regarding the adoption of health care interventions. The lack of compelling evidence necessary to guide investment suggests that provider organizations should be allowed to invest in a manner that makes the most sense for them. For example, instead of being mandated to invest millions of dollars in a specific safety intervention, providers should be allowed and expected to pursue safety improvements that they can support with a compelling business case and that consider the unique characteristics of that organization and its financial condition. Alternatively, if a particular intervention is deemed critically important, all constituents that realize a return on that investment must share financial responsibility for its cost.

References

1. Kohn LT, Corrigan JM, Donaldson MD, eds. Committee on Quality of Health in America, Institute of Medicine. *To Err Is Human: Building a Safer Health System.* Washington, DC: National Academy Press; 1999.

2. Devers KJ, Pham HH, Liu G. What is driving hospitals' patient-safety efforts? *Health Affairs.* 2004;23(2):103-115.

3. Heffler S, Smith S, Keehan S, Clemens MK, Won G, Zezza M. Health spending projections for 2002–2012. *Health Affairs.* 2003(Jan-Jun); Suppl Web Exclusives: W3-54-65. Posted February 7, 2003.

4. General Accounting Office. Glossary of IT Investment Terms. Available at: www.gao.gov/policy/itguide/glossary.htm. Accessed April 20, 2004.

5. Oetgen WJ, Oetgen PM. A business case for patient safety. *Physician Exec.* 2003;Sept/Oct:39-42.

6. Massaro R. Investing in patient safety: an ethical and business imperative. *Trustee.* 2003;56(6):20-23.

7. Cassalino LP. Markets and medicine: barriers to creating a "business case for quality." *Perspect Biol Med.* Winter 2003;46(1):38-51.

8. Joint Commission on Accreditation of Healthcare Organizations. Patient Safety: Instilling Hospitals with a Culture of Continuous Improvement. Testimony before the Senate Committee on Government Affairs. June 11, 2003. Available at: www.jcaho.org/news+room/on+capitol+hill/. Accessed June 14, 2004.

9. Ohio Patient Safety Institute. *OPSI Patient Safety Bulletin.* October 2002. Available at: www.ohiopatientsafety.org/Bulletins/OPSIOctober2002Bulletin.pdf. Accessed June 5, 2004.

10. Agency for Healthcare Research and Quality. *Making Health Care Safer: A Critical Analysis of Patient Safety Practices.* Evidence Report/Technology Assessment, No. 43. AHRQ Rockville, MD: AHRQ; July 2001. AHRQ publication 01-E058. Available at: www.ahrq.gov/clinic/ptsafety/. Accessed April 15, 2004.

11. Rosenthal MB, Fernandopulle R, Song HR, Landon B. Paying for quality: providers' incentives for quality improvement. *Health Affairs.* 2004;23:127-141.

12. Gold MR, Siegel JE, Russell LB, Weinstein MC, eds. *Cost-Effectiveness in Health and Medicine.* New York: Oxford University Press; 1996.

13. Woolhandler S, Himmelstein DU. Paying for national health insurance—and not getting it. *Health Affairs.* 2002;21(4):88-98.

14. The Leapfrog Group. About Us—General Principles and Assumptions. Washington, DC: Leapfrog Group. Available at: www.leapfroggroup.org/governance1.htm. Accessed January 13, 2004.

15. Birkmeyer JD, Dimick JB. The Leapfrog Group's Patient Safety Practices, 2003: The Potential Benefits of Universal Adoption. Washington, DC: Leapfrog Group; February 2004.

16. Freudenheim M. Many hospitals resist computerized patient care. *New York Times.* April 6, 2004. Available at: www.nytimes.com/ref/membercenter/nytarchive.html.

17. Kuperman GJ, Gibson RF. Computer physician order entry: benefits, costs, and issues. *Ann Intern Med.* 2003;139:31-39.

18. Landis NT. Pharmacies gain staff time as new "employee" lends a hand. *Am J Health-Syst Pharm.* 1993;50:2236-2242.

19. Johnson JA, Bootman JL. Drug-related morbidity and mortality and the economic impact of pharmaceutical care. *Am J Health-System Pharm.* 1997;54:554-558.

20. American Society of Health-System Pharmacists. CPOE, bedside technology, and patient safety: A roundtable discussion [special feature]. *Am J Health-Syst Pharm.* 2003; 60:1219-1228.

21. May EL. The case for bar coding: Better information, better care, and better business. *Healthcare Exec.* 2003;18(5):8-13.

22. Berger RG, Kishak JP. Computerized prescriber order entry: helpful or harmful? *J Am Med Informatics Assoc.* 2004;11(2):100-103.

23. Ash JS, Gorman PN, Seshadri V, Hersh WR. Computerized prescriber order entry in U.S. hospitals: results of a 2002 survey. *J Am Med Informatics Assoc.* 2004;11(2):95-99.

24. Devers KJ, Liu G. Leapfrog Patient-Safety Standards Are a Stretch for Most Hospitals. Issue Brief No. 77. Washington, DC: Center for Studying Health System Change; February 2004. Available at: www.hschange.org/CONTENT/647/#ib5. Accessed December 21, 2004.

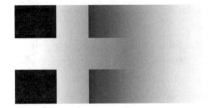

CHAPTER 4

Blueprint for a Culture of Safety

Joanne E. Turnbull

Introduction to a Culture of Safety

For improvements in patient safety to endure, there must be radical changes in the health care culture. This chapter describes the fundamental elements that need to be in place to instill a culture of safety in every component of the health care delivery system, irrespective of type or size of organization, location, or population served. The chapter begins by defining a culture of safety and by examining some of the barriers to a culture of safety in the existing health care environment. The second part of the chapter lays out a blueprint for a culture of safety. It introduces the notion of *complexity*, a concept that both characterizes health care organizations and guides assumptions that underlie and inform a culture of safety. The chapter also focuses on the importance of aligning the multiple cultures and subcultures that make up today's complex health care systems and influence the delivery of care. A case study illustrates a cultural intervention related to safe medication use. The chapter ends with a discussion of the new type of leadership that will be needed in the coming culture of safety.

WHY IS A CULTURE OF SAFETY SO IMPORTANT?

Three recent reports have documented the need for a culture of safety in health care and made efforts to outline the characteristics of such a culture. In 1999, the publication of the Institute of Medicine (IOM) report *To Err Is Human: Building a Safer Health System* marked a watershed for the politics and practice of health care in the United States.[1] The patient-safety movement was well under way when this report appeared and it was based on a few studies that were the subject of debate. Nonetheless, the IOM report produced two remarkable and immediate changes. First, it broke the secrecy that had long surrounded harm to patients. Second, the report captured the attention of both the public and professionals worldwide by estimating that as many as 98,000 deaths per year in the United States may be attributed to preventable adverse events. Preventable adverse events, the report stated, are the eighth leading cause of death in the United States, ahead of car accidents (43,000 deaths per year), breast cancer (42,300), and AIDS (16,516). Following the publication of *To Err Is Human*, patient safety became a top priority on the national agenda.

The years immediately following publication of the IOM report were marked by the introduction of a number of "transforming concepts"—messages that are so powerful that they can cause an individual's cognitive paradigm to shift. With respect to medication safety, two transforming concepts stand out. The first is that most errors occur not because of flawed humans but because of flaws in poorly designed systems.[2] The concept is that design of safer systems of care is contingent on substantial change in the culture of health care.[3]

In 2001, the IOM issued a second seminal report, *Crossing the Quality Chasm: A New Health System for the 21st Century*.[4] This report captured less attention than the 1999 report did; however, its message was equally powerful. In addition to condemning several failures in the current health care culture (e.g., the failure to translate knowledge into practice, to apply new technology in a safe and effective manner, to make the best use of resources, and to restructure clinical services to meet the needs of patients), this report describes what happens when a health care delivery system embraces new technology but fails to adapt its culture to accommodate it. Practitioners are inundated with information from vast, continually expanding knowledge bases, and the number of drugs, medical devices, diagnostic techniques, and other technological supports continues to grow.

Crossing the Quality Chasm is more practical than the 1999 IOM report, and it goes beyond mandating fundamental change in the organization and delivery of health care in America and sets the groundwork for a road map to a safe health care culture. Noting that outmoded systems of work must be redesigned to protect both patients and caregivers, the report sets forth six specific quality aims for care: It must be safe, effective, patient centered, timely, efficient, and equitable.[4]

From a cultural perspective, the report's greatest contribution may be that it calls for health care leaders to commit themselves to a shared agenda of improvement. The report places responsibility for creating a culture of safety squarely on the shoulders of health care's administrative and clinical leaders. While the first report generated worldwide publicity, this second report changed the nature of patient-safety activity. Having lived with the burden of medical accidents while bound by the fear and secrecy of the health care culture, leaders now were being encouraged to acknowledge the problem and ask for help.

A third report, produced by the National Quality Forum (NQF) and entitled *Safe Practices for Better Healthcare: A Consensus Report,* moved the field to a new level by offering an initial set of 30 best practices for safer patient care.[5] The goal of this report is to ensure that the American people have the highest-quality, safest health care possible. The report notes that health care encompasses an exceedingly complex set of activities that rely heavily on the actions of human beings and combines a variety of technologies that are capable of both healing and causing significant harm. It is this combination—complex processes, dependence on human performance, and powerful technologies—that makes health care a high-risk and error-prone enterprise.

Although medical error has been increasingly recognized for several decades, the health care community has been slow to address improvement of health care or to make patient safety a priority. Compared with practices of other risk industries, health care's approach to safety, the report contends, is lackluster at best. Culture is the major barrier to change. Thus, the first practice listed in the *Safe Practices Report* is the creation and promotion of a culture of safety in all health care settings.[5] The remaining 29 patient safety practices rely on the first.

The promotion of a culture of safety is declared the single most important change called for in the NQF report. The health care industry must embrace the high-risk nature of modern medicine and assume collective responsibility for risk reduction. Transparency, that is, free and open communication and nonpunitive reporting of adverse events and full disclosure to injured patients and their families, must become the norm. Organizational objectives and incentives must be aligned with the goal of improving patient safety.

The *Safe Practices Report* lists the minimum specifications for a health care culture of safety. These specifications include standardized policies and procedures that rank reportable patient-safety events and situations a top priority and that support the analysis of these reported events. These policies and procedures should also guide the implementation of remedial actions, evaluate their effectiveness, and ensure that they do not cause unintended adverse consequences. Organizational leaders must be kept knowledgeable about patient-safety issues. They must ensure that the issues are appropriately addressed and that patient safety is continually improved. Leaders must oversee the coordination of patient-safety activities, provide feedback to frontline health care providers about lessons learned, publicly disclose data on implementation of and compliance with all applicable NQF-endorsed safe practices, and train all staff in techniques of team-based problem solving and management.

WHAT IS A CULTURE OF SAFETY?

The current health care culture has not made patient safety a priority.[3] Thus, it is not surprising that a formal, widely accepted definition of a "culture of safety" has yet to be formulated. Characteristics of a culture of safety can, however, be deduced from research on high-reliability organizations and from the initiatives of cutting-edge health care organizations. Key characteristics of high-reliability organizations, which may be defined as organizations that perform high-risk activities with low accident rates, include blameless, voluntary reporting systems, rigorous analysis of accidents and near misses, open communication about safety and error that includes the patient and family, a focus on individual accountability, and an unflagging commitment to patient safety from the leadership of the organization.[6] A safety culture rests on trust, knowledge, and appropriate system design.

Vulnerable System Syndrome

James Reason,[7] one of the major thinkers in human factors and safety, and his colleagues, have identified a group of core pathological elements—denial, blame, and pursuit of the wrong kind of excellence—that cause organizations to be susceptible to adverse events. Each of these pathologies interacts with and increases the strength of the other two, creating what these authors call the vulnerable system syndrome. Forming a self-sustaining cycle that is a malignant and undermines influence on any patient-safety program, these core pathologies cause an organization to be vulnerable, rather than resilient, to patient harm. The tendency to place blame when an accident occurs, along with denial that health care is a high-risk industry, are outgrowths of the myth of perfection, often mentioned as a cultural barrier in the *Safe Practices Report*.[5] The pursuit of the wrong kind of excellence refers to pursing management goals such as efficiency, cost savings, and patient satisfaction with ancillary services (e.g., a hospital's decor or menu) at the expense of pursuing excellence in the area of preventing harm to patients.

Pathological, Bureaucratic, and Generative Cultures

One indication of an organization's culture is the way in which it handles information. Westrum[8] identifies three types of organizational cultures that are distinguished by the way in which they pursue and respond to safety-related information. He categorizes these cultures as pathological, bureaucratic, or generative (see **Figure 4-1**).

Pathological Culture	Bureaucratic Culture	Generative Culture
Don't want to know.	May not find out.	Actively seek it.
Messengers (i.e., whistle blowers) are "shot."	Messengers are listened to if they arrive.	Messengers are trained and rewarded.
Failure is punished or concealed.	Failure leads to local repairs.	Failures lead to far-reaching reforms.
New ideas are discouraged.	New ideas often present problems.	New ideas are welcomed.

A safety culture is generative, constantly "uneasy," seeking, learning, changing.

Figure 4-1. How Different Organizational Cultures Handle Safety Information

Pathological organizations do not want to know about safety problems. Such cultures punish those who report or are involved in accidents and near misses. They cover up failures and discourage new ideas. Generative cultures lie at the other end of the spectrum. They boast features that resonate with a culture of safety. In generative cultures, all members of the organization are alert and vigilant; they constantly seek information about how the organization and all its parts, systems, processes, and people are performing. Hazards and vulnerabilities are identified and examined; if they cannot be eliminated, they are at least made visible, and strategies are put in place to militate against them. Individuals are trained to identify and report risks, errors, failures, near misses, and similar events. Employees are not only trained to report but encouraged to do so. Leaders publicly thank and celebrate reporting and hazard identification.

A bureaucratic culture falls between generative and pathological. Most health care organizations fall into this category. A bureaucratic culture compartmentalizes safety management (e.g., by naming a patient-safety officer rather than holding senior leadership accountable for safety), deals with error on an isolated, local basis, and does not integrate lessons from failures throughout the organization. Reporters are not penalized, but the organization lacks an effective means of evaluating and accommodating new ideas. Health care organizations must nurture generative cultures in order to become high-reliability organizations.

Edgar Schein, a noted theorist and researcher on organizational culture, defines organizational culture as *"a pattern of shared basic assumptions that the group learned as it solved its problems of external adaptation and in internal integration that has worked well enough to be considered valid and therefore, to be taught to new members as the correct way to perceive, think, and feel in relation to those problems."* [9]

Following the logic of Schein's definition and adding to it the unacceptable number of accidents, we can surmise that health care's pattern of shared assumptions is based on perceptions, thoughts, and feelings that no longer work.

BARRIERS TO A CULTURE OF SAFETY IN HEALTH CARE
Many barriers unique to improving safety for patients are unique to health care. None is more potentially damaging than the myth that "good" health care professionals will also perform perfectly and, conversely, that adverse events are caused by human carelessness, negligence, or incompetence. Unfortunately, this myth is very much alive not only within the health care professions but also among the public at large. A second barrier occurs in the intersection of the medical culture and the legal system. Legal and liability concerns stifle open communication about safety problems and data sharing. A third barrier is the lack of data or the failure to use data to effect improvement. Most health care organizations lack effective reporting systems, and there is no law to create a national reporting system. There is still ignorance in the health care industry about systems thinking and inadequate knowledge about the systemic nature of health care accidents, particularly among those who control the resources. Finally, there is a lack of leadership regarding patient safety among health care leaders.

One of the greatest barriers to a culture of safety is the "blame and shame" mentality. When an error occurs, the immediate reaction is to blame, criticize, and sanction the individual who happened to be closest to the failure or accident. The cultural ramifications of this mentality are chilling. Personal feelings of guilt are compounded by the isolation, shame, and secrecy that surround errors. All learning stops, and the conditions that produced the accident persist. A similar failure is likely to occur.

Societal judgment mirrors and reinforces the health care culture. Regulatory and legal systems emphasize individual culpability or harm to patients and rarely address vulnerabilities inherent in system and process failures. Licensing boards in medicine, nursing, and pharmacy focus on individual action or inaction and look to limit or remove licenses to practice, an approach that jeopardizes the livelihood of professionals and perpetuates fear. The result is an environment in which most errors are driven underground.

The hierarchical nature of medical practice is another major barrier to safety. Hierarchical relationships, as opposed to collaborative partnerships, characterize many of the interactions between physicians and nurses, nurses and nurses' aides, physicians and pharmacists, pharmacists and nurses, and pharmacists and pharmacy technicians. A hierarchy also exists between patients and their health care providers, with the provider as the expert and the patient as a recipient of services, rather than a partner in care.

The *authority gradient*, a term that refers to the interpersonal dynamics present in any situation of real or perceived power, is a characteristic of hierarchical cultures. The authority gradient exists in other high-risk organizations, such as the armed forces and the airline and shipping industries. In any situation governed by the authority gradient, communication patterns are altered in a way that increases the probability of accidents. Truth, especially bad news, may be withheld or watered down. Statements from subordinates to the individuals perceived to be in positions of superior authority tend to be vague and indirect. In an effort to overcome the negative effects of the authority gradient, the airline industry has trained pilots and copilots in clear, collaborative communications. In this process, dubbed "crew resource management training," crew members are not only trained to communicate with each other more directly but also are empowered and obligated to report observed system or process vulnerabilities that might lead to an accident.[10]

Blueprint for the Culture of Safety

The blueprint for the culture of safety is neither a detailed set of plans, such as those developed by an architect, nor a linear formula, such as a prescription or protocol. The journey to a culture of safety is full of rough, entwined, and twisting roads filled with daunting challenges. Concepts from complexity theory can help those concerned with safety understand the nature of both the journey and the blueprint.[11]

Health care is a complex, adaptive system, and as such, it exhibits certain characteristics common to all such systems, whether they be the immune system, a colony of termites, the financial market, or just about any collection of humans, such as a committee or even a family.[12] Like these other systems, health care is a collection of individual agents that have freedom to act in ways that are not always totally predictable and whose actions are interconnected so that one agent's actions change the context for others.

COMPLEX, SIMPLE, COMPLICATED

The words *simple, complicated*, and *complex* describe three different domains of problems or work within the complex adaptive systems that make up organizations.

Simple domains are those that can be managed by a protocol that brings stakeholders close to agreement and certainty. Following a recipe to bake a cake is a simple procedure. A simple approach may not use many resources or require much effort but still have great impact in a complex system.[13]

Complicated domains require multiple steps of analysis and multiple perspectives for system design and control. A complicated problem introduces greater variability, less certainty, and a broader zone in which agreement must be negotiated. Examples of complicated problems include performing open-heart surgery or managing a quality-improvement project. In a complex system, a complicated approach may use many resources and require effort yet have little impact or sustainability.[13]

The word *complex* is applied to systems characterized by nonlinear, interactive components, emergent phenomena, continuous and discontinuous change, and unpredictable outcomes. Although there is at present no one accepted definition of complexity, the term is applied across a range of different yet related system features, such as chaos, adaptivity, neural nets, nonlinear dynamics, and far-from-equilibrium conditions.[11] These ideas from complexity theory are better understood through illustration than through concrete definition. Table 4-1 illustrates the characteristics of simple, complicated, and complex domains.

Table 4-1. Simple, Complicated, and Complex Domains

Simple (e.g., following a recipe)	Complicated (e.g., sending a rocket to the moon)	Complex (e.g., bringing up a child)
The recipe is essential.	Formulas are critical and necessary.	Formulas have limited utility.
Recipes are tested to ensure easy replication of success.	Sending one rocket increases probability of future success.	Raising one child provides experience but no assurance of future success.
No particular expertise is required, although practice can improve the success rate.	High expertise in a variety of fields is essential.	Expertise can be helpful but is neither necessary nor sufficient to contribute to success.
Recipes produce standardized, predictable results every time.	There is a high degree of outcome predictability.	Every child is a unique individual; outcomes are unpredictable.

Source: McCandless K, Zimmerman, B. Simplicity on the Other Side of Complexity. Patient Safety Fellowship Workbook, American Hospital Association Health Forum, 2003-2004.

Examples of complex domains include raising a child and creating a culture of safety. Compared with solving simple problems, solving a complex problem requires more individual freedom and more sharing and understanding of deviations from protocol. Complexity may mean ambiguity; it is associated with dynamic and changing interactions of parts that combine and propagate in unpredictable ways, with nonlinear effects. Disagreement is high. Continual trade-offs and negotiations are required.[6] Complexity-inspired approaches are likely to have the highest probability of success in complex systems. Small changes can have big effects in complex systems because of nonlinearity. A single event can engender big results, whereas big initiatives can effect very little change. Multiple sources of information—people, events, and relationships—continually provide input into decision making.[13]

In its ideal state, a culture of safety constantly learns not only from failure but also from anticipation of failure and from mental simulations of possible-failure scenarios. The culture explicitly encourages and supports the reporting of any situation or circumstance that threatens, or may threaten, the safety of patients or caregivers. It views near misses and adverse events as opportunities to make the health care system better.

One primary characteristic that distinguishes generative safety cultures from other organizations is *mindfulness*. A term coined by psychologist Karl Weick,[14] mindfulness is an ongoing scrutiny of existing expectations, a continuous refinement and differentiation of expectations based on newer experiences, a willingness and capacity to invent expectations that make sense of unprecedented events, a nuanced appreciation of context and ways to deal with it, and an identification of new dimensions of context that improve foresight and current functioning. In everyday terms, mindfulness can be defined as alertness or hyperawareness. Mindfulness allows workers to react to very weak signs when change or danger is approaching. The willingness and ability to organize in a complex manner is what allows workers in a safety culture to deal with a complex environment that produces unexpected events.

Health care organizations can learn to be more mindful by adopting certain practices. These include an obsession with failure, a commitment to resilience, sensitivity to operations, managerial attention focused on the front line where the work really gets done, awareness of the importance of listening to the workers, deference to expertise, refusal to simplify, and cultivation of a greater response repertoire on the team. One strategy to develop mindfulness is to encourage workers to actively bring observations about safety and risk to the attention of higher management.

TRANSFORMING ASSUMPTIONS TO CREATE A CULTURE OF SAFETY

Kuhn[15] notes that health care is in the throes of a paradigm shift. A *paradigm shift* is a change in thinking, structures, and processes that is so radical that "before" and "after" appear to have little relationship to one another. The change from before to after is not linear or incremental, but rather jarring and discontinuous. Integrating Kuhn's notion of paradigm shift with the concept of first and second "curves" put forth by Ian Morrison,[16] Martin Merry[17] contrasts the structures of 20th-century health care (the "first curve") with an entirely new second-curve health care paradigm that is now in its infancy. Different assumptions and beliefs underlie the two curves. These differences cause shifts in behavior that are so rapid that they are experienced as dramatic, revolutionary, and traumatic (see **Figure 4-2**).

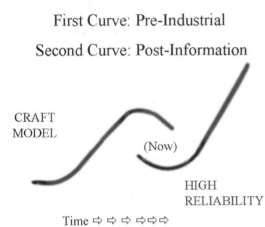

First Curve: Pre-Industrial

Second Curve: Post-Information

CRAFT MODEL

(Now)

HIGH RELIABILITY

Time ⇨ ⇨ ⇨ ⇨⇨⇨

Figure 4-2. First and Second Curves in Health Care

Source: *Morath JM, Turnbull JE.* To Do No Harm: Ensuring a Culture of Safety in Health Care. *San Francisco, CA: Jossey-Bass; 2004.*

Health care's first curve dates to a 1910 report by Flexner[18] that transformed America's "diploma-mill" medical education system into an academic medical education model and summoned an escalating technical capability in American health care. Unfortunately, health care failed to develop a systems infrastructure to support the burgeoning complexity that accompanied technology. As a result, unfortunate, unintended consequences are evident today: tremendous complexity, fragmentation, and a propensity to cause harm go hand in hand with the miraculous medical and surgical innovations of the past century. Health care's rapid advance in technology spawned a complex industry built on an eighteenth-century, pre–Industrial Revolution craft model—

a *Concorde* engine in a Wright Brothers chassis.[19]

One prominent feature of a pre–Industrial Revolution craft model of health care is that it separates operations from clinical care, leaving much of the design of actual patient care up to the craftspeople: training physicians, nurses, and pharmacists; licensing them; allocating resources; and then letting them alone as they care for patients. In contrast, the second curve does not isolate clinical practice from the management of resources. Rather, leadership purposefully designs essential organizational infrastructures to support the complexity of practice that accompanies advanced technology. Key assumptions that distinguish the second from the first curve are depicted in **Table 4-2**.

New systems designed with second-curve assumptions and beliefs can be measured against the beliefs and assumptions of the first curve.

Table 4-2. Key Assumptions that Distinguish the First and Second Curves in Health Care

First Curve: Pre–Industrial Revolution	Second Curve: Postinformation Age
Organized around needs of providers.	Designed around needs of those served, including those of caregivers.
Asks community to come to provider.	Providers reach out to the community.
Reacts only to individual (e.g., a person with diabetes); pays little attention to needs of population (e.g., all persons with diabetes).	Plans for population, reduces need for individual care, but retains ability to respond to needs of the individual.
Defines quality in terms of morbidity and mortality and resists publication of data.	Users add to definition of quality, including satisfaction with service, functionality, and value; insist on actual information to choose, using appropriately case mix–adjusted information.
Defines quality mainly in terms of professional skills; pays little attention to support systems.	Understands that carefully designed quality infrastructure is essential to reduce risk and optimize skills of professionals.
Assumes that providers' intentions are impeccable and that their performance will be error free.	Assumes that humans are inherently fallible and that harm occurs despite providers' best intentions.
Reality: Human error generates harm; threat of punishment is a deterrent.	Reality: System is error-tolerant and accepts human error as inevitable; designs errorproofing strategies.
Complexity makes it easy to do things wrong, hard to do things right.	Well-designed latent workplace conditions make it easy to do things right and hard to do things wrong.
Solution to problems entails censuring professionals and provider institutions.	Solution to problems translates to redesigning systems to become more error-tolerant and supportive of workers.
System is fragmented; patients must fend for themselves.	Seamless system coordinates needs of complex patients, using case managers for especially difficult cases.
Ultimate definition of quality endlessly debated, thus avoiding adequate measurement, management, and improvement.	Consensus regarding a variety of key measures, including access to care, clinical outcomes, functionality, satisfaction, and value received.
Medical record fragmented and idiosyncratic to particular "silo"; Individual caregivers work from unconnected, often contradictory "scripts."	Electronic medical record instantly updated and available for all relevant caregivers.
Information centralized and hierarchical; physician seen as a "supreme source of knowledge, dictator of therapy."	Information dispersed and all caregivers and patients have direct access to it. Physician may serve as integrator or facilitator of choices.
Insurance monolithic, not enrollee sensitive, with only a few choices for individuals.	Insurance mass customized; Web-based options chosen by individuals on the basis of specific needs.
Billing and payment systems arcane, confusing, virtually impossible to understand.	Coverage and copayment clear, Web-facilitated, and easy to navigate.

First Curve: Pre–Industrial Revolution	Second Curve: Postinformation Age
Payment system blind to quality and value and rewards volume, even that generated by poor quality and error.	Payment system fine-tuned to value; rewards superior performance as defined by value equation.
Huge resources consumed in "reimbursing" inefficient systems, human error, litigation, and "cost-plus" models.	Huge resources freed up for innovation and quality improvement, with "cost-plus, value-blind reimbursement" a distant memory.
Health care as an isolated, quirky "high-tech, organizationally primitive" industry, a throwback" to pre-18th-century human organizational development.	Health care as a vibrant participant in the best that learnings from the industrial/information revolution can offer.
"Crashes" common; iatrogenic death/injury headlines a regular, predictable occurrence.	Crashes rare, with iatrogenic death equivalent to that of airline industry.
As of 2005, trust in system increasingly shaky and falling.	As of 200?, trust in system high and rising.
Extremely high, probably incalculable cost of poor quality.	Minimal cost of poor quality.

Source: Merry M. Health Care's Need For Revolutionary Change. Quality Progress 2003; 36(9): 31-35.

ALIGNING CULTURES AND SUBCULTURES

The culture of the health care system is made up of embedded systems, each with distinct cultures and subcultures. The culture of each system must be aligned toward a goal of safety in order for the culture of safety to become a reality. **Figure 4-3** depicts how these different systems and cultures are embedded.[20]

The term *onion model* has been used in diverse fields, ranging from computers to religion, to describe multilayered phenomena that are embedded within a complex system.[20] The onion model can illustrate how culture can change through socialization of the various subcultures of the health care system. Each of these embedded, dynamic systems is complex in its own right, and each system needs to be understood in order to grasp the whole picture. Each system can have more than one subculture, and no single layer can be considered in isolation.

Each concentric circle represents a system or culture that has direct socialization effects on the adjacent culture. Cultural changes at the organizational level have direct effects on the culture of the practice level, and vice versa. For example, an organization's decision to disclose adverse events has direct effects on the subcultures of the practice level. The direct effects of disclosure on health care professionals might range from fear of exposure and increased litigation to feelings of betrayal. Patients and their families, in contrast, might react with disbelief or feel less adversarial.

Systems or cultures that are distant from one another, for example, the media culture at the social layer and the patient and family culture at the innermost circle, influence each other via filtered effects. An example would be patients responding to sensationalized stories of accidents by bringing video cameras to nursing units in order to document activities, or slanted media reports based on an interview with a disgruntled employee.

Interactions between patients and families and the practice subcultures in health care are changing drastically. For example, patients and families are now seeking meaningful involvement in their care, and are doing so in a respectful way. Recognizing patients and families as partners in the system of care, not as passive recipients of care, brings an abundance of expertise and safety nets to the clinical encounter. As the patient and practice cultures become

Onion Model: Health Care Cultures and Subcultures

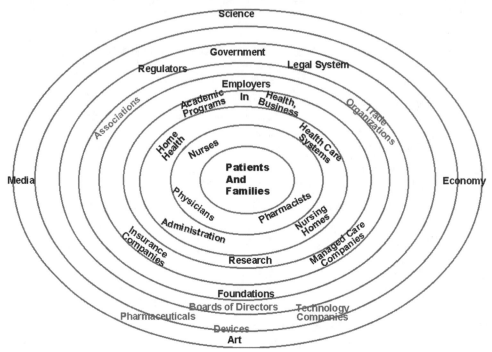

Figure 4-3. *Onion Model*

Source: *J. Turnbull , The Onion Model, adapted from Veroff, J. and Douvan, E. Unpublished manuscript for the Patient Safety Fellowship Workbook, American Hospital Association Health Forum; 2003-2004.*

better aligned, professionals are meeting with families of victims of medical error to hear their concerns. This approach helps heal grieving people who in the past have had their suffering compounded by anger at an unresponsive system. As professionals embrace consumer involvement, they increasingly recognize patients and their families as a source of wisdom, resilience, and capacity, that enhances the skill, compassion, and resourcefulness of the workforce and enables providers to identify what works and what does not work for patients.[6,21]

The practice culture is known in patient safety language as the "sharp end."[22] The practice culture contains multiple subcultures. For example, the subculture of pharmacists is very different from that of physicians, yet both are components of the practice culture. For the culture of safety to become a reality, change has to happen at cultural level, and every subculture of the health care system has to be aligned.

Education holds great promise for aligning the patient, practice, and organizational cultures and subcultures. Health care professionals educated under the new paradigms will influence, and eventually replace, their senior colleagues. All training programs in the health professions will integrate elements of safety science into their curricula, and instruction in human factors and organizational analysis will provide a consistent foundation for all disciplines in patient safety.

But even more radical change may be on the horizon. For example, future professionals in pharmacy, nursing, and medicine may undergo the first two years of training together with a unified curriculum. When this happens, a more unified practice culture will emerge.

At the organizational level, culture is changing as the role of the department yields to a multidisciplinary approach that is organized on the basis of the needs of different patient populations. Many organizations have longstanding experience with group dynamics and team building and believe that they have been practicing it all along. Team *learning*, however, differs from team *building*. Team learning is not about improving team members' communication skills but about creating alignment, the goal of which is to enable the team not to agree on everything but to function as a whole.[23] Building alignment is concerned with enhancing a team's capacity to think and act in new, synergistic ways, with full coordination and a sense of unity because team members know and respect each other; they do not have to bury their disagreements. Rather, the team develops the capacity to use differences of opinion to enrich its collective understanding.[23]

A SAFETY CULTURE IS A JUST CULTURE

The systems approach that underlies the safety culture in no way obviates individual, organizational, or social accountability. A safety culture is a "just culture."[24] The systems approach requires that processes in high-risk delivery systems be designed to prevent solitary human missteps (i.e., single-point failures that stem from unintentional error) from leading to a catastrophic result. Any intentional rule violation, by contrast, requires timely and appropriate actions that are carried out equitably with respect to everyone, irrespective of position. Intentional rule violations are not necessarily related to risk taking, but they do demonstrate that an individual purposely violated a rule, procedure, or duty in the course of performing a task. These are "blameworthy behaviors" that violate standards of conduct and practice.[6] They are relatively rare circumstances that require confirmation by evidence such as the consultation of knowledgeable colleagues. Blameworthy actions include those carried out by individuals who are impaired, whether because of the influence of drugs or alcohol, diminished capability due to illness or changes with aging, engaging in reckless behavior, or showing a failure to learn over time.

CULTURAL INTERVENTIONS

Transforming a culture is a long and arduous process. However, transformation vehicles now exist that are moving forward transformation of the culture. Among them are simulations, blameless reporting systems, and learning partnerships or collaborations.

Simulations range from sophisticated laboratories that train anesthesia residents to sustain life during surgical emergencies[25] to spontaneous role plays conducted by team members in an emergency department to prepare for situations of high risk to mental rehearsals of what can go wrong conducted by individual practitioners. The objectives of such simulations are to create an environment of thoughtful and intelligent adherence rather than thoughtless or routine compliance, to develop discipline and guidance around communication and teamwork, and to create the expertise to cope with unexpected problems. An organization on its way to the culture of safety has training as a priority and it invests in training that is particular to the work situation.

A safety culture uses a blameless reporting system infrastructure to identify sources of system vulnerability that become the focus of improvement and risk-mitigation efforts. The system prospectively captures information about system performance, latent conditions, and vulnerabilities. Its voluntary, nonpunitive nature helps create a culture that does not view individuals as the source of harm but instead recognizes that professionals continuously create safety and prevent harm to patients by intercepting error and compensating for faulty and risk-prone systems. Therefore, a voluntary reporting system is focused on systems, not on people, and it provides the vehicle for systematically collecting and learning from frontline wisdom.

A patient-safety learning partnership goes beyond the basic reporting system. It contains all the tools and processes needed for organized learning about patient safety. These tools can be stored in an organization's data warehouse or in regional or national learning laboratories. Learning systems begin with a computer database with intelligent query capability, such as that available in data warehouses and decision-support systems.[6]

Collaborations and partnerships for the purposes of seeking and sharing information exist at both the state and national levels. Examples include the National Patient Safety Foundation's listserv, the Institute for Health Care Improvement's collaboratives, the American Hospital Association Health Forum's patient safety fellowship, and the many collaborations that are emerging at the state and regional levels.

Case Study: Pharmacists as Cultural Change Leaders

The following case study illustrates not only how pharmacists can be leaders in the transformation to the culture of safety but also the essential cultural contributions they have to make to such a culture.

A team from the Joint Commission on the Accreditation of Healthcare Systems (JCAHO) arrived at Smithville Hospital two weeks after the tragic death of a six-week old infant from a digoxin overdose. Following disclosure of this sentinel event in the opening conference, the surveyor asked that the hospital provide an analysis of the number of medication events that had been prevented during the past year. The analysis was due the following day.

At first, the pharmacy leadership stated that no such data existed. But as the dialogue progressed, one of the pharmacy leaders mentioned the pharmacy consultation program, an initiative under which Smithville Hospital pharmacists contacted physicians regarding medication orders that were prescribed in such a way that an adverse outcome might be likely. The pharmacists had been documenting calls to physicians concerning orders with toxic or subtherapeutic doses for more than two years. The data had never been analyzed because of the negative responses of physicians to the pharmacists' warnings. The pharmacy leadership, along with performance-improvement staff, worked through the night to analyze the data in order to submit them to the JCAHO team. They found that 30 percent of the orders had the potential to produce adverse outcomes.

On hearing the results of the analysis of the data in the pharmacy consultation program, the hospital's medical director stepped in. He encouraged the pharmacy staff to call physicians and he intervened with verbally abusive physicians, counseling them to welcome the calls and to be grateful for this valuable input. Stickers were placed on every patient's chart that outlined a new prescribing policy. Under this policy, pharmacists were authorized as approved countersigners for high-risk medications ordered by resident physicians. This was a huge cultural shift.

Initially, the rate of physician compliance with the new ordering policy was 58 percent; within a year, compliance rose to 98 percent. The real cultural change was revealed in the attitude of the physician leadership, which declared that 98 percent compliance was not good enough. They would accept nothing less than 100 percent as the goal for the following year (see **Figure 4-4**).

Medical Staff Reminder for Writing Medication Orders

- All orders must be accompanied by DATE, TIME, and BEEPER NUMBER.
- Write out full drug name.
- Spell out "microgram" and "units."
- Did not use trailing zeros.
- Use a zero before a decimal point.

Guidelines for Pediatric Orders

- Write dose: (dose per weight or body surface area [BSA]) x (weight or BSA) = final dose or maximum or age-appropriate dose.

- Secure co signature for orders written by house staff for the following high-risk drugs: Intravenous (i.v.) digoxin, i.v. vasoactive drugs (norepinephrine, epinephrine, dopamine, dobutamine, and phenylephrine), i.v. potassium, chemotherapy, insulin, magnesium sulfate, calcium gluconate.

- Approved cosigners: Pharmacist, senior resident, fellow, or attending physician.

Figure 4-4. *Prescribing Guidelines*

Source: *Morath JM, Turnbull JE.* To Do No Harm: Ensuring a Culture of Safety in Health Care. *San Francisco, CA: Jossey-Bass; 2004.*

New Types of Leaders

The call for a new type of leadership is as pressing as is the call for a culture of safety. In a culture of safety, positional authority gives way to leadership based on expertise. Health care is in desperate need of leaders who can begin to think in terms of the second and first curves: leaders who bring along the best values of the first curve as they begin to solve problems and design innovative systems in the context of second-curve assumptions and beliefs.[17] If leaders put these beliefs and assumption into practice, a coherent vision of a second-curve health care system will emerge. A safe culture requires that management assume major responsibility for safety and that it implement changes that will make the delivery of care safer. This includes monitoring and feedback strategies that foster and reinforce practice change by focusing the organization on meeting evolving frontline needs.

New roles in the culture of safety revolve around leaders creating, managing, and, in some cases, destroying culture.[9] Creating, managing, and destroying culture requires moral courage and leadership. Another important leadership role is to tell the truth and create hope.[26] In the culture of safety, telling the truth means dismantling myths and acknowledging that practitioners face increased process complexity, unrelenting change, and information overload. Creating hope means believing that harmfree care is possible.

Conclusion

The three seminal reports that articulate the need for a new culture in health care—two from the Institute of Medicine[1,4] and one from National Quality Forum[5]— list cultural barriers and articulate minimum specifications for creating a culture of safety. These are important first steps, but health care's entrenched culture requires deeper transformation. For example, deep and diverse problems must be confronted in order to align the many subcultures of the health care system and to enable them to work together to bring the vision of a high-reliability, safe culture to reality. Transparency, i.e., the free and open communication and nonpunitive reporting of adverse events, including reporting to patients and families, must become the norm. Organizational objectives and incentives must be aligned with the top-priority goal of improving patient safety. Only a culture in which patient safety is the top priority will achieve this. The high-risk nature of modern health care and the collective responsibility for risk reduction must be recognized and accepted in all health care settings and within all cultures that make up the health care delivery system.

Moving health care culture from its current state to a culture of safety is a massive undertaking that requires new leadership. It may not come to full fruition in our lifetimes. In the coming culture of safety, the considerable forces at work to discourage the evolution of a health care culture of safety will slowly disappear. These include destruction of silos and hierarchies and the replacement of the "train, name, blame, and shame" mentality with mindfulness that welcomes near misses as learning opportunities.

References

1. Kohn LT, Corrigan JM, Donaldson MD, eds. Committee on Quality of Health in America, Institute of Medicine. *To Err Is Human: Building a Safer Health System.* Washington, DC: National Academy Press; 1999.

2. Leape LL, The epidemiology of patient safety. Paper presented at: Salzburg Seminar on Patient Safety and Medical Error; April 25–May 2, 2001; Salzburg, Austria.

3. Manasse HR, Turnbull JE, Diamond LH. Patient safety: a review of the contemporary American experience. *Singapore Med J.* 2002;43:254-262.

4. Committee on Quality of Health Care in America, Institute of Medicine. *Crossing the Quality Chasm: A New Health System for the 21st Century.* Washington, DC: National Academy Press; 2001.

5. National Quality Forum. Safe Practices for Better Healthcare: A Consensus Report. Washington, DC: National Quality Forum; 2003.

6. Morath JM, Turnbull, JE. *To Do No Harm: Ensuring a Culture of Safety in Healthcare.* San Francisco: Jossey-Bass; 2004.

7. Reason J, Carthey J, de Leval M. Diagnosing vulnerable system syndrome: an essential prerequisite to effective risk management. *Qual Health Care.* 2001;10(suppl II):1121-1125.

8. Westrum R. Cultures with requisite imagination. In: Wise JA, Hopkin VD, Stager, P, eds. *Verification and Validation of Complex Systems: Human Factors Issues.* Berlin: Springer-Verlag; 1992.

9. Schein E. *Organizational Culture and Leadership.* 2nd ed. San Francisco: Jossey-Bass; 1992.

10. Helmreich R. On error management: lessons from aviation. *Br Med J.* 2000;320:781-785.

11. Zimmerman B, Lindberg C, Plsek P. *Edgeware: Insight from Complexity Science for Health Care Leaders.* Irving, TX: VHA Health Foundation; 1998.

12. Plsek PE, Greenlagh T, eds. Complexity science: the challenge of complexity in health care. *Br Med J.* 2001;323:625-638. Available at: http://bmj.bmjjournals.com/cgi/content/full/323/7313/625. Accessed January 17, 2005.

13. McCandless K, Zimmerman B. Simplicity on the Other Side of Complexity. Patient Safety Fellowship Workbook 2003–2004. American Hospital Association Health Forum. Chicago: American Hospital Association; 2003.

14. Coutu D. Sense and reliability: A conversation with celebrated psychologist Karl E. Weick. *Harvard Business Review.* April 2003.

15. Kuhn T. *The Structure of Scientific Revolutions.* Chicago: University of Chicago Press; 1996.

16. Morrison I. *The Second Curve. Managing the Velocity of Change.* Del Ray, CA: Ballantine Books; 1996.

17. Merry M. Health care's need for revolutionary change. *Qual Progress.* 2003;36(9):31-35.

18. Flexner A. *Medical Education in the United States and Canada.* Boston: Merrymount Press; 1910.

19. Denham C. The economics of honesty: Is there a business case for transparency and ethics? Paper presented at: National Patient Safety Foundation Congress; March 15. 2003; Washington, DC.

20. Turnbull J. The Onion Model. Patient Safety Fellowship Workbook 2003–2004. American Hospital Association Health Forum. Chicago: American Hospital Association; 2003.

21. National Patient Safety Foundation. Nothing about me without me. White paper produced by the NPSF Patient and Family Advisory Council. McLean, VA: National Patient Safety Foundation; 2003.

22. Reason JT. *Human Error.* Cambridge, England: Cambridge University Press; 1990.

23. Kleiner A, Roberts C, Ross RB, Smith BJ. Strategies for team learning. In: Senge P, Kleiner A, Roberts C, Ross RB, Smith BJ (eds). *The Fifth Discipline Fieldbook.* New York: Doubleday; 1994.

24. Marx D. Patient Safety and the "Just Culture": A Primer for Health Care Executives. New York: Columbia University; 2001. Available at: www.mers-tm.net/support/Marx_Primer.pdf. Accessed June 2004.

25. Gaba DM, Howard SK, Fish KJ, Smith BE, Sowb YA. Simulation-based training in anesthesia: a decade of experience. *Simulation and Gaming.* 2001;32:175-193.

26. Grace W. *Ethical Leadership: In Pursuit of the Common Good.* Seattle, WA: Center For Ethical Leadership; 1999.

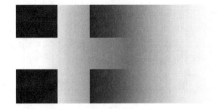

CHAPTER 5

What to Focus on First— Prioritizing Safety-Improvement Initiatives

Michael D. Sanborn

Pharmacist Leadership in Medication Safety

The primary tenet of pharmaceutical care is that the pharmacist is directly responsible to the patient for the quality of his or her medication therapy.[1] Medication use, however, is inherently dangerous. Drugs have been reported to be the leading cause of medical injury in hospitals, accounting for 19.4 percent of injuries.[2] The Institute of Medicine (IOM) report *To Err Is Human: Building a Safer Health System* estimates that 7,000 or more Americans die each year as a result of medication errors.[3] Pharmacy departments in health systems coordinate drug delivery to patients. Even though pharmacists often understand the impact and magnitude of medication errors, they may find it difficult to answer a basic question: "How do I begin my effort to make the medication-use process in my hospital safer?"

Efforts to improve medication safety should be approached both proactively and reactively. For the purposes of this chapter, a *medication error* is defined as any preventable event that may cause or lead to inappropriate medication use or patient harm. A medication error could be further defined as any variance from the established medication-use process. *Adverse drug event* is a broader term that includes medication errors as well as adverse drug reactions or other unanticipated events resulting from drug use. It is essential to aggressively investigate errors and to understand the contributing factors and root causes using techniques such as root-cause analysis and failure mode and effects analysis (FMEA). These practices are the hallmark of many health care systems' approach to reducing medication errors. Once an error occurs, a team is assembled, the error is studied, and safety measures are implemented. Because of the legal and regulatory requirements surrounding a medication error and the recognition that it may uncover specific weaknesses in an institution's processes, examining the causes of errors is imperative. The Joint Commission on Accreditation of Healthcare Organizations (JCAHO) requires that these types of techniques be used for all sentinel events.[4]

Techniques such as FMEA also play a critical role in improving the safety of the medication-use process. It is necessary to review pharmacy operations and hospital practices to identify opportunities for errors *before* they occur. In fact, Cohen[5] states that the primary means of reducing adverse drug events is to ensure that they do not occur in the first place. A proactive operational review and subsequent improvements can prevent medication errors from occurring. Instituting safe practices in advance is critical, and most hospitals have some proactive measures in place. Pharmacy information systems that perform dose-range check-ing and drug protocols for administration of high-risk medications are examples of proactive measures. Drug formularies, unit dose dispensing, independent double checks, and technol-ogy solutions such as computerized prescriber order entry (CPOE) or positive patient identi-fication are other proactive methods that can prevent errors.

Pharmacies and health care systems must prioritize medication-safety-improvement ini-tiatives on the basis of their own unique capacities and patient populations. Resources needed to effect process change may include human, financial, and technological components. It is also imperative to foster a nonpunitive environment. Medication errors are rarely the result of one individual's behavior; more often, they indicate a flaw in system design or a process breakdown. In order to improve the safety of the medication-use process, it is critical to implement system and process changes that reduce the possibility of human error.

So, where *do* you start? This chapter reviews safe-practice recommendations in key areas of hospital pharmacy practice and discusses tools that may be used to prioritize patient-safety-improvement efforts. It also describes some medication-safety initiatives that a phar-macist can influence outside of the hospital pharmacy. It is critical to integrate each best practice discussed in this chapter into the day-to-day operation of the pharmacy. Although some of the improvements will take time, pharmacists can also achieve results very rapidly if they focus on areas that are completely within their sphere of influence.

Understanding Spheres of Influence

The medication-use process is complex and involves many steps (**Figure 5-1**). Medications are typically ordered by physicians, evaluated and dispensed by pharmacists, and adminis-tered by nurses. Monitoring, another component of medication use, can be performed by a variety of health care professionals, including physicians, pharmacists, and nurses. Members of other professional disciplines, such as respiratory therapists, may also be involved in the process. Thus, all efforts to improve the medication-use process must be collaborative and multidisciplinary in order to be fully effective.

It is easier to influence processes that are under one's direct control than those that are under the control of others. Thus, from a pharmacist's perspective, it is much less complicated to address all process improvements and error reductions individually or within the pharmacy department than to take a broader focus. In many instances, however, the results of such efforts are inferior to those achieved as a result of the collaboration of multiple health care professionals. This reality can be further complicated by the fact that other hospital depart-ments or committees may have their own medication-safety initiatives. Because the pharma-cist does not control the entire medication-use process, a recognition and understanding of spheres of influence is critical to the success of any improvement effort.

A pharmacist's sphere of influence traditionally includes all activities that occur within the confines of the central pharmacy. In some settings, it includes other areas, such as phar-macy satellites. Nurses typically have influence over the medication-administration process, while physicians control the process of prescribing. When the pharmacy is prioritizing im-provements in the medication-use process, it is important to evaluate the complexity of the improvement by asking, "How much influence do we wield over the process that is targeted for change?"

In the simplest of terms, the pharmacy department is in control of all aspects of dispens-ing and of medication procurement. When the dispensing process is further examined, how-ever, it often becomes evident that pharmacy does not have complete control. For example, pharmacies that cannot provide 24-hour service often rely on nurses to dispense medications when the central pharmacy is closed. Physicians and nurses frequently acquire medications

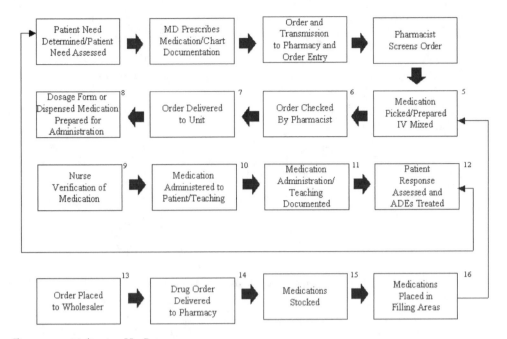

Figure 5-1. Medication-Use Process
Reprinted with permission, McKesson Medication Management

from floor stock in other areas, such as the operating room and emergency department. In these situations, the pharmacist essentially relinquishes control of patient-specific dispensing to another health care professional. This reduces the pharmacist's sphere of influence over the entire process.

When trying to identify a starting point in the improvement of the medication-use process, pharmacists must determine those factors that are truly under their direct influence. The responsibilities of medication procurement, storage, preparation, and delivery usually fall under the control of the pharmacy, with minimal influence from outside entities. In these areas, safety can be enhanced relatively quickly using some of the approaches described in this chapter. In areas where the pharmacist exerts less influence, such as prescribing and administration, improvements must be ranked in order of priority and addressed as part of a multidisciplinary effort in which the pharmacist is a key participant.

Pharmacy Processes

Health-systems pharmacists must make the improvement of practices within their own departments the top priority. For most pharmacies, this is the first step is to foster a culture of medication safety within the department. Pharmacy employees should be encouraged to recognize and report practices within the department that may be prone to error. Workflow in each area of the pharmacy should be analyzed for risk. Particular emphasis must be given to areas where the consequences of error pose the greatest patient risk. Examples of such areas include chemotherapy admixture, neonatal parenteral nutrition compounding, preparation of vasoactive intravenous products, and the dispensing of high-alert medications.

The work environment cannot be overlooked as a potential catalyst for medication errors. In *Medication Errors*, Cohen lists a set of critical steps that apply to each pharmacy-based process (see **Table 5-1**).[5,6] The authors recommend that distractions (such as telephone calls and unnecessary conversation) that can occur during order processing be reduced to a minimum. The pace and volume of work for which each pharmacist is responsible should be appropriate for the type of work being performed. For both pharmacists and technicians, appropriate training to ensure proficiency in required tasks is also critical to reducing work-place errors.

Table 5-1. Critical Steps for Pharmacist Processing of Orders

Activity	Critical Steps
Order Review	• Review and assessment of the prescription
	• Verification of questions with the prescriber
Order Processing	• Computer data entry
	• Review of patient profiles
	• Selection of proper medication in the computer
	• Review and assessment of computer alerts
Preparation	• Selecting and preparing the medication
	• Verifying the product expiration date
	• Counting, measuring, or compounding the product
	• Affixing the correct label
	• Double-checking the prescription
	• Returning stock containers to their proper locations
Dispensing	• Assessing/taking the patient's history
	• Delivering the product to the correct nurse or patient
	• Providing patient counseling or nurse education

Adapted from Davis and Cohen.[6]

As noted above, pharmacy-owned processes include inventory management, order pro-cessing, drug preparation, product delivery, and pharmacist review and monitoring of drug therapy. It is impossible to illustrate all the process improvements that could be considered in each of these areas since each pharmacy department is unique. Many improvements, how-ever, can be generally applied quickly to all pharmacies.

In each of these areas, as described in the paragraphs that follow, policies and procedures should be developed to incorporate the stated best practices. More important, day-to-day pharmacy activities should mirror these policies and procedures. Employees should be trained using these policies, and performance of these activities should be periodically observed to ensure that they are being followed.

INVENTORY MANAGEMENT

Management of drug purchases and inventory control are areas that are commonly over-looked with respect to patient safety, even though many techniques can be implemented in these areas to reduce the likelihood of error. For example, par levels (i.e., minimum and maximum levels of products to keep on hand) should exist for at least the top 80 percent of medications. This will not only prevent a shortage of medications but also reduce the like-lihood that those medications will expire. Daily review of inventory levels, as well as fre-quent checks for expired medications, is a requisite for maintaining a safe and adequate drug supply.

In many facilities, the individual who purchases pharmaceuticals is not a pharmacist. In this case, it is important that a licensed pharmacist review orders to the vendor to assess the necessity and appropriateness of the items being ordered. This is especially true in large institutions where the buyer often receives a multitude of requests for product from a variety of sources. This review will also ensure that drug products are purchased in the proper quantities and strengths. For example, dosing errors resulting from inappropriate procurement and storage of a concentrated morphine product that is not on the hospital formulary can be avoided by having a pharmacist review the order and discuss potential formulary alternatives with the physician.

Pharmacy personnel should also review each order for accuracy when the product is received from the wholesaler or manufacturer. To guarantee that the ordered items were received, delivered medications should be compared to the invoice or to the confirmation report received at the time of the order. Many prime vendors offer bar-code technology that can automate and expedite this process using bar-code technology.

Medication-storage practices can be designed to enhance safety. In most pharmacies, different dosage forms of medications are stored in separate areas. This practice allows for rapid retrieval of a particular type of medication and functions as a safety measure that prevents the unintended selection of the wrong dosage form. Shelf labels, bar codes, and numbering systems should also be used to identify stocked items. It is also important to separate look-alike and sound-alike medications (**Figure 5-2**) or to label them in a way that draws any similarities to the attention of the person picking the medication. Stock should be rotated to further prevent the potential for expired medications. When drugs do expire or are subject to a recall, these medications should be quarantined and disposed of according to established policies and procedures.

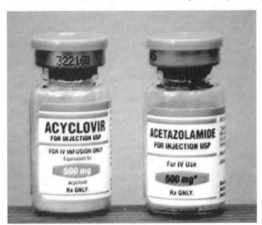

Figure 5-2. Look-alike medication vials.

ORDER PROCESSING

Institutions can receive and process medication orders in several ways. Some facilities receive orders via fax; others receive them via a scanned image, a tube system, or as carbon copies from the original order. Traditionally, the pharmacy staff is responsible for the review and processing of medication orders into the pharmacy information system. This task can be accomplished by a pharmacist or an appropriately trained pharmacy technician. In some hospitals, nonpharmacy personnel—for example, a physician using CPOE, a nurse, or a unit secretary—enter orders into the hospital information system. In each facility, the pharmacist must assess the process for receiving and managing medication orders and implement effective safeguards or process improvements to reduce the potential for error.

The variety of order-processing scenarios can result in systems that are very complex. For example, in a university teaching hospital, the majority of medication orders was being processed by unit secretaries or nursing personnel, using a hospital information system that interfaced with the pharmacy information system. Approximately 5 percent of the orders were received via CPOE as printed documents. A pharmacist manually entered these orders into the information system. Pharmacists were responsible for reviewing medication orders received in the pharmacy system against faxed copies of the originals. The orders were verified prior to dispensing. Internal audits and trained nonpharmacy observers identified a transcription-error rate of 5 percent to 12 percent in this setting, meaning that thousands of orders had to be corrected each year. The complexity of this order-processing system cannot be completely resolved immediately, but resources have been allocated to move toward pharmacist order entry and CPOE that is electronically interfaced with the pharmacy information system.

Despite the systems variations that can occur, many safety measures apply to every type of order-processing situation. For instance, each medication order should be reviewed to ensure that it is for the right patient and that the dosage, dosage form, and route of administration are correct. Pharmacists should also review the order for clinical appropriateness. Many pharmacy information systems can assist with this review by screening orders for therapeutic duplications, drug interactions, allergies, or doses that are not within an acceptable range. The patient's renal, liver, and metabolic function should also be considered where appropriate. Some pharmacy systems can assist with this process by using algorithms and advanced screening of laboratory data. For example, metformin orders can be screened electronically against the patient's renal function and blood gases to reduce the risk for lactic acidosis.

Order review by the pharmacist should also include prioritizing medications on the basis of urgency (e.g., stat, now, as soon as possible, routine). The order should also be reviewed to ensure that it is legible, for the correct patient, and appropriate for the disease state or diagnosis. Attention should be given to the frequency of administration as well as to administration instructions. Changes should be made only after direct consultation with the prescriber. Corrections should be repeated to the prescriber for accuracy, and the appropriate clarification must be written in the patient's chart.

If therapeutic interchange is employed, all appropriate policies and procedures should be followed. A new order for the therapeutic alternative should be placed in the patient's chart and a note should also be placed in the patient's medication administration record to alert the prescriber and nurse of the substitution.

Orders should include instructions relating to such matters as the time over which the drug is to be administered, flow rates for infusion pumps, duration of therapy, or reconstitution information. All "as-needed" orders should be reviewed to ensure that the dose range is appropriate and that the administration times and indications for use are included. If technician order entry is employed, technicians should have only conditional order-entry privileges that are contingent upon verification by a pharmacist.

PRODUCT PREPARATION

Activities associated with medication preparation pose one of the greatest opportunities for error within the pharmacy. Preparation includes the selection, compounding (sterile or nonsterile), packaging, and labeling of the product. For each of these steps, it is critical that technical and professional staff understand the importance of following appropriate procedures and double-checking their work. All products should be dispensed in unit dose packaging and delivered in a ready-to-use form.

Errors in medication selection are the most common type of errors that other health care professionals and the general public associate with the pharmacy. Both lay and professional publications are full of examples of dire patient consequences that have resulted from the selection of an incorrect medication, dosage strength, or formulation. Many safeguards must be instituted to ensure that the appropriate medication is selected 100 percent of the time. Some practices, such as separating look-alike and sound-alike medications and checking the product expiration date, are necessary for accurate product selection.

Certain forms of technology, such as robotics and bar-coded carousel storage technology, have improved the safety associated with medication selection. These technologies automate portions of the selection process and can add a level of electronic confirmation at the point of drug selection; however, they are not fail-safe. Indeed, they themselves can contribute to multiple errors. If the incorrect medication is placed in the bar-coded storage bin or package, it can result in repeated selection of the incorrect product without any warnings from the system.

Product selection is only the first step in the preparation phase. A large percentage of medications require further manipulation or labeling. In addition, safeguards must be instituted for sterile and nonsterile compounding. Both activities often require calculations to determine the amounts of medications and other ingredients to be used. Care should be taken when performing these calculations and, when appropriate (e.g., with chemotherapy), calculations should be subject to a pharmacist double-check. The pharmacist should also evaluate the compound for stability, compatibility of ingredients, and suitability for the patient. An appropriate expiration date for the product should be determined and included on the label. Products should not be compounded that are identical to commercially available products. Finally, pharmacists should work with only one compound at a time to eliminate potential switching of ingredients or containers.

All sterile compounding should be performed in a clean environment that is maintained in accordance with recommended guidelines.[7] Professional and technical staff should be trained in aseptic technique and product handling. This training should be documented and competencies reassessed at least annually. Prior to the compounding process, all necessary materials should be collected, including the medication(s) selected, diluent, container for the final product, and any items needed during the compounding process (tubing, syringes, filters, needles, etc.). After compounding, all products should be quarantined until they undergo a final check by the pharmacist. Because of their potential for harm, antineoplastic agents require even greater safeguards.[8]

Nonsterile compounding requires adherence to many of the same precautions. Standard formulation instructions should be maintained for compounded products that are commonly needed. Compounding logs should be maintained for products that are compounded in batches or compounded in advance of patient need. If a technician performs nonsterile compounding, a pharmacist must check all calculations, ingredients, and measurements before they are mixed and do a final check afterward.

PRODUCT DELIVERY

The order-delivery process also poses the potential for error. As with selecting and compounding, standard safeguards can be employed to decrease the likelihood of errors.

Pharmacy personnel should ensure that medications are delivered to the correct patient care unit and are stored in a secure, patient-specific area labeled with the patient's name. If a medication is needed urgently, a nurse should be notified that it has arrived. In certain situations (e.g., with new formulary drugs), it is important to ensure that nursing personnel understand how the medication is to be administered and monitored. Any medications that are discontinued should be returned to the hospital pharmacy.

Pneumatic tube stations, while convenient, pose a patient-safety threat unless policies are implemented to guarantee their proper use. With pneumatic tubes, it is possible for medications to sit unattended in the receiving station unless someone is assigned to monitor the receipt of medications. Such medications may also be transported to an incorrect unit. In some instances, their integrity can be damaged by the motion (e.g., certain biologics and other medications are sensitive to shaking). At a minimum, these situations can delay therapy. Most pharmacists have experienced missing dose calls resulting from "tubed" medications that seemingly never made it to the nursing unit.

PHARMACIST REVIEW AND MONITORING

A number of studies has shown that that pharmacist interventions can reduce costs and improve patient safety.[9,10] In these studies, increased pharmacist involvement in the review of patient allergies, trends in laboratory test results, and review of medication orders for appropriateness was shown to significantly reduce adverse events. Additionally, pharmacist review can improve medication selection through evaluation of drug indications, patient age, weight, and organ function. Types of errors prevented in these studies included prescribing errors (inappropriate dose, nonformulary agent, medication errors related to transfer), administration errors (inappropriate timing of dose, transcription errors, missed doses, extra doses given, doses administered after discontinuation), pharmacy errors (inappropriate dose recommendations, pharmacokinetic levels not evaluated, incomplete dispensing instructions), and discharge errors. For these reasons, every hospital pharmacy should have an active intervention program that includes documentation and monitoring various types of pharmacist involvement over time.

At a minimum, pharmacists should routinely screen medication orders against the criteria listed in the previous paragraph. First doses should not be administered until such screening has taken place. Pharmacist provision of patient education can help reduce errors that may occur after discharge because the patient does not understand how to take a medication. This is especially true for patients who are discharged with complex drug regimens.

PHARMACY AUTOMATION

Over the past two decades, there have been significant advances in pharmacy automation. Pharmacists today can choose from automated compounders for i.v. admixtures, unit-based dispensing devices for medications, robotic picking systems, and automated high-capacity storage devices, to name just a few. A recent survey showed that 66 percent of hospitals use either robotics or automated dispensing cabinets (ADC) to assist in the dispensing process.[11] Many of these technologies are engineered to assist the pharmacy department in reducing medication errors, and when implemented correctly, they can do so to some degree. However, they should by no means be considered fail-safe, and appropriate checks and balances should be incorporated into their daily use. Poor implementation of proved technology can introduce new opportunities for error.

For example, unit-based ADCs such as Pyxis®, AcuDose®, and Omnicell® have long been used by pharmacy departments and nursing personnel to automate the drug-delivery process. One study demonstrated that ADC technology can reduce the frequency of medication errors, especially missed doses and errors caused by a delay in therapy.[12] ADC technology, however, is not foolproof. For instance, restocking an area of the cabinet that is programmed to contain heparin 20,000 units/500mL with heparin 40,000 units/mL could result the administration of a much higher-than-desired concentration of this product. In one study, Pyxis® users found that 2.3 percent of drawers contained incorrect unit dose medications, many of which had the potential to cause serious medication errors.[13] Other studies have also found increased error rates with this technology.[14,15]

To prevent these types of errors, some vendors of ADC technology have developed bar-code scanners that can be used at the site of the cabinet to assist in accurate restocking (see **Figure 5-3**).

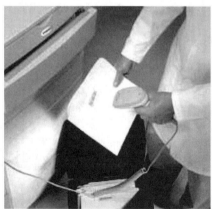

Figure 5-3. *Bar-code scanning system for unit-based dispensing cabinets.*

When restocking, the pharmacist or technician scans the bar code using a device that is integrated with the cabinet. The ADC software recognizes the code and opens the appropriate bin or drawer for that product. When possible, pharmacists should use such point-of-delivery bar-code verification or newer technologies such as radio frequency identification. If this technology is not available, some hospitals have reduced the incidence of incorrect restocking by implementing a second check of technician-refill activities.[16]

Despite the interest in automated technology and patient safety, few controlled, published studies have confirmed an association with automation and the reduction of medication errors.[17] Further study of such technologies is necessary. More important, it is necessary to document effective implementation strategies that will prevent medication errors. People, systems, and technology must be integrated to deliver a highly reliable medication-use system.

Multidisciplinary Processes

Although focusing on internal pharmacy processes is the first step to improving safety, pharmacist participation in multidisciplinary efforts is also necessary. Today, most hospitals have an organization-wide performance-improvement process whose purpose is to identify and analyze medical errors, medication errors, and near misses. The reporting of such adverse events should be nonpunitive, and each report should be reviewed and investigated.

The pharmacy and therapeutics (P&T) committee has a key role in multidisciplinary safety-improvement activities. Its importance cannot be understated. By design, the P&T committee is a team consisting of pharmacists, physicians, nurses, hospital administrators, and other health care professionals. The committee should have a leadership role in the hospital's medication-safety efforts. Improvement initiatives should be a major part of every P&T agenda. Some P&T committees have developed institution-wide standards that summarize hospital policies, medical staff rules, and national recommendations designed to enhance safe medication practices.[18]

Many hospitals have established a medication-safety committee that is often a subcommittee of the P&T committee. The medication-safety committee can review and evaluate current literature, national error reports, internal reporting, and hospital processes to assist with recommendations for improvement. Membership on this committee should also be multidisciplinary and should include representatives from the hospital's risk-management and quality-control departments. In some hospitals this committee has been charged with forming risk-reduction teams and developing auditing systems to investigate patterns of medication errors; on the basis of such findings, they then identify and recommend system-based changes.[19]

The Pharmacist's Role in Reducing Prescribing and Administration Errors

Errors associated with medication prescribing and administration are the most common types of error found in the literature. They can make up to 93 percent of all errors reported.[3] In most cases, the pharmacist is responsible for these functions, but the pharmacist can assist the health care team in developing system improvements that can reduce the potential for error.

A good place to start is simply ensuring that drug information references are available and up to date (electronic format is ideal). Active pharmacist participation in information-systems teams that are responsible for the selection and implementation of new patient-safety technologies is highly advisable. Pharmacists can also promote the use of other safeguards that reduce or prevent errors associated with prescribing and administration.

PRESCRIBING

Pharmacist review of medication orders prior to the administration of the first dose is an invaluable safety measure. Policies should also be in place that require drug indications and complete prescription orders. These policies should require the prescriber to enter the generic name of the drug and its strength, the dosage form, and complete directions for use. The order should have a legible prescriber signature (or name stamp). Medical staff policies should also prevent the use of ambiguous orders such as "May take home meds" or "Resume preop orders."

Guidelines, protocols, and preprinted order forms are helpful and can be pharmacist-driven through the P&T committee. The metric system should be used for all medication orders. Orders for vials, amps, tablets, and bottles should be clarified with the prescriber, since many products are available in multiple sizes and strengths. Other important safeguards include eliminating the use of potentially ambiguous or confusing abbreviations (**Table** 5-2).

Table 5-2. Examples of Ambiguous Abbreviations and How to Avoid Them

Abbreviation	Potential Problem	Preferred Term
U (for unit)	Mistaken as zero, four, or cc.	Write "unit."
IU (for international unit) or 10 (ten)	Mistaken as i.v. (intravenous).	Write "international unit."
Q.D., Q.O.D. (Latin abbreviation for once daily and every other day)	Mistaken for each other. The period after the Q can be mistaken for an "I," and the "O" can be mistaken for "I."	Write "daily" or "every other day."
Trailing zero (X.0 mg), Lack of leading zero (.X mg)	Decimal point is missed.	Never place a zero by itself after a decimal point, and always place a zero before a decimal point (0.X mg).
MSMSO$_4$MgSO$_4$	Confused with one another. Can mean morphine sulfate or magnesium sulfate.	Write "morphine sulfate" or "magnesium sulfate."
mg (symbol for microgram)	Mistaken for mg (milligrams), resulting in 1,000-fold overdose.	Write "mcg."
D/C (for discharge)	Interpreted as "discontinue" whatever medications follow.	Write "discharge."

Adapted from National Patient Safety Goals, Joint Commission on Accreditation of Healthcare Organizations. Available at: www.jcaho.com/accredited+organizations/patient+safety/04+npsg/04_faqs.htm Accessed October 31, 2004.

Verbal orders should be avoided whenever possible and, if allowed, should be repeated to the prescriber in their entirety to ensure correct transmission. All verbal orders should immediately be transcribed in the patient's medical record and should include the time, the date, and the signature of the person taking the verbal order. Verbal orders should never be accepted for high-risk medications (e.g., chemotherapy).

CPOE is gaining support as a method to improve prescribing and patient safety. Many hospitals are using, implementing, or evaluating CPOE technology. The IOM, the Leapfrog Group, and patient-advocacy groups have recommended CPOE as a patient-safety enhancement. Some believe that CPOE could be the single most effective means to reduce medication errors and have estimated that it could prevent as many as 500,000 serious medication errors annually.[20] CPOE might also prevent errors associated with transcription, misidentification of the prescriber, and delays in order transmission. Finally, the information-exchange and decision-support capabilities incorporated into many CPOE systems can potentially reduce adverse events caused by incorrect doses, drug-drug interactions, and allergic reactions.

CPOE is not a panacea, as evidenced by the experience of the U.S. Army health clinics, which have used it for more than a decade. A three-year study identified that in the ambulatory setting, one in every 100 prescriptions still contained an error.[21] After CPOE implementation, the Thomas Jefferson University Hospital actually measured an increase in the number of pharmacist interventions, especially in those related to dose inconsistency and duplicate orders. This suggests that while some types of prescribing errors may decrease with CPOE, others, which are associated the technology, may increase.[22] Pharmacists should take active roles in the development of the various CPOE decision algorithms necessary to ensure enhancement of patient safety. Even after CPOE has been successfully implemented, the pharmacist should continue to monitor physician orders for appropriateness.

MEDICATION ADMINISTRATION

In many hospitals, medication administration is the step in the process that has the fewest safeguards. It typically relies on a single health care professional to execute it correctly; there are generally no double checks prior to administration. Some hospitals do require a second check of medications such as insulin and other high-alert drugs, and this practice should be encouraged. Infusion pumps should require a double check to ensure accurate programming and admixture placement. All hospitals should require a double check of chemotherapy medication prior to administration.

One of the most effective ways to prevent administration errors is to provide all medications used within the hospital in ready-to-administer form. The unit dose system is tantamount to this premise, and i.v. preparations are no exception. All medications should remain intact in their labeled packaging until the point of administration. Maintenance of an accurate medication administration record (MAR) is also critical, and procedures must be in place to periodically review the accuracy of the MAR. Policies that regulate the storage of medications in patient care areas should also exist.

The "five rights" of medication administration (right patient, right drug, right dose, right route, and right time) should be observed at all times. Practice should be monitored periodically as a validation. The pharmacy should provide appropriate administration instructions for each medication (e.g., "Take with food," "Do not crush," or "Administer via slow i.v. push over at least five minutes."). Oral liquids should be provided in medication cups or oral syringes that are incompatible with i.v. tubing ports.

Pharmacists should be readily available at all times to answer questions related to a particular drug or its administration. They should also participate in the design of a medication administration course for nursing staff and other health professionals responsible for drug administration. Participation in this course should be documented.

Automated bedside point-of-care (BPOC) scanning is a relatively new process that uses bar-code technology to guarantee that the five rights are followed. Using a handheld scanner, the nurse scans the patient's name badge and the medication to be administered, and then scans the patient. Because the system is electronically integrated with the MAR, it will alert the nurse if an error is detected (e.g., wrong patient, wrong administration time). These systems are now considered to be best practice because of their ability to reduce medication errors associated with drug administration by 65 percent to 86 percent.[23] The IOM report cited bar-code technology as a way to reduce medication errors by "ensuring that the identity and dose of the drug are as prescribed, that it is being given to the right patient, and that all of the steps in the dispensing and administration processes are checked for timeliness and accuracy."[3]

The pharmacist should be an active participant in the selection and integration of BPOC technology within the hospital. The implementation of BPOC is complex and requires careful consideration of interface requirements, bar-coding capabilities, handheld screen design, and training needs. To prevent the potential for bypassing BPOC system safeguards, pharmacists must be committed to providing all medications in bar-coded form to realize all of the benefits of BPOC.

Putting It All Together—Where Do I Start?

One of the most important strategies for improving patient safety is making it a priority. The commitment to improve patient safety must start at the top, with the hospital administrator and the director of pharmacy. A culture of safety must exist throughout the hospital. Health care professionals must be able to report errors without fear of retribution. Errors and opportunities for error must be identified. With challenges such as rising drug costs, inadequate staffing, technology implementation and maintenance, and daily assignments, pharmacists often have other priorities that can prevent medication-safety initiatives from moving forward. Many of the process improvements suggested in this chapter require little time to implement. Rather, implementation of these techniques is a matter of making a commitment to instituting them as daily practices.

There are also many resources to assist with recommendations regarding safe medication use. Organizations such as the Institute for Safe Medication Practices (ISMP), the Leapfrog Group, the Healthcare Advisory Board, the Institute for Healthcare Improvement, the National Quality Forum, and many state hospital and pharmacy organizations provide valuable resources to assist in the identification and development of safe medication-use practices. Pharmacists should also familiarize themselves with the American Society of Health-System Pharmacists (ASHP) guidelines on preventing medication errors in hospitals.[24]

Every organization is at a different point along the continuum of improving medication-use safety. Therefore, it is important to first identify which hospital efforts are currently under way to improve patient safety. For example, in their book, *Medication Safety and Cost Recovery: A Four-Step Approach for Executives*, Caldwell and Denham discuss a method to implement a 100-day plan that enables health care organizations to reduce medication errors and adverse drug events.[25] Table 5-3 lists the four steps that these authors suggest are necessary to implement the 100-day plan. Hospitals may have similar specific plans to address patient-safety issues. Pharmacy should be a key player in these efforts.

Table 5-3. 100-Day Plan Management Method[25]

Step	Process
1	Generate an organizational will to reduce medication errors.
2	Conduct a comparative data and gap analysis.
3	Implement idealized design change concepts and, if necessary, execute the knowledge and management loop.
4	Hold the gains.

Pharmacists should develop their own departmental medication-improvement plans in a similar way. The first step in the development of such a plan should be to review existing practices throughout the department. An accurate self-assessment is the key to any performance-improvement plan. This review should focus on day-to-day processes in key areas such as inventory management, order processing, drug preparation, product delivery, and ongoing pharmacist review and monitoring. As part of this process review, it is important to observe pharmacists and support staff completing their daily activities. Simply reviewing existing written policies and procedures is important, but not adequate. A thorough evaluation of both policy and practice will increase the effectiveness of the safety plan.

Several tools can be used to assist in this evaluation. Perhaps the most extensive tool available is the Medication-Use-System Safety Strategy (MS3) developed by ASHP.[26] This tool is designed to facilitate a system-based approach to the development of safe medication-use systems. Another tool is the Medication Safety Self-Assessment, available from the ISMP.[27] It was designed to establish a baseline of hospital efforts surrounding the safe use of medications, but it is also useful in identifying specific opportunities for improvement. Another useful tool is the Medication Error Prevention Program: Checklist for Hospitals available from Bridge Medical, Inc.[28] This comprehensive tool includes a Likert-based scoring system that can assist in the prioritization of identified improvements.

When completing any tool, it is important to objectively evaluate the department's true performance against the characteristics. For example, if 100 percent of the mnemonics in the pharmacy information system have not been reviewed for look-alike drug names, then this should be noted as an opportunity for improvement. Likewise, if pharmacists already review 100 percent of all medication orders prior to medication administration, then this would not necessarily be an improvement opportunity.

Once a list of improvement opportunities has been created, an implementation plan should be developed. Each improvement should be listed and ranked on the basis of the risk it poses to patient safety and the frequency at which an error may occur. It is also worthwhile to characterize initiatives on the basis of impact and feasibility. It is often helpful to begin by picking some initiatives that are highly feasible. This will build momentum. High-impact initiatives are also a good choice. Special consideration should be given to opportunities that have been shown to create the largest potential for harmful error. Argo et al.[29] identified the 10 most common lethal medication errors in hospitalized patients, which included medications in concentrated form and those with narrow therapeutic indexes. Factors such as inadequate knowledge, lack of access to patient information, the need to calculate drug doses, special dosage formulations, and ambiguous nomenclature have also been shown to create a high potential for prescribing errors[30] and should be considered from a pharmacy perspective.

The next step is to set reasonable but aggressive deadlines for achieving each of the identified improvements. The director of pharmacy or an appropriate designee should be responsible and held accountable for the execution of the safety plan. The director should regularly monitor performance against the plan, but this does not mean that he or she must implement every improvement. Responsibility for certain improvements should be delegated to other department supervisors or staff members. Teams can be formed to use a continuous quality improvement model for complex improvements. These tactics will increase medication-safety awareness throughout the department and can accelerate the implementation of process improvements.

Consideration should also be given to the ease with which the improvement can be accomplished. As noted earlier, some improvements will take longer than others. As an example, if pharmacists do not routinely screen medication orders for allergies, a screening process could be implemented rather quickly. Pharmacists should be reeducated on the importance of allergy screening and the steps required with the new process. Even if allergy screening is often bypassed because the pharmacy information system does not receive allergy information via an electronic interface, a reliable and up-to-date allergy resource must be identified and made accessible to the pharmacist during medication-order processing.

Fostering a Culture of Continuous Improvement

Improving medication-use safety is a continuous process. Crane[31] has described a three-step process to improve error reporting and to develop methods to improve patient safety (see Table 5-4). The process focuses on eliminating blame, investigating errors, and developing specific improvement strategies. The concepts of this methodology are central to fostering a proactive medication-safety culture.

Table 5-4. Three-Step Process for Reducing Medication Errors and Adverse Drug Events[31]

Step 1. Stop using the medication-error reporting system primarily for punishment and shift the emphasis to using it for improvement.

Step 2. Recognize that current approaches to preventing medication errors and adverse drug events are inadequate, and shift the emphasis to a scientific investigation of preventable patient harm.

Step 3. Understand the complexity of human performance in the medication-use cycle, and develop strategies that enhance, rather than restrict, human performance.

Improving medication-error detection, reporting, and analysis is critical to the identification of opportunities for error as well as to the measurement of the overall performance of the organization with respect to patient safety. Analyzing errors that actually occur, both internally and outside the facility, is paramount to any error-reduction strategy. Merely focusing the hospital on improved medication-error reporting can serve as an impetus for a change in the organizational culture surrounding medication errors.[32]

A commitment to patient safety and error prevention must be a covenant between every member of the pharmacy staff and the patients they serve. Every process should be scrutinized for error potential. Staff members who identify new safety strategies should be recognized and rewarded. Pharmacists should be both active participants and leaders in multidisciplinary efforts to improve patient safety. Where to start will be different for every facility, but the imperative is shared: to demonstrate the leadership and intensity necessary to advance medication safety for all patients.

References

1. Hepler CD, Strand LM. Opportunities and responsibilities in pharmaceutical care. *Am J Hosp Pharm.* 1990;47:533-542.

2. Bates DW, Cullen DJ, Laird NM, et al. Incidence of adverse drug events and potential adverse drug events: implications for prevention. *JAMA.* 1995;274:29-34

3. Kohn LT, Corrigan JM, Donaldson MS, eds. Subcommittee on Quality of Health Care in America, Institute of Medicine. *To Err Is Human: Building a Safer Health System.* Washington DC: National Academy Press; 1999.

4. Joint Commission on Accreditation of Healthcare Organizations. *Comprehensive Accreditation Manual for Hospitals.* Oak Brook Terrace, IL: JCAHO; 2003.

5. Cohen MR, ed. *Medication Errors.* Washington DC: American Pharmaceutical Association; 1999.

6. Davis NM, Cohen MR. Sterile cockpit. *Am Pharm.* 1995; NS35(12):11.

7. American Society of Health-System Pharmacists. Quality Assurance for Pharmacy-Prepared Sterile Products: Best Practices for Health-System Pharmacy. Bethesda, MD: ASHP;2003:28-46.

8. American Society of Health-System Pharmacists. ASHP Guidelines on Preventing Medication Errors with Antineoplastic Agents. *Am J Health-Syst Pharm.* 2002;59:1648-1668.

9. Leape LL, Cullen DJ, Clapp MD, et al. Pharmacist participation on physician rounds and adverse drug events in the intensive care unit. *JAMA.* 1999;282:267-270.

10. Scarsi KK, Fotis MA, Noskin GA. Pharmacist participation in medical rounds reduces medication errors. *Am J Health-Syst Pharm.* 2002;59:2089-2092.

11. Pedersen CA, Schneider PJ, Scheckelhoff DJ. ASHP national survey of pharmacy practice in hospital settings: dispensing and administration—2002. *Am J Health-Syst Pharm.* 2003;60:52-68.

12. Borel JM, Rascati KL. Effect of an automated, nursing unit-based drug-dispensing device on medication errors. *Am J Health-Syst Pharm.* 1995;52:1875-1879.

13. Klibanov OM, Eckel SF. Effects of automated dispensing on inventory control, billing, workload, and potential for medication errors. *Am J Health-Syst Pharm.* 2003;60:569-572.

14. Barker KN, Allan EL. Research on drug-use-system errors. *Am J Health-Syst Pharm.* 1995;52:400-403.

15. Sutter TL, Wellman GS, Mott DA, et al. Discrepancies with automated drug storage and distribution cabinets. *Am J Health-Syst Pharm.* 1998;55:1924-1926.

16. Lucas AJ. Improving medication safety in a neonatal intensive care unit. *Am J Health-Syst Pharm.* 2004;61:33-37.

17. Oren E, Shaffer ER, Guglielmo BJ. Impact of emerging technologies on medication errors and adverse drug events. *Am J Health-Syst Pharm.* 2003;60:1447-1458.

18. Shaw-Phillips MA. Institutionwide medication safety program. *Am J Health-Syst Pharm.* 2003; 60:2198-2200.

19. Simmons RL. Reducing medical errors: An organizational approach. *P & T.* 2003;28:780-782.

20. Birkmeyer J, Birkmeyer C, Wennberg D, et al. Leapfrog Safety Standards: Potential Benefits of Universal Adoption. Washington, DC: Leapfrog Group; 2000.

21. Ballentine AJ, Kinnaird D, Wilson JP. Prescription errors occur despite computerized prescriber order entry. *Am J Health-Syst Pharm.* 2003;60:708-709.

22. Senholzi C, Gottlieb J. Pharmacist interventions after implementation of computerized prescriber order entry. *Am J Health-Syst Pharm.* 2003;60:1880-1882.

23. Neuenschwander M, Cohen MR, Vaida AJ, et al. Practical guide to bar coding for patient medication safety. *Am J Health-Syst Pharm.* 2003;60:768-779.

24. American Society of Health-System Pharmacists. Guidelines on Preventing Medication Errors in Hospitals: Best Practices for Health-System Pharmacy. Bethesda, MD: ASHP; 2003:153-161.

25. Caldwell C, Denham C. *Medication Safety and Cost Recovery: A Four-Step Approach for Executives.* Chicago: Health Administration Press; 2001.

26. American Society of Health-System Pharmacists Center on Patient Safety. The Medication-Use-System Safety Strategy. Introduction and Task Analysis. 2001. Available at: http://www.ashp.org/patient-safety/MS3-1.pdf. Accessed December 3, 2003.

27. Institute for Safe Medication Practices. Medication Safety Self-Assessment. Available at: http://www.ismp.org/Survey/SurveyTool31_pass3.html. Accessed January 19, 2004.

28. Bridge Medical Inc. Medication Error Prevention Program: Checklist for Hospitals. Available at: www.mederrors.com/pdf/hospital_checklist.pdf. Accessed December 3, 2003.

29. Argo AL, Cox KK, Kelly WN. The ten most common lethal medication errors in hospital patients. *Hosp Pharm.* 2000;35:470-474.

30. Lessar TS, Briceland L, Stein DS. Factors related to errors in medication prescribing. *JAMA.* 1997;277:312-317.

31. Crane VS. New perspectives on preventing medication errors and adverse drug events. *Am J Health-Syst Pharm.* 2000;57:690-697.

32. Stump LS. Re-engineering the medication error-reporting process: removing the blame and improving the system. *Am J Health-Syst Pharm.* 2000;57(suppl 4):S10-17.

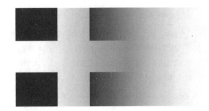

CHAPTER 6

Thinking about Accidents and Systems

Richard I. Cook and
Michael F. O'Connor

Introduction

Accidents and the threat of accidents are the primary motivators for work on safety. Take away accidents, and concern about safety diminishes and attention shifts toward production. Virtually all safety work takes place in the shadow of accidents, and experience with accidents—both our direct experience and the experience we acquire by hearing about the accidents that happen to others—shapes our general and specific approaches to safety.

How do accidents happen, and what do they mean? Are accidents foreseeable? If so, are they preventable? What are the implications of accidents in one place for operations taking place elsewhere? What role does technology play in accidents? What role does human performance play? Are accidents evidence of systemic problems, or are they isolated failures? If accidents are systemic, how can the system be fixed to prevent them?

Pharmacists are not alone in asking these questions. Over the past 30 years, the same questions have been asked by those trying to understand accidents in aviation, nuclear power generation, telecommunications, unmanned and manned space flight, railroad transport, shipping, and many other fields. Although there are important differences between these fields and health care, our current health care safety efforts draw heavily on experience in these fields.

Both accidents and postaccident investigation and analysis take place within a complex system that includes many elements: people, goals, technology, incentives, rules, knowledge, and expertise. Whenever we begin to explore one component of the system we immediately find it is connected to another, and that one to yet another, and so on. This should not be surprising; after all, it is the operation of the *system* that produces the results—both the desired and undesired ones—and therefore failure must necessarily have the same connections as success.

The connectedness within the system is a major obstacle to investigating and analyzing accidents. It also makes it hard for us to foresee future failures. Because we have difficulty seeing how future accidents will occur, we have difficulty in planning work on safety. We want to use our experience with past accidents to make the system safer. We aspire to improve safety by eliminating accidents. But the relationship between past accidents and the way in which the system will fail in the future is seldom clear.

Health care accident investigations are almost exclusively conducted by insiders and stakeholders. Investigators bring their own experience and biases to investigations, often in ways that are imperceptible, yet the results of accident investigations are treated as though they were independent, objective, and unbiased. Experienced practitioners recognize that the results of investigations into health care accidents are often quite narrow and sometimes misleading. What may come as a surprise, however, is that the same narrowness of view can be found in other fields, including some domains where accident investigation is thought to be quite sophisticated. The reason is that accident investigations tend to be framed and directed, and therefore limited, by the very same systemic factors that produced the accident in the first place. The realization that both accidents and their investigation reflect the workings of the system in which they take place has deep theoretical and practical implications.

Complex System Failure, Not Pilot Error: The Case of Air Ontario Flight 1363

On March 10, 1989, a Fokker F-28 commuter jet aircraft took off from Dryden, Ontario, on the last leg of a series of round trips between Winnipeg, Manitoba, and Thunder Bay, Ontario. During the brief stopover in Dryden, the aircraft had been refueled. The temperature was hovering near freezing, and it had been raining or snowing since the aircraft had landed. Several passengers and at least one crew member had noticed that slush had begun to build up on the wings.

Flight 1363 began its takeoff roll but gathered speed slowly and only barely cleared the trees at the end of the runway (see **Figure 6-1**). The plane never became fully airborne. It crashed less than 1 kilometer beyond the end of the runway. The aircraft, loaded with fuel, was destroyed by fire. Twenty-four people on board, including the pilot and copilot, were killed.

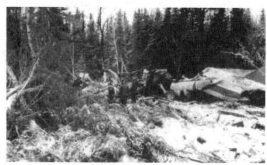

Figure 6-1. Wreckage of Flight 1363 near Dryden, Ontario.

The initial assessment was that pilot error, specifically the decision to take off despite the slush that was forming on the wings, was the cause of the accident. That decision was not in keeping with the pilot's record or reputation. The pilot was experienced and was regarded by others as a thoughtful, cautious, and competent man who operated "by the book." Nevertheless, he had chosen to take off in the presence of hazardous conditions that a competent pilot should have known were unacceptable.

The reactions to this accident might well have ended there. Human error by practitioners is known to be the proximate cause of 80 percent of accidents. At first, the Dryden crash seemed to be just another instance of the unreliability of humans in technological settings. If the pilot had been inexperienced or physically or mentally impaired (e.g., if he had been drinking alcohol before the crash), it is likely that attention would have turned away and that the crash would be remembered today only by the survivors and the families of those who died.

But the Canadian federal government commissioned an unprecedented investigation, under the direction of retired Supreme Court Justice Virgil Moshansky, into all the factors surrounding the accident. Why it did so is not entirely clear, but at least three factors seem to have played roles. First, the event was national in scale; it was too large to be treated in ordinary ways. Images of the charred wreckage and the firsthand accounts of survivors captivated the entire country.

Second, the accident "fit" hand in glove into a set of concerns about Canadian aviation that had been growing slowly over several years. Those years had seen substantial change in Canadian commercial aviation. Deregulation had produced a significant increase in airline operations. New aircraft were being brought into service, and new routes were being opened.

In addition, the aviation industry itself was in turmoil. Once-small companies were expanding rapidly, and larger companies were buying up smaller ones. Significantly, instead of keeping pace with the growth of commercial aviation, the Canadian government's regulatory-oversight body for aviation was shrinking as the government sought to reduce its budget deficit. There was no obvious connection between any of these large-scale factors and the accident at Dryden, Ontario. But the small waves of concern about aviation safety that had been rippling across the surface of the country now appeared to be harbingers of the large wave that came from the accident.

The third factor was the collection of new insights that flowed from the aftermath of the nuclear reactor meltdown at Three-Mile Island (TMI) in Pennsylvania that had occurred 10 years earlier. TMI was a watershed event that spawned a renaissance in research on safety, accidents, and human factors. This research formed the basis for a new understanding of accidents and human error, providing new insights into how accidents happen and what role human operators have in accident genesis and recovery. This new understanding was captured, in part, at North Atlantic Treaty Organization conferences in the early 1980s and popularized separately by Charles Perrow[1] in his 1984 book *Normal Accidents*. The research did not directly explain the Dryden crash. Instead, it showed how an investigation of the system in which the accident took place might lead to an explanation that went *behind* human error.[2] This systems view of accidents requires detailed examination of the variety of contributors—the factors and the actors—that made the accident possible.

The investigation took almost two years to complete and became the most exhaustive, most extensive examination of an aviation accident ever conducted. Well more than 200,000 pages of documents and transcripts were collected and analyzed. The investigators explored not just the mechanics of flight under icing conditions but details about the running of the airport and the air-transportation system, including its organization and regulation. All these factors were linked in the commission's four-volume report. The report does not identify a single cause, or even multiple causes, of the accident. Instead, it makes clear that the aviation system contained many faults that together created an environment that would eventually produce an accident, if not on the tenth day of March in Dryden, Ontario, then on some other day in some other place.[3]

Bad weather at the Dryden airport was just one of many problems that came together on March 10, 1989. The airline itself was a family operation without strong management. It had traditionally relied on smaller, prop aircraft and had only recently begun jet operations. The operating manual for the Fokker F-28 had not yet been approved by Canadian regulators. The company's safety manager, an experienced pilot, had recently resigned because of disputes with management. There were deferred maintenance items, among them fire sensors in the small engine the Fokker carried that would allow it to start its main engines. Company procedures called for the engines to be shut down for deicing of the wings but there was no convenient way to restart them at Dryden because the company did not have ground starting equipment for its new jet aircraft at the Dryden airport. To deice the aircraft would have required turning off the engines, and once they were turned off there was no way to restart them.[1] Bad weather at Dryden caused snow and ice to build up on the aircraft wings. The Dryden refueling was necessary because the airline management had required the pilots to remove fuel before taking off from Thunder Bay for the trip to Winnipeg. The pilot had wanted to leave passengers behind in Thunder Bay to avoid the need to refuel, but management had ordered him to remove fuel instead, creating the need for refueling in Dryden.[2] The takeoff of Flight 1363 from Dryden was further delayed when a single-engine plane urgently requested use of the one runway in order to land because the snow was making visibility worse. Ultimately, more than 30 discrete contributing factors were identified, including characteristics of the deregulation of commercial aviation in Canada, management deficiencies in the airline company, and lack of maintenance and operational equipment.

No single one of these problems was sufficient in itself to cause a crash. Only in combination could these multiple *latent conditions*[5,6] create the conditions needed for the crash. In hindsight, there were plenty of opportunities to prevent the accident. But the fact that the multiple flaws are necessary to create disaster has the paradoxical effect of making each individual flaw seem insignificant. Seen in isolation, no flaw appears dangerous. As a result, many such flaws may accumulate within a system without raising alarm. When they do occur simultaneously, they present the operator with a situation that teeters on the edge of catastrophe or indeed becomes catastrophic (see **Figure 6-2**). The latter was the situation in the case of Flight 1363.

The pilots were not so much the instigators of the accident as the recipients of it. Circumstances had combined (some would say conspired) to create a situation that was rife with pressures, uncertainty, and risk. The pilots were invited to manage their way out of the situation but were offered no attractive opportunities to do so. Rather than being a choice among several good alternatives, the system produced a situation where the pilots were forced to choose among bad alternatives under conditions of uncertainty. They made an effort to craft a safe solution but were obstructed by managers who insisted that they achieve production goals.

Unlike many postaccident inquiries, the investigation of the crash of Flight 1393 was detailed and broad enough to show how the situation confronting the pilots had arisen. The investigation provided a fine-grain picture of the kinds of pressures and difficulties that operators at the sharp end of practice confront in daily work.[7] It showed how the decisions and actions throughout the aviation system had brought these pressures and difficulties together in the moments before the crash. This is now recognized as a systems view of the accident. A *systems view* is a picture of the system that shows, in detail, how the technical characteristics of

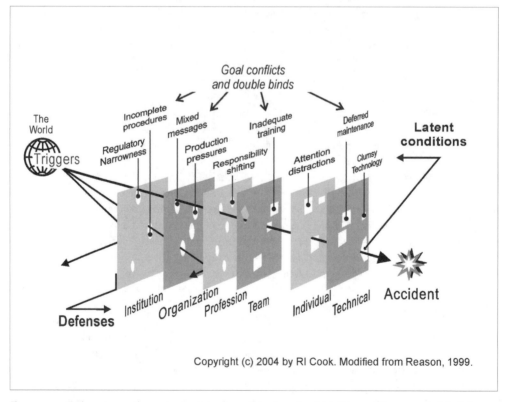

Copyright (c) 2004 by RI Cook. Modified from Reason, 1999.

Figure 6-2. Failures in complex systems require the combination of multiple factors. The system is defended against failure, but these defenses have defects or "holes" that allow accidents to occur.

the workplace, the technical work that takes place there, and the pressures and difficulties that workers experience combine to create a situation that produces an accident. Rather than attributing the accident to a discrete cause or causes, the investigation works toward providing a detailed account of the interactions between the factors that created the situation.

Detailed investigations of health care accidents are the exception rather than the rule. In part this is because creating a systems view is difficult and takes substantial time and resources. Instead, most accident investigations end with the conclusion that they were caused by "human error."

Why are we critical of operators after accidents? Why do accidents such as the crash of Flight 1393 appear to be preventable? One reason is that hindsight bias makes the accident seem likely and that we believe that the operators could have and should have anticipated this likelihood. A second reason is that the human-operator aspects of the accident seem to be the variable (and therefore correctable) element of the system while other elements appear to be relatively fixed.

HINDSIGHT BIAS

Hindsight bias is the effect of knowing that an outcome has occurred on our estimate of how likely that outcome was.[8] The fact that an outcome has occurred biases our judgment. What is now obvious *after* the fact we think should have been obvious *before* the event occurred. Put another way, the occurrence of an event changes our view of how likely it should have seemed to have been before it occurred. This bias makes us believe that events that have happened were potentially foreseeable (see **Figure 6-3**).

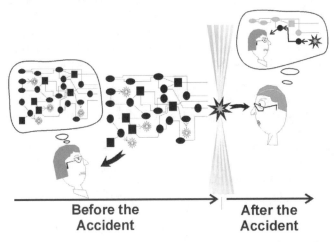

Before the Accident → **After the Accident**

Figure 6-3. Hindsight bias. Knowledge of the outcome leads accident investigators to believe that the event should have been foreseen.

This bias is deeply ingrained, and we are usually not aware of its effect on our assessments.[3] Its effect is subtle, so much so that even though people may recognize it in others, many of them (including experts!) often assert that it is not a part of their own cognition. Yet hindsight bias is heavily engaged when we confront past events, and it is particularly pernicious when we search for the "cause" of accidents. The apparent likelihood of past events leads us to believe they were so likely that they should have been anticipated.

Accidents have profound consequences, and this makes us think that they were foreseeable and therefore should have been foreseen. After accidents, we can identify the multiple contributors to accidents. Hindsight bias leads us to believe that they should have been foreseen by those who were involved. This is the reason that investigations of accidents so often "discover" that human operator "error" caused the accident.

FIXED VERSUS VARIABLE ELEMENTS OF THE SYSTEM

Human performance appears to be the variable element of the system. It seems to be the point in the system where there is some opportunity to intervene in the accident sequence. By contrast, other aspects of the system appear to be fixed. Accident analysis is a practical endeavor, not a theoretical one, and we would expect it to focus on things that can be changed. We do not expect aircraft crash investigators, for example, to "discover" that gravity caused the accident, although this is literally true! Instead, we expect accident investigators to concentrate on the factors that are amenable to change. Because human activity seems to be a leverage point for change, most accident analyses stop when they encounter a human with presumed freedom of action. Other aspects of the system are likely to be regarded as forces of nature—things that are outside the boundary of what can be controlled. The intense focus on worker performance serves as a signal that most of the health care system, including the incentives, economic factors, organizational elements, and technology, are outside that boundary and, therefore, uncontrollable.

Focus on operator error seems to be a particular, although not exclusive, problem for locally conducted analyses. Workers and managers within a system tend to view almost everything about that system as unchangeable except for the most superficial local factors. This is mainly because their scope of action is largely limited to local conditions. Because humans appear to be the most controllable components within the system, most analytical attention gets directed at these potential targets of corrective action. The situation is not unlike the old joke about the drunk who, at midnight, decided to look for his lost car keys under the streetlamp because that is where the light was better.

The success of the Dryden crash investigation owes much to a deep understanding of the ways in which accidents are so often misunderstood. The accident happened because multiple, individually small faults combined to create conditions that were sufficient to cause a catastrophe. The accident investigation succeeded where it might have failed because of the independent, deliberate, thorough, and time-consuming work of the investigating team and its ability to achieve a systems view that encompassed these contributing factors. The Dryden accident was required in order to make such a deep look possible. The tragedy of the accident is that the passengers and crew paid the price for the economic and social efficiency that produced the accident.

Investigations into health care accidents are rarely as insightful as the Air Ontario crash investigation was. The few detailed investigations that are available demonstrate that accidents in intensive-care units, operating rooms, and pharmacies happen in the same way. More often than not, health care accident investigation halts with the diagnosis of human (operator) error, and all subsequent work is directed toward preventing this type of error from recurring. Health care accidents tend to be investigated and analyzed locally in ways that play into hindsight bias and focus on the apparently variable elements of the system. Deep systems views of accidents are the exception rather than the norm because they are difficult, time-consuming, expensive, and organizationally dangerous to produce. The independence and insight needed to produce these systems views are usually beyond the capacity of those with the responsibility for the investigation and analysis.

Realizing that a system is vulnerable and prone to failure amplifies the shock of the accident itself. Detailed investigations of accidents frequently show that the system was managed *toward* catastrophe, often for a long while. Accidents are not anomalies that arise from isolated human error. Instead, they are normal events that arise from deeply embedded features of the systems of work.[1] The 1999 bonfire tragedy at Texas A&M University in College Station, described in the next section of this chapter, is a case in point. The accident revealed a system that was profoundly out of control and that had, over a long period, been marching toward disaster.

Marching into Disaster: The Texas A&M Bonfire Tragedy

On November 18, 1999, a multistory stack of logs that was to be burned in a traditional football bonfire collapsed while being built by students at the Texas A&M University (see

Figure 6-4). Twelve students working on the structure were crushed to death and 27 others were injured. It was the worst such disaster at a college campus in the United States, and it had a devastating effect within the tight-knit community that prided itself on its engineering college.

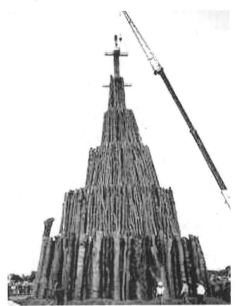

Figure 6-4. Texas A&M University bonfire structure before the collapse, which killed 12 people. A partial collapse five years earlier did not change the approach to building this large structure.

An independent commission was established to investigate the causes of the collapse. Extensive and expensive engineering studies were conducted that showed that the collapse was the result of specific aspects of the structural design of the bonfire. The studies revealed that the collapse occurred because the bonfire had evolved from being a conventional bonfire into a large-scale construction project. That project had never been competently designed or analyzed and was largely carried out by unsupervised amateurs.

The investigating board's report is available on the Internet[9] and the report itself has been reviewed.[10] The bonfire was a Texas A&M football tradition extending over many years. It began in 1928 as a haphazard collection of wooden pallets. It grew gradually, increasing in scale and complexity each year until the 1990s, when it required a crane to erect. In 1994, a partial collapse occurred but was attributed to shifting ground underneath the structure rather than to structural failure.

The 1999 catastrophe overwhelmed the medical facilities of the area. The response to the failure made it clear that no one imagined that this sort of disaster was possible, let alone likely. In hindsight, it seems incredible that this should have been the case. Even here, hindsight misleads us into believing that the inevitability of this particular sort of accident should have been apparent. Nonetheless, it was not at all obvious before the fact. The relative lack of failure over many years produced a sense that failure was unlikely, even though the growing size of the structures was taking the system in that direction. Each increment in complexity and scale was too small to signal that the system was becoming dangerous in new ways. The bonfires of the late 1990s reached new heights without anyone understanding what those heights meant. The inability to recognize that the system was unsafe was a property of the system itself, a property essential to the development of the accident situation.

Complex systems have a tendency to move incrementally toward unsafe operations.[11] Because such systems are expensive to operate, there is a constant drive to make their operations cheaper or more efficient. Because they are complex, it is difficult to project how changes in the operations will create opportunities for new forms of failure.[12] Because many of the changes are difficult to reverse (e.g., when they involve new technology or significant organizational change), there may be little opportunity to return to the old ways of doing things.[13]

The desire for early warnings that our systems are becoming dangerous has led to interest in incident and near-miss reporting systems. The value of these systems remains speculative. Even relatively strong danger signals, such as the partial collapse of the bonfire in 1994 or the partially burned O-rings from shuttle boosters before *Challenger*, can be misinterpreted.[14]

Equally strong counterbalancing forces usually exist, most notably the pressure to make systems economically efficient. Until overt failure occurs, it is easy to rationalize away warnings, especially when the system is operating near the margins of economic failure, as is often the case with hospitals and other health care facilities.

Before an accident, proponents of safety measures find themselves in a difficult position. The various warning signals usually do not herald a specific failure. Because of this, efforts to improve safety appear diffuse and general in character. Paradoxically, the costs of these measures are easily calculated while their potential benefits remain unknown and unknowable. Together, these characteristics tend to channel organizational work on safety toward low-cost ventures that do not affect production. Because failure is rare, warning signals may be separated from the accidents themselves by long periods of time. This may make the warning signals seem uninformative. System managers may come to believe that dismissing these warning signals reflects good judgment rather than successful gambling. The Texas A&M bonfire tragedy is a telling case of a process that incrementally grew well beyond the boundaries of safety without the danger of the situation ever being recognized by those who managed the process. Repeated success with larger and larger bonfires led everyone to believe that the system was not hazardous and actually encouraged further growth.

Against this backdrop of success, warning signals such as the partial collapse could be discounted. The partial collapse was treated as an incident. It was not large enough to garner the sort of attention needed for the kind of detailed examination that would show how dangerous the increasingly large bonfires were. Only a truly catastrophic failure was enough to produce a new look at what the bonfire had become. The people managing the bonfire had marched into tragedy with their eyes open, but they were unable to interpret what they were seeing.

The same march into disaster can be identified in the Dryden Air Ontario crash, although the complexity of that system makes it harder to see. The people in Air Ontario and at the Texas A&M University were, in a sense, conducting a series of experiments that explored the failure boundaries of their systems.

The Systems View of Health Care Accidents: The MAR Knockout Case

During the Friday night shift in a large tertiary-care hospital, a nurse called the pharmacy technician on duty to report a problem with the medications just delivered in a unit dose cart for a patient on her ward. The call was not usual; the hospital occasionally had problems with the medications delivered to the floor, especially if a new order was made after the unit dose fill list had been printed. In this case, however, the pharmacy had delivered medicines that had never been ordered for that patient. The medicines delivered, however, did match the patient's newly printed medication administration record (MAR). This was discovered during a routine reconciliation of the previous day's MAR with the new one. The MAR that had just been delivered was substantially different from the one from the previous day, but the patient's chart had no indication that these changes had been ordered. The pharmacy technician consulted a computer screen that showed the patient's medication list. This list corresponded precisely to the new MAR and to the medications that had been delivered to the ward.

While the technician was trying to understand what had happened to this patient's medication, the telephone rang again. It was a call from another ward where the nurses had also discovered something wrong. For some patients, the unit dose cart contained drugs their patients were not taking; in others, the cart did not contain drugs the patients were supposed to get. Other calls soon came in from other areas in the hospital, and all were reporting the same situation. The problem seemed to be limited to the unit dose cart system; the intravenous medications were correct. In each case, the drugs that were delivered matched the newly printed MAR, but the MAR itself was wrong. The pharmacy technician notified the on-call pharmacist who realized that, whatever its source, the problem was hospital-wide.

By early Saturday morning, the pharmacists knew they were confronting a crisis. First, the pharmacy's computer system was somehow generating an inaccurate fill list. Neither the MARs nor the unit dose carts already delivered to the wards could be trusted. There was no pharmacy computer–generated fill list that could be relied on. Second, the wards were now without the right medications for the hospitalized patients, and the morning medication-administration process was about to begin. No one knew what was wrong with the pharmacy computer. Until it could be fixed, some sort of manual system was needed to provide the correct medications to the wards. Across the hospital, the unit dose carts were sent back to the pharmacy.

A senior pharmacist realized that the previous day's hard-copy MARs as they were maintained on the wards were the most reliable available information about what medicines patients were supposed to receive. By copying the most recent MARs, the pharmacy could produce a manual fill list for each patient. For security reasons, there were no copying machines near the wards. Each ward did, however, have a fax machine. The pharmacy staff organized a ward-by-ward fax process to get hand-updated copies of each patient's MAR. Technicians used these faxes as manual fill lists to stock unit dose carts with the correct medications. Ordinarily, MARs provided a way to track and reconcile the physician orders and medication administration process on the wards. In this instance, they became the source of information about what medications were needed. Because the hospital did not yet have computerized physician order entry, copies of handwritten physician orders were available. These allowed the satellite pharmacies to interact directly with the ward nurses to fill the gaps.[4]

As pharmacy staff worked to ensure that patients received the appropriate medications, the source of the failure was still unknown. There had been a problem with the pharmacy computer system during the previous evening. The pharmacy software detected a fault in the database integrity. The computer specialist had contacted the pharmacy software vendor, and they had worked together to fix to the problem. This fix was unsuccessful, so they reloaded a portion of the database from the most recent backup tape. After this reload, the system had appeared to work perfectly.

The computer software had been purchased from a major vendor. After a devastating cancer chemotherapy accident in the institution, the software had been modified to include special dose-checking programs for chemotherapy. These modifications worked well, but pharmacy management had been slow to upgrade the main software package because it would require rewriting the dose-checking add-ons. Elaborate backup procedures were in place, including frequent "change" backups and daily "full" backups onto magnetic tapes.

Working with the software company throughout Saturday morning, the computer technicians discovered why the computer system had failed. The backup tape was incomplete. Reloading had internally corrupted the database.[5] The problem was not related to the fault for which the backup reloading was necessary. The solution to the problem was to reload the last "full" backup (now more than a day-and-a-half old) and to re-enter all orders made since that time. The pharmacy technicians collected all the handwritten order slips from the past 48 hours and began to enter these.[6] The manual system was used all day long on Saturday.

The computer system was restored by the end of the day. The managers and technicians examined the fill lists produced for the nightly fill closely and found no errors. The system was back online. As far as pharmacy and nursing management could determine, no medication misadministration occurred during this event, although some doses were delayed.

Several factors contributed to the hospital's ability to recover from this event. First, the accident occurred on a Friday night, which meant that the staff had all day Saturday to recover and all day Sunday to observe the restored system for new failures. Few new patients are admitted on Saturday, and the relatively slow tempo of operations allowed the staff to concentrate on recovering the system. Second, the hospital had a large staff of technicians and pharmacists who were called in to restore operations. The ability to quickly bring together a large number of experts with operational experience was critical to success. Third, the availability of the manual, paper records allowed these experts to "patch up" the system and make it work in an unconventional but effective way. The paper MARs were the basis for new fill lists, and the paper copies of physician orders provided a paper trail that made it possible to replay the previous day's data entry, essentially fast forwarding the computer until its "view" of the world was correct. Fourth, the computer system and technical processes contributed. The backup process, while flawed in some ways, was essential to recovery because it provided the full backup needed. In addition, the close relationship between the software vendor and hospital information technology staff made it possible for the staff to diagnose the problem and devise a fix with little delay.

Other features of this event are worth noting. First, it was not immediately clear what had happened, only that something was wrong. Such a situation is common. This was an event with systemwide consequences that required decisive and immediate action. This action was expensive and potentially damaging to the prestige and authority of those in charge. An effective response required simultaneous, coordinated activity by experienced, skilled people.

The role of information technology in this event was conflicted, as it continues to be throughout health care. Technology that is introduced to improve safety, such as the dose-checking software in this case, may actually make it harder to achieve safety, for example, by making it difficult to upgrade to new software. Information technology makes it possible to perform work efficiently by speeding up much of the process. But technology can also make it difficult to detect failures and recover from them. It introduces new forms of failure that are hard to appreciate before they occur. These failures are foreseeable, but not foreseen.

Finally, the resilience of this system resides in its people rather than in its technology. It was people who detected the failure, planned a response, devised the work-arounds needed to keep the rest of the system working, and restored the pharmacy system. A large cadre of experienced operations people—mainly pharmacy technicians—was available to assist in the recovery. The consequences of this event were far less than those of Flight 1363 or of the Texas bonfire collapse. The potential for disaster, however, was larger than that of these two other cases. What kept the MAR knockout case from being a catastrophe was the ability of workers to recover the system from the brink of disaster.

Thinking about Systems *Before* Accidents

Accidents lead us to think about ways to anticipate and prevent accidents. But accidents are surprises, and large-scale accidents are fundamental surprises,[15] that is, events that were regarded as impossible before they occurred. The history of complex systems is littered with such events: the TMI nuclear meltdown, the *Challenger* explosion, and the terrorist attacks of 9/11, to name but a few. Interestingly, the technical details of these events were all more or less well understood before the events occurred. What was lacking was the ability to foresee that circumstances would conspire to create the conditions needed to make these technical features active and lethal.

In the accidents described in this chapter, the technical details matter a great deal, but the organizational and social details matter as well. Neither the technical nor the organizational details make sense alone. Instead, the technical, organizational, and social details are connected in a dense mesh that makes it impossible to analyze them separately. Although it is convenient for us to model systems with distinct and separate sharp (technical) and blunt (organizational and institutional) ends, it is the connections among these components that produce accidents and that require analysis. Successful accident investigation requires both a knowledge of technical and organizational characteristics and an understanding how these characteristics interact.

In an attempt to obtain systems views of accidents, various authorities have stressed the importance of going beyond the superficial by repeatedly asking "why" the event happened.[7] These three accidents suggest that it may be more useful to ask "how." How did the conditions that permitted the accident arise? How did the people involved with the accident recognize the potential for it? How did they react to it once it began to evolve? How did incentives in the world lead the system to march toward, rather than away from, disaster? How did the workers recognize that disaster was brewing, and how did they know what actions needed to be taken to avert it?

Accident investigation serves many needs, but one of its primary goals is to aid in the prevention of future accidents. Although it is relatively easy to design countermeasures to forestall recurrence of the most recent accident, making the system itself safer is much harder. There is little chance that the most recent accident will be repeated. The next accident is likely to occur in a different place or in a different way. Using experience with accidents to prevent future events requires that we learn and apply the more general lessons that accidents contain (see **Table 6-1**). The apparent clarity that accident investigation can provide is not the same thing as foresight. What we would like to do is use our experience with past accidents to predict—and prevent—future ones.

Anticipating Health Care Accidents

Predicting the next accident is difficult and, in some sense, impossible. The specific accidents we foresee clearly are prevented. It is the ones we cannot foresee that occur. *The next accident will be different from the last one.* Accidents occur because multiple factors combine to create the necessary conditions for them. Because the pattern of factors in health care work is constantly changing, the accident characteristics of the system are also changing. Even if we cannot predict the next accident, we may be able to anticipate some characteristics of future accidents.

Health care technology changes constantly. Much of the new technology in pharmaceutical operations is intended to play a role in preventing accidents. Information technology is at the heart of these changes. Much of this information technology is intended to couple the parts of the system more tightly and to eliminate intermediate steps involving workers. This tighter coupling will change the ways in which the system fails and the ways in which failures present themselves to workers. It also will reduce the time and restrict the ability of workers to derail accidents-in-the-making. The result is a shift toward fewer, but higher-consequence, failures and an accompanying reduction in the ability of workers to recover from accidents in progress. The paradox is that the use of information technology to couple all the system components is likely to reduce the *number* of accidents but to increase the *severity* of the accidents that do occur. The one-at-a-time, hand filling of prescriptions is itself prone to fail, but each failure tends to be independent, with the effects limited to that particular patient. Robotic systems will eliminate much of the person-to-person variability of dispensing, but accidents with robots may involve many patients.[8] Such systems usually demonstrate increased resistance to low-consequence failure and therefore display lower rates of these failures even as they create the opportunity for new forms of large, spectacular failures.

Increased coupling is part of nearly all new pharmacy systems. Using the computer to link physician order entry with medicine delivery to patients involves coupling the parts of

Table 6-1. Lessons from Three Accidents

Accident	Observation	Interpretation	Implications for Pharmacy Practice
Air Ontario crash in Dryden	Multiple flaws in operations / Problems with equipment / Lack of oversight by government regulators / Production pressure / Inherent hazards of aviation	Complex system failure	Pharmacy systems are complex. Accidents in these systems involve multiple contributors, including technical factors, human performance, management, and regulators.
	Accident initially regarded as "pilot error." / Detailed investigation needed to reveal multiple contributors.	Hindsight bias	Because investigation and analysis of pharmacy accidents are usually conducted in-house, hindsight bias will likely lead to the conclusion that human error by practitioner(s) was the cause of the accident.
Texas A&M bonfire collapse	Incremental growth over time allowed builders to take repeated success as indications that the construction was well managed.	Erosion of safety margin	Pharmacy operations may become hazardous long before overt failure occurs.
	Accident was unanticipated, despite precursor event.	Fundamental surprise	Minor incidents signal presence of hazard but may go unnoticed until an accident occurs.
Pharmacy computer failure	Failure pathway created by attempt to recover computer system using backup. / Floor nurses were first to detect the failure. / Failure involved "safety" software.	Information technology failure	Vulnerability of pharmacy systems shifting toward information technology failures. Information technology failures may be hidden from view of operators. Technology intended to increase safety may open new pathways to failure.
	Recovery involved many people and innovative use of paper records.	Recovery from failure	The ability to recover from failures is an important part of the pharmacy system; resilient responses depend on worker expertise.

this process tightly. The use of bar coding for medication administration is an example. In addition to the many work changes that come with the new technology,[17] the technology adds new dependencies. Use of dose-checking software, for example, changes the role of the pharmacy and the significance of pharmacy computing.

The pharmacy accident described in this chapter had limited consequences because workers were able to revert, at least partly, to manual operations. Some opportunities to recover using manual operations will always be present, but they will be increasingly limited. Recovery was possible in this case because a large number of skilled workers were available to read orders, fill carts, and handle immediate needs while simultaneously working to restore the system. Future systems are unlikely to have these recruitable resources and will present fewer opportunities to intervene. The novel strategy of faxing old medication administration reports to the pharmacy to be used as surrogate fill lists depended on the presence of paper artifacts. At the time of this event, physicians wrote out orders on multipart paper forms. Copies of these orders were used to reenter orders into the pharmacy computer system once the day-old backup was restored. Computerized physician order entry systems, in contrast, will rely on entirely electronic records, making recovery more difficult or impossible.

Much thinking about the future of pharmacy operations envisions smooth-running, sophisticated, and easy-to-manage computer systems doing the bulk of what used to be manual work, with pharmacists supervising the computers. Whether such systems can be developed and kept running is not yet known. Experience with other complex computer systems indicates that these systems may be harder to build and maintain than their proponents believe. Maintaining the hardware, software, and the stored information, such as rules related to warnings and alerts, the pharmacy formulary, limits on dosing, and so forth, is likely to be difficult and expensive. These systems are likely to be used differently than their proponents envision. Little attention has been paid, for example, to the reliability of information and to system-maintenance tasks. Because so much of the work of maintaining these systems is left to the individual facility, critical information-maintenance functions may be left in the hands of pharmacists and technicians, paradoxically producing new opportunities for human error.

Along with this change in the nature of accidents will come a change in the skills and expertise needed to analyze them. As pharmacy operations become internalized within information technology, accident investigations will require that pharmacists acquire more computer forensic expertise. This is unfamiliar territory for those already in practice, but it seems likely that future health-systems pharmacists will have training in information technology on par with what they already receive in therapeutical chemistry.

Because devastating failures are increasingly rare and recovery from failure is increasingly difficult, planning for failure and recovery of modern, information technology–based systems is both more difficult and more important than was the case for yesterday's manual-work systems. Changing information technology–based systems is time-consuming and expensive. It is imperative that pharmacists play increasingly active roles in the design of all the elements of these systems as they seek to make them robust and resilient. Many aspects of the design of future systems can benefit from pharmacist involvement. Experience with accidents shows the value of anticipating the new forms of failure and of designing and testing recovery approaches *before* the failures occur. This is an activity for which health-systems pharmacists are uniquely qualified.

Conclusion

Accidents are powerful reminders of the vulnerability of the systems in which they occur. Rather than being simple events in complex systems, accidents are themselves complicated events with multiple contributors. They arise out of the same systemic complexity that makes them difficult to investigate in detail. Close study of accidents can reveal many of these contributors. It can reveal how, over time, systems can march toward accidents. Close study also reveals how workers detect accidents in progress and work to limit their impact and consequences.

Accidents are signals sent from deep within a system about the sorts of vulnerability and potential for disaster that lie within. Our capacity to make safe systems depends on our ability to connect our experience with accidents to productive work on all the connected elements of the system: people, goals, technology, incentives, rules, knowledge, and expertise. This is a daunting task, but it is also an essential one. Pharmacists have deep knowledge of medication and medication administration and an understanding of the variety and complexity of the processes that bring together medicines and patients. They are uniquely prepared for this work. This gives them the opportunity to make patients safer and the responsibility to do so.

Acknowledgements

Preparation of this chapter was made possible in part by Agency for Healthcare Research and Quality grants R18 HS11816 and UC1 HS14126 and by National Library of Medicine grant R03 LM07947. The authors gratefully acknowledge the many pharmacists and pharmacy technicians who generously shared their experiences and Christopher Nemeth, Ph.D., for many suggestions. The views expressed are those of the authors alone.

Footnotes

[1] The F-28 aircraft had an auxiliary starting engine located in the tail to allow the aircraft to start its own jet engines using internal power. The pilots believed this engine was unusable because certain sensors were not working. In fact, the auxiliary engine was operable.

[2] The situation was even more complex than indicated here and involved weather at expected and alternate airports, the certification of the pilot for operation of the Fokker, and detailed characteristics of the aircraft. For a complete description, see Moshansky.[4]

[3] There is a large body of literature on hindsight bias. Interestingly, hindsight bias cannot be overcome by warning people that it exists: Even if I tell you that your judgment of the likelihood of an event is influenced by knowing that it has happened, the bias remains. Disentangling the effects of cognitive biases from post facto reasoning about accidents is extremely difficult. For more details, see Woods and Cook.[8]

[4] Among the interesting features of this event was the absence of typewriters in the pharmacy. Typewriters, discarded years before in favor of computer label printers, would have been useful for labeling medications. New technology displaces old technology, making it harder to recover from computer failures by reverting to manual operations.[13]

[5] The backup was corrupted because of a complex interlocking process related to the database management software that was used by the pharmacy application. Under particular circumstances, tape backups could be incomplete in ways that remained hidden from the operator.

[6] The process was considerably more complex than is indicated here. For example, in order to bring the computer's view of the world up to date, its internal clock had to be set back, the prior day's fill list regenerated, the day's ordered entered, the clock time set forward, and the current day's morning fill list rerun.

[7] See Joint Commission on Accreditation of Healthcare Organizations.[16]

[8] Such failures have almost certainly occurred, but there is no standard for reporting of these events.

References

1. Perrow C. *Normal Accidents: Living with High-Risk Technologies.* Princeton, NJ: Princeton University Press; 1999.

2. Woods DD, Johannesen L, Cook RI, Sarter N, Cook RI. *Behind Human Error: Cognitive Systems, Computers, and Hindsight.* Dayton, OH: Crew Systems Ergonomic Information and Analysis Center, Wright-Patterson Air Force Base; 1994.

3. Maurino DE, Reason J, Johnston N, Lee RB. *Beyond Aviation Human Factors.* Aldershot, UK: Ashgate Press; 1999.

4. Moshansky VP. Commission of Inquiry into the Air Ontario Crash at Dryden, Ontario. Final Report. Ottawa, Canada: Ministry of Supply and Services. Catalog number CP32-55/1-1993E. 1992.

5. Reason J. *Human Error.* Cambridge, UK: Cambridge University Press; 1990.

6. Reason J. *Managing the Risks of Organizational Accidents.* Aldershot, UK: Ashgate Press; 1997.

7. Cook RI, Woods DD. Operating at the sharp end: the complexity of human error. In: Bogner MS, ed. *Human Error in Medicine.* Mahwah, NJ: Lawrence Erlbaum Assoc; 1994:255-310.

8. Woods DD, Cook RI. Perspectives on human error: hindsight bias and local rationality. In: Durso RS, et al., eds. *Handbook of Human Cognition.* New York: Wiley; 1999:141-171.

9. Texas A&M University. Special Commission on the 1999 Bonfire. 2000. Available at: www.tamu.edu/bonfire-commission/reports. Accessed November 22, 2004.

10. Petroski H. Vanities of the bonfire. *American Scientist.* 2000;88:486-490.

11. Rasmussen J. Risk management in a dynamic society. *Safety Science.* 1997;27:183-213.

12. Woods DD, Cook RI. Nine steps to move forward from error. *Cognition Tech Work.* 2002;4:137-144.

13. Cook RI. Observations on risks and RISKS. *Comm ACM.* 1997;40:22.

14. Vaughan D. *The Challenger Launch Decision: Risk Technology, Culture, and Deviance at NASA.* Chicago: University of Chicago Press; 1997.

15. Lanir Z. *The Fundamental Surprise and Conceptual Learning in the Army.* Tel Aviv: Praxis; 1998.

16. Joint Commission on Accreditation of Healthcare Organizations. Sentinel Event Policy and Procedures. Rev. July 2002. Available at: www.jcaho.org. Accessed November 22, 2004.

17. Patterson ES, Cook RI, Render ML. Improving patient safety by identifying side effects from introducing bar-code medication administration. *J Am Med Informatics Assoc.* 2002;9:540-553.

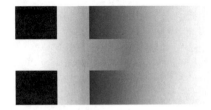

CHAPTER 7

Building an Effective Medication-Safety Team

Sondra May

Attention to Safety: Driving Influences Focused on Building Effective Teams

The Institute of Medicine (IOM) report *To Err Is Human: Building a Safer Health System*, published in 1999, has been credited with the intensified focus on patient safety.[1] Specifically, its finding that medication errors are the largest single cause of medical errors in hospitals prompted many health care organizations to reexamine their medication-use processes with a focus on quality improvement.

The momentum generated by the IOM report has now become far-reaching. The public is more aware of the risk of errors in health care, and regulatory and accrediting bodies are ramping up efforts to develop standards for error reduction. Purchasers of health care are providing incentives and rewards for patient-safety initiatives, patient-advocacy groups are developing evidence-based medication safety strategy recommendations, and professional societies are leading initiatives aimed at improving patient safety. Although these collective efforts to reduce medication errors sometimes differ in their specifics, they all emphasize the need for an organization-wide model of shared accountability for developing and implementing effective, system-based solutions to medication-error reduction. The culture of an organization is the key factor that influences its ability to be successful in creating a safety culture, i.e., one that supports shared responsibility and accountability by building interdisciplinary teams that focus prevention efforts on weaknesses in the system and not on individual care providers. The Joint Commission on Accreditation of Healthcare Organizations (JCAHO) has defined essential elements of a safety culture as part of its standards that support patient safety and medical and health care error reduction (see **Table 7-1**).[2]

Table 7-1. Elements of a Safety Culture[2]

- A collaborative, integrated organizational approach to patient safety.
- Leadership fosters a safety environment through accountability and personal example.
- Staff is oriented to patient-safety issues, and opportunities for organizational learning are encouraged.
- The environment encourages recognition of patient-safety risks from a process and systems perspective and supports disclosure and initiation of actions to reduce risks.
- Mechanisms are in place and adequate resources are allocated for supporting ongoing, proactive patient-safety initiatives.

Experience in the airline industry and other industries has proved that an integrated systems approach that supports safety is far more effective at minimizing negative outcomes than the traditional "blame-and-shame" culture. By focusing on systems rather than on individuals, health care organizations create a nonpunitive environment that encourages recognition of patient-safety risk.[3] These risks are the driving influence for building effective teams with a commitment to safety as a top priority.

Safe Medication-Use Systems: Building an Effective Medication-Safety Team

PURPOSE OF THE TEAM

The medication-use process (see **Figure 7-1**) is complex and error-prone. Errors may occur at any step of the process, and each step brings new opportunities for organizational efforts to ensure safety.[4] To effectively deal with medication-safety issues and problems, organizations are encouraged to create medication-safety teams. The chief benefit of a collaborative, systematic approach to evaluating and promoting the safety of the medication-use process is that it supports achievement of optimal clinical outcomes while eliminating patient harm. All too often, individual providers try to manage error in professional or departmental silos, working to eliminate the causes of only those errors that are most familiar to them. This approach does not take into consideration the culture, infrastructure, or clinical practices of the institution as a whole. As a result, long-lasting improvements in patient safety are not only difficult to achieve but also difficult to maintain.

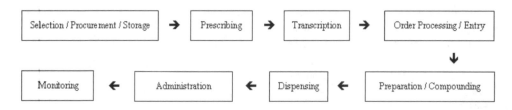

Figure 7-1. Steps in the Medication-Use Process

Although the purpose of a team is consistent, the specific principles that guide it may vary on the basis of the organization's needs and experiences related to patient safety. Medication-safety teams generally are charged with five responsibilities: (1) building and fostering a safety culture within the organization; (2) improving and maintaining effective medication incident–reporting procedures; (3) reviewing high-alert drugs and processes; (4) actively engaging practitioners in implementing positive changes regarding medication-use and patient safety; and (5) achieving regulatory compliance related to patient safety.

TEAM COMPOSITION

An effective team must allow for participation by individuals at all levels of the organization, yet still be able to take frequent action. Success of the team and of the organization's safety initiatives is dependent on the ability to achieve this balance.[5] The exact composition of the team may differ, depending on the organization's needs and experiences related to patient safety, but all teams must have multidisciplinary representation. Additionally, all teams must possess three characteristics: leadership, influence, and authority.

A physician, nurse, and pharmacist are the most important team members, as they have personal knowledge of the medication-use process. Additional patient care providers, including staff from the radiology department, dietary department, the laboratory, and physical and respiratory therapy departments, may be included as necessary. Staff members who seem enthusiastic about reporting and resolving process problems in their respective practice areas are well suited for membership. Department supervisors, managers, or directors (e.g., directors of pharmacy and nursing, nurse managers, nurse educators, medical directors) are important members as they oversee the day-to-day operations of the organization and can assess staff response to change. Senior administrative leaders (e.g., president of the medical board, vice president of patient services, chief nursing officer, chair of the pharmacy and therapeutics [P&T] committee) who lead by example, keep management informed, and remind others of safety's importance to administration are key participants in sustaining a culture of safety. Additional members may include individuals who interact with the medication-use process (e.g., consumer representative, information systems analyst, risk/quality/safety manager, human resources staff, patient educator). Process-improvement initiatives will succeed only if all departments feel that they are part of the process.

Although everyone involved in the medication-use process shares responsibility for the development and outcomes of safety initiatives, delegating supervision of these initiatives to a single individual is critical for ensuring overall success. The individual should be charged with coordinating medication-safety efforts across the departments and committees that function within the organization.[3] This individual is an excellent choice to chair the medication-safety team and to lead the organization's strategic initiatives to improve patient safety.

In addition to having the right members, teams must possess baseline knowledge of human factors, of principles of error reduction, and of issues surrounding the culture of safety, systems thinking, and the use of technology in improving safety. It is also important that the organization invest time and resources to promote team building among members of the medication-safety team.[6] Team-building activities help build trust and acknowledge individual members' unique skills, contributions, and ideas. This enables the group to reach its goals more quickly and effectively.

REPORTING STRUCTURE

An organization must provide oversight for the medication-safety team's initiatives in order to demonstrate to its customers that it supports a culture of risk identification and reduction, encourages open communication about medication errors and unsafe conditions, and is committed to preventing patient injury. Methods for reporting progress on patient-safety initiatives vary, depending on the organization's size and management philosophy. A medication-safety team may be a stand-alone entity that reports directly to the organization's quality council, medical board, and board of directors, or it may be a subcommittee of a larger group, such as a patient-safety committee or a pharmacy and therapeutics (P&T) committee (see **Figure 7-2**).

Many organizations have a layered approach to patient safety. In this arrangement, several groups or committees work independently on separate tasks and responsibilities, but share ideas via members who sit on the multiple committees. Additionally, a reporting structure may include work groups that have been formed by the medication-safety team. These ad hoc groups often include individuals who are experts in a particular area and who assist the medication-safety team in addressing particular areas of concern. Their work is done in parallel with, but coordinated and overseen by, the medication-safety team. The group is disbanded after accomplishing its objectives.

The specific reporting structure used by an organization is not as important as is ensuring that information is effectively disseminated and applied. Additionally, reporting structures may need to change over time to meet the evolving needs of the organization.

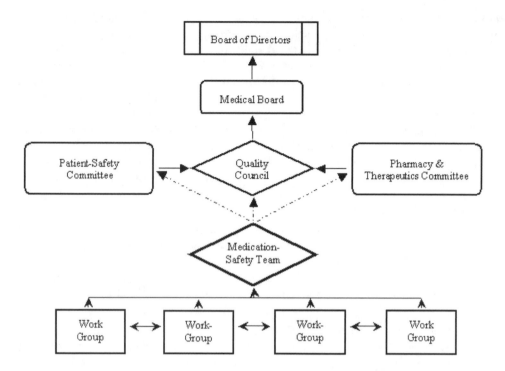

Figure **7-2.** *Medication-Safety Team Reporting Structure*

MEETING LOGISTICS

To address ongoing responsibilities, the medication-safety team must meet regularly. The success of these meetings is dependent on many factors, among the most important of which are discussed in the following paragraphs.

Establish a Meeting Time and Place

Meeting planners should choose an appropriate meeting date and time that are convenient for all members. Early-morning meetings or meetings scheduled around mealtimes often work best for health care providers, especially if food or refreshments are provided. Set a time limit for the meeting and adhere to it. Additionally, it is important to determine the frequency with which meetings will be held.

The meeting location should be convenient for all members or should be rotated among various locations if necessary. The meeting location should be suitable to the team's size and equipment needs.

Create and Distribute the Agenda

The agenda is a road map for the meeting. It gives the meeting a sense of purpose and direction. The agenda should be created with input from members. This will not only increase attendance and participation but also ensure that all issues important to the team are being addressed.[7] Agenda items should correlate with the charges of the team and should be action oriented (e.g., decide, discuss, select, announce, vote). Specific amounts of time should be allotted for each agenda item, and the name of the individual(s) responsible for presenting the information should be included.

Productive meetings depend on members being prepared. Therefore, the agenda and supporting materials should be distributed as far in advance of the meeting as possible, and a reminder of the meeting time and place should also be sent.

Start and End the Meeting on Time
Members are more likely to attend meetings if they are productive and predictable. The time lines outlined on the agenda should be followed as closely as possible.

Introduce Guests
Guests will often be invited to participate in discussions or make presentations. It is important that their roles be clearly defined and that the team acknowledge their work.

Work through the Agenda
An agenda item should be introduced with appropriate background information provided. Time should be allowed for sufficient discussion of the item; an appropriate action should then be agreed on and, in some circumstances, voted on. It is important to encourage participation by all members. To facilitate discussions and open communication, it is essential that the confidentiality of the meeting's proceedings be maintained. Often a confidentiality statement is included on the meeting attendance record as a reminder of the private nature of the proceedings; members' signatures signify their attendance at the meeting and their acknowledgment of its confidential nature.

Maintain Meeting Minutes
One team member should be assigned responsibility for taking minutes. The minutes are the official record of the meeting and should include agenda items, summaries of discussions that took place and recommendations made or actions taken by the team, and any follow-up that is necessary, including the names of responsible individuals. Minutes from the preceding meeting should be distributed in a timely manner to members, guests, and other committees as required.

Minutes can also be an effective tool for bringing new members and other interested parties up-to-date with the guiding principles of the team and its past and present initiatives.

It takes effort to increase the chance for team success, but with good planning and committed follow-through, successful meetings will facilitate teamwork.

Creating a Strategic Plan

The JCAHO Patient Safety Standards expect that safety will be integrated into the design of processes, functions, and services across the organization.[2] To accomplish this, an organization's mission, vision, and values must support a safety culture that is backed by a well-defined strategic plan for medication safety.[8] This plan should not only describe how the organization will strive to manage the short-term safety needs of patients but also define where the organization wants to be in the future. The plan must have the full support of key organizational leaders as well as the members of the medication-safety team. The team must then identify goals that clearly align with the organization's initiatives to establish a framework for measuring and attaining medication-safety improvement. Careful preparation and significant resource allocation are necessary to ensure that the team's strategic plan will move forward.

Selecting Improvement or Change Initiatives

GUIDING PRINCIPLES
Guiding principles of a medication-safety team are specific recommendations that shape the way in which safe medication-use programs are designed, implemented, and maintained. Such principles establish the backbone for what the team wants to accomplish. A variety of resources may serve as templates for establishing a team's guiding principles.[1,9-16] These resources contain similar recommendations, but often differ in the amount of detail and direction they offer an organization that is beginning to undertake process-improvement initiatives.

One principle that remains constant is the need for a systems-oriented approach. This approach does not look to individuals to achieve ultimate patient safety on their own, but instead provides a framework for organizations to redesign care delivery by effectively integrating individual components of the medication-use process to support one another.

With its numerous recommendations, the IOM report *To Err Is Human: Building a Safer Health System* brought increased national attention to issues surrounding patient safety.[1] One of its specific aims was to implement safety systems in health care organizations through the adoption of practices that have been shown to reduce error and improve safety. These practices include improving standardization, using technology, and establishing environments that support convenient access to relevant patient and medication information at the point of care.

The Massachusetts Coalition for Prevention of Medical Errors published a set of principles and best practices for reducing medication errors.[9] These were based on the Massachusetts Hospital Association's (MHA's) medication error–prevention project and include adopting a systems-oriented approach to medication-error reduction that is nonpunitive and supports open communication and learning from errors. Eight of the coalition's twelve best practices focus on reducing human error and are recommended for immediate implementation. The remaining four practices incorporate the use of technology and are recommended for implementation over a longer period of time.

The National Coordinating Council for Medication Error Reporting and Prevention has published a variety of recommendations for system approaches to reducing medication errors in the prescribing, dispensing, and administration phases of the medication-use process.[10] The council's recommendations for minimizing the risk for error are grounded in an evidence-based approach that encourages collaboration within and among health care organizations, health care professionals, patients, industry, standard setters, and regulators.

The Institute for Safe Medication Practices (ISMP) developed a Medication Safety Self-Assessment™ to guide organizations in assessing their medication-use systems.[11] The tool is divided into key elements thought to most strongly influence safe medication use. Each element is defined by one or more distinguishing characteristics of safe medication systems. Organizations can use these characteristics to compare experiences and identify opportunities for improvement through individual scoring methods.

The Regional Medication Safety Program for Hospitals, launched by the Health Care Improvement Foundation, identified 16 action goals aimed at improving medication safety.[12] The program was designed to involve all organizational stakeholders, including members of the board of directors, administrators, medical staff, employees, patients, and community members. The program focuses on four main areas: organizational culture, infrastructure, clinical practice, and technology. Safety tools have been developed to assist organizations with implementing the specific goals and for measuring progress related to medication safety.

One of the most comprehensive strategies for achieving a safe medication-use system was developed by the American Society of Health-System Pharmacists and is known as the Medication-Use-System Safety Strategy (MS³).[13] Similar to the key elements outlined in the ISMP's Medication Safety Self-Assessment™, the MS³ delineates 13 categories of multidisciplinary job responsibilities that include 84 different tasks necessary to ensure a safe medication-use system (see **Table 7-2**). The strategy outlines a systematic, interdisciplinary approach to improving medication safety that is based on both well-established and theorized principles.

Table 7-2. MS³ Categories of Job Responsibilities[13]

Patient and medication information

Prescribing and monitoring

Communication of medication orders

Medication labeling, packaging, and nomenclature

Medication standardization and storage

Medication preparation, distribution, dispensing, and administration

Medication-delivery-device acquisition, use, and monitoring

Environmental factors

Staff competency and education

Patient education

Quality processes and risk management

Legal and regulatory compliance

Management and organizational and public liaison

In its Pathways for Medication Safety[SM] series, the American Hospital Association, the Health Research and Education Trust, and the ISMP suggest seven long-term goals that make up a model strategic plan for medication safety (see **Table 7-3**).[14] These goals represent demonstrated best practices for improving medication safety and are applicable to a wide variety of practice settings. Unique to this set of goals is the inclusion of potential barriers or threats that could impede an organization's progress related to each goal. Although not all-inclusive, these barriers and threats are often as important to the success of a strategic initiative as are the guiding principles themselves. They therefore should be part of every medication-safety team's planning efforts.

Table 7-3. Goals for a Model Medication-Safety Strategic Plan[14]

1. Create, communicate, and demonstrate a leadership-driven culture of safety.
2. Improve error detection, reporting, and use of the information to improve medication safety.
3. Evaluate where technology can help reduce the risk of medication errors.
4. Reduce the risk of errors with high-alert medications prescribed and administered to high-risk patient populations or at vulnerable periods of transfer through the health care system.
5. Establish a blamefree environment for responding to errors.
6. Involve the community in medication-safety initiatives and medication self-management programs.
7. Establish a controlled formulary in which the selection of medications is based more on safety than on cost.

Unlike the voluntary recommendations from patient-safety advocates and professional societies, JCAHO's recommendations are obligatory for all organizations that wish to obtain or maintain accreditation. The National Patient Safety Goals and the Medication Management Standards are examples of evidence- and expert-based practices that JCAHO uses to measure compliance during its survey process.[15,16] Although some organizations place greater priority on JCAHO medication-safety recommendations than on those described above, the majority of the recommendations closely mirror those described elsewhere, in both philosophy and design, and therefore serve as an excellent template for designing an organizational strategy for improving medication safety.

Because of the breadth and depth of the recommendations highlighted, organizations must carefully consider the availability of resources and committed personnel when selecting their guiding principles. Success in transforming an organization's practices to those that support principles of medication safety is also dependent on interdisciplinary collaboration and communication.

In addition to using external models, an organization must assess its own strengths and weaknesses related to medication safety in order to establish clear, concise, measurable goals and to identify tasks that should be overseen by the team.[17] Depending on an organization's current status with respect to medication safety, the information for such assessments may be prevalent or sparse. Although it is important to analyze available information, teams should not spend too much time creating sources for information that do not currently exist. Opportunities to collect specific types of data can be established once a set of guiding principles has been formed on the basis of information initially available.

Conducting a survey to assess staff perceptions and organizational commitment to medication safety is often an important starting point.[18] Surveys can identify deficiencies within the system and aid in establishing policies on issues such as reporting and analyzing medication-safety events. They also identify opportunities for education and training at all levels of the organization and provide good baseline measurements on which comparisons can be made to measure progress. Medication-safety information can be collected and analyzed from a number of data sources, including direct observation, chart review, computerized monitoring using rules and triggers, incident reports, and documented interventions. Lessons learned from proactive (failure mode and effects analysis) and reactive hazard analysis (root-cause analysis) can also assist teams in designing plans for removing or decreasing potential and actual system failures. Finally, many organizations find it useful to solicit informal feedback from staff on their perceptions of unsafe practices observed in their day-to-day activities. This feedback can be obtained through focus groups, suggestion boxes, telephone safety hotlines, and safety rounds where frontline providers can share concerns.[19]

After reviewing all available information, the team identifies those long-term goals or guiding principles that not only compliment the organization's strategic plan but also match identified opportunities for improvement. The goals must be measurable and be able to withstand an ever-changing health care system. They must reflect the values and interests of the individuals responsible for overseeing their achievement while challenging the organization to provide the safest and highest level of care possible. Most important, they must force improvement in the safety of the medication-use process.

ASSOCIATED TASKS

Process-improvement strategies often target practices that are high-volume, high-risk, or problem-prone.[20] Because of the complexities of the medication-use process, many aspects of medication management fulfill these criteria. Therefore, developing a strategy for planning and prioritizing associated tasks that the medication-safety team will oversee is critical to designing, implementing, and maintaining a safe medication-use system.[13] Each of the tasks must address the needs identified in the guiding principles selected by the team. Additionally, the tasks should be accomplishable in a defined period of time, should balance the benefit to the organization with the resources necessary to accomplish them, should focus on improving the system, and should contribute to the ultimate the goal of improved medication safety.[20] As with the guiding principles, the tasks must be measurable and practical. Selecting relevant tasks at the outset will assist the team in establishing focus and ensuring that its efforts are guided by evidence-based practices.

As with all process-improvement initiatives, efforts may need to be reprioritized over time. Organizations cannot afford to address only errors that have occurred within their own four walls; they must continuously follow the safety literature to keep the team's efforts aligned with local, state, and national medication-safety initiatives. Specific guiding principles or associated tasks may need to be modified or eliminated on the basis of new information, including lessons learned from the experience of others. Valuable sources of information include presentations at recent professional meetings, publications in professional journals, the general news media, ISMP newsletters, JCAHO Sentinel Events ALERTS, FDA MedWatch™ Safety Alerts, and HCPro, Inc. Briefings on Patient Safety.

A Continuous Quality Improvement Model

Once the medication-safety team has selected its improvement or change initiatives, it must test the changes by planning for them, doing them, checking them, and acting on the results. These steps compose the cyclical, four-stage process of the Plan-Do-Check-Act (PDCA) continuous quality improvement (CQI) model (see **Figure 7-3**).[21] The PDCA model supports action-oriented learning through a process of continuously making changes and reflecting on the consequences of those changes. (For examples of how the model can be used to achieve specific medication-safety goals, see the Case Studies at the end of this chapter.) Because of the complexities of today's health care environment, management of medication-safety initiatives by a single individual is neither feasible nor in the best interest of patients. A team-based approach is the only mechanism for systematically implementing, evaluating, and, as necessary, modifying the multiple initiatives that need to be occurring simultaneously to achieve a safe medication-use system in an efficient and effective manner.

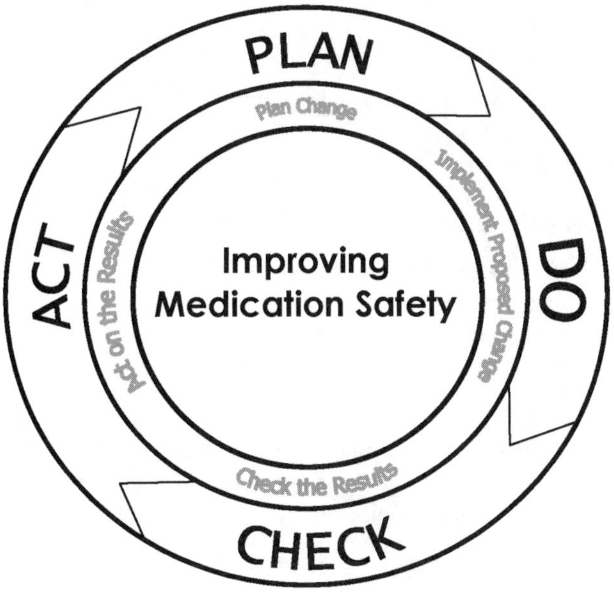

To prepare themselves to apply CQI principles, team members may find it helpful to attend a course that addresses the basics of team development and describes the tools necessary for following performance-improvement and patient-safety activities. Teams that effectively apply CQI principles accept the notion that processes and products can always be improved and that deficiencies signify opportunities for change.[22]

Figure 7-3. *PDCA Continuous Quality Improvement Model*

PLAN CHANGE

The team must plan for change by matching a measurable objective with the specific change initiatives that will be used to achieve that objective. Responsibility for the test must be assigned and a time line for the initiative should be established.

IMPLEMENT PROPOSED CHANGES

New ideas can sometimes have a negative effect on the quality of care. Therefore, it is important that they be properly evaluated prior to systemwide implementation. A small-scale study or pilot test can place boundaries on tests of proposed changes by limiting the number of people involved or the location or duration of the test. Following implementation of the proposed change, data should be collected to determine its impact.

CHECK THE RESULTS

Effective measurement is fundamental to evaluating system performance and improvement.[23] Measuring improvement requires transforming data into information.[16] Medication-safety data can be aggregated and analyzed using tools that measure how change has modified the medication-use process and affected the potential for patient harm. It is important to track both process and outcome measures to determine whether or not performance expectations related to process stability and outcome predictability are being met.[24] Measuring the impact of change in areas such as a specific step in the medication-use process or within the process for reporting medication errors will assist the team in determining whether or not the changes are leading to overall improvements in the medication-use system (see **Table 7-4**). Likewise, measuring specific outcomes can help the team determine whether or not the improved medication-use system is reducing patient harm from medication errors (see Table 7-5).

Table 7-4. Process Measurements[24]

Percentage of staff completing training in medication safety

Pharmacist interventions per 100 admissions

Number of self-reported medication errors

Dispensing errors detected by machine-readable cart-fill technology

Number of potential or near-miss medication errors with high-alert drugs

Table 7-5. Outcome Measurements[24]

Percentage of emergency department visits caused by adverse drug events

Number of preventable adverse drug events per 1,000 doses

Average length of stay for a patient experiencing an adverse drug event

Severity of adverse drug event (i.e., serious, life-threatening, or fatal)

Patient-satisfaction scores

Teams may use a variety of tools to analyze and display data to identify specific performance patterns or trends.[25] Most commonly used are bar graphs, which display patterns of occurrence over time and pie or radar charts, which display before-and-after data. The Pareto chart is a specific type of bar graph that can be used to measure progress (see **Figure 7-4**). The Pareto distribution focuses efforts on problems that offer the greatest potential for improvement. The tallest bars are the biggest contributors to the problem. This is often referred to as the "80/20" rule (i.e., 80 percent of an organization's problems are due to 20 percent of the deficiencies in the system). Comparing before and after data in Pareto charts assists in assessing changes in patterns over time. These charts also identify whether changes improve certain problems yet worsen others. Run charts can also be very effective for tracking trends over a specified period of time (see **Figure 7-5**). They can be used to compare the performance of a process before and after specific changes in order to determine the value of those changes.

Regardless of which tools are used, the team must review and evaluate the results of change and compare findings against its improvement goals. One of the team's most impor-

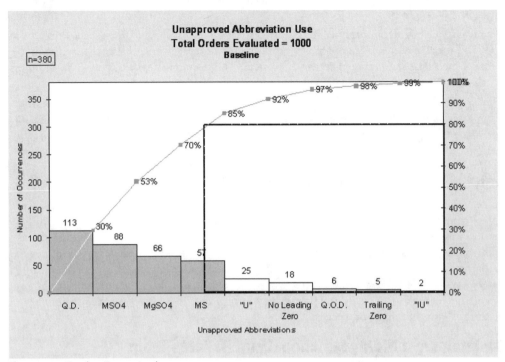

Figure 7-4. Baseline Pareto Analysis

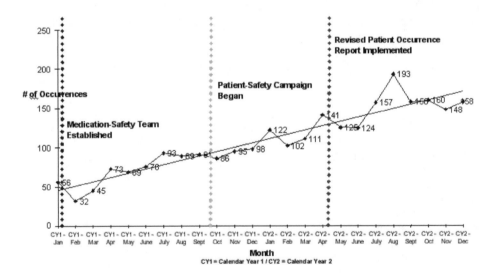

Figure 7-5. Run Chart

tant responsibilities is to make sure that improvement initiatives are having the desired effect. Assigning an individual sole responsibility for monitoring the impact of change can result in an assessment that reflects only the limited view and expertise of that person. An interdisciplinary, team-based approach to medication-use safety is necessary for accurately assessing outcomes from a systems perspective.

ACT ON THE RESULTS

The team now has an opportunity to reflect on what it has learned and, if necessary, to repeat the PDCA cycle with redesigned changes. If change initiatives meet expectations, the same process should be standardized across the system. The team must have a strategy for holding the gain and a plan for future evaluation.

The PDCA model is an efficient tool for decreasing the time between lessons learned from errors and applying corrective action to prevent future errors.[26] It applies a systematic approach to improving the quality of care that is easily modified to address individual organizations' needs for preventing errors.

Tracking and Communicating Progress

In order to keep medication safety highly visible within the organization, the medication-safety team must demonstrate success and communicate progress to everyone, from frontline staff to hospital administrators. Establishing oversight of long-term goals and specific change projects, as well as celebrating small achievements along the way, will assist with keeping initiatives on track (see **Figure 7-6**).[17] Developing effective mechanisms for communicating safety solutions (e.g., e-mail, newsletters, posters, storyboards, in-service training) that also encourage feedback from staff and patients about how change is affecting them will increase the probability of long-term success.

Maintaining a Highly Functional and Reliable Team

Realistic expectations are the final key to maintaining an effective and reliable medication-safety team. An organization cannot set an expectation of zero errors, but must support a model of shared accountability that promotes safety through the redesign of medication-use systems.[26] The expectations of the organization must clearly match the guiding principles established by the team and allow influence and authority to be applied when necessary. Additionally, because consistency breeds reliability, expectations of the organization must be consistent with what the team believes it is responsible for achieving.

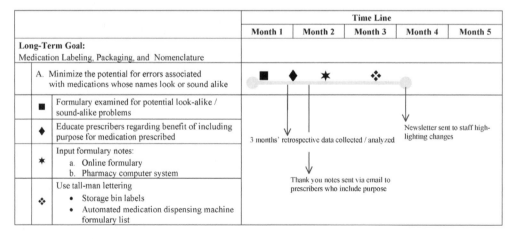

Figure 7-6. Timeline for Tracking an Example Medication-Safety Initiative

Case Studies

Case Study 1

GOAL

To minimize the potential for errors associated with medication names that look or sound alike.

PLAN

Drugs whose names look or sound alike increase the risk for error at all steps of the medication-use process. Therefore, the medication-safety team examined all medications on the formulary for potential look-alike or sound-alike problems. Team members identified the following opportunities for implementing safeguards: (1) encourage prescribers, through education, to include the purpose for which a medication is prescribed; (2) enter formulary notes in both the online formulary and pharmacy computer system to alert providers when a look-alike or sound-alike threat is present; and (3) use "tall-man" lettering (i.e., DOBUTamine, DOPamine) on storage bin labels and in automated medication-dispensing machine formulary lists to help differentiate products. Retrospective baseline data were collected to determine the number of actual and potential errors involving look-alike or sound-alike drugs.

DO

Because of the number of drug pairs identified, the team elected to implement and test safeguards for only a limited number of drugs that were considered to be high-alert (i.e., products known to have a high potential for causing harm when used incorrectly). After implementation, the team reviewed three months' worth of patient-occurrence reports to determine the number of events involving look-alike or sound-alike drugs.

CHECK

The team used pie charts to analyze before-and-after data. They found a statistically significant decrease in the number of occurrences involving high-alert look-alike or sound-alike drugs. The aggregate number of occurrences involving other look-alike or sound-alike drugs remained relatively stable. Staff provided positive feedback related to the benefits of the safeguards. No patients were harmed by high-alert drugs that had look-alike or sound-alike drug names.

ACT

The expectations for error reduction were met. The team decided to implement the safeguards for the remaining look-alike and sound-alike drugs on the formulary. A suggestion was made to develop a plan for proactive risk assessment of formulary-addition requests for look-alike and sound-alike drug-name problems to allow for safeguards to be continually implemented as formulary additions were made.

EXAMPLE TEAM MEMBER RESPONSIBILITIES

All Members: Review formulary, collect and analyze data, communicate changes to staff.

Physician: Provide education to prescribers, including e-mail thank you notes.

Pharmacist and Nurse: Enter formulary notes and implement tall-man lettering.

Case Study 2

GOAL

To facilitate a systemwide nonpunitive approach to medication-error reporting.

PLAN

The team determined that to encourage employees to report actual and potential medication errors without fear of disciplinary action, a safety culture that focused on system-based causes of error, not individuals, must be established. As part of a patient-safety campaign, the team designed a survey to solicit information from health care providers about the current reporting culture.

DO

The team developed a 12-question survey and distributed it to all health care providers. Data were collected anonymously and stratified on the basis of occupation.

CHECK

A 56 percent response rate was achieved. Using a Pareto chart, the team analyzed survey responses to determine areas with the greatest potential for improvement. The team discovered that a large percentage of respondents either "strongly agreed" or "agreed" with the following statement: "The process for reporting errors at my hospital is cumbersome."

ACT

Analyzing data generated by the organization's patient-occurrence reporting program is important for improving the medication-use system. Therefore, the team decided to revise the form used for reporting such occurrences as part of a larger process for facilitating a nonpunitive approach to error reporting. The redesigned form would focus more on system-based causes of error.

Example Team Member Responsibilities

All Members: Create survey questions that are applicable to all health care providers, encourage participation in completing the survey, collect and analyze data, communicate results.

Physician: Encourage prescribers to complete the survey.

Pharmacist: Encourage pharmacists to complete the survey.

Nurse: Encourage nurses to complete the survey.

Case Study 3

GOAL

To ensure that methods for the communication of medication orders minimize the risk of errors.

PLAN

Abbreviations can make order communication particularly challenging. They may be misunderstood for a variety of reasons, resulting in medication errors. The team determined that the organization should maintain a reasonably comprehensive list of abbreviations, acronyms, and symbols that must be avoided and that this list should be continually enforced.

DO

Team members developed a list of unapproved abbreviations. They used information from the literature and data from the organization's occurrence-reporting program to generate the list. The list was approved by the medical board, and its use became policy. Before the policy was implemented, 1,000 prescription orders were reviewed to determine the rate of unapproved abbreviation use. All providers who completed any form of clinical documentation were educated regarding the list. A provider-specific feedback letter was developed and sent to all providers who had used an unapproved abbreviation. All preprinted orders were reviewed, and unapproved abbreviations were eliminated.

CHECK

Monthly audits of unapproved abbreviation use were conducted. The number of letters sent was tracked by provider, service, and type of abbreviation misuse. Run charts were used to measure progress over time, until an unapproved abbreviation use rate of less than 10 percent was achieved. Service directors and individual prescribers determined to be in continued noncompliance were contacted by a representative of the medical board or a board designee.

ACT

The team agreed that in addition to ongoing educational initiatives, a system for obtaining evidence of confirmation of the intended meaning of an unapproved abbreviation prior to carrying out the order needed to be established. In addition to identifying alternative mechanisms for achieving 100 percent compliance with the policy, the team also continually assessed the need for revisions to the unapproved list. Implementation of computerized prescriber order entry and an electronic medical records system will further help the organization minimize the risk of errors related to communication of medication orders.

EXAMPLE TEAM MEMBER RESPONSIBILITIES

All Members: Review literature and organization data, establish list of unapproved abbreviations, eliminate unapproved abbreviations in preprinted orders, revise policy, provide ongoing education, and write feedback letters, collect and analyze data.

Physician: Obtain medical board approval, work with providers to minimize the use of abbreviations, provide peer review and appropriate follow-up.

Pharmacist: Perform audits, send provider-specific feedback letters, track literature, provide periodic updates to the team.

Nurse: Work with providers at the point of order writing to minimize the use of abbreviations.

References

1. Kohn LT, Corrigan JM, Donaldson MS, eds. *To Err Is Human: Building a Safer Health System.* Subcommittee on Quality of Health Care in America, Institute of Medicine, Washington DC: National Academy Press; 1999.

2. Joint Commission on Accreditation of Healthcare Organizations. Revisions to Joint Commission Standards in Support of Patient Safety and Medical/Health Care Error Reduction. Oak Brook Terrace, IL: JCAHO; 2002.

3. Senholzi C, Fricker MP. Improving the quality of care: a regional medication-safety effort. *P&T.* 2002;27:341-344.

4. Meyer TA. Improving the quality of the order-writing process for inpatient orders and outpatient prescriptions. *Am J Health-Syst Pharm.* 2000;57(suppl 4):S18-22.

5. Creating an Alert and Active Team. Medication Safety Issue Briefs. Series II, no 2. *Hospitals and Health Networks.* July 2003;77(7). Available at: www.ashp.org/patient-safety/issuebriefs.cfm.

6. Cohen MM, Eustis MA, Gribbins RE. Changing the culture of patient safety: leadership's role in health care quality improvement. *Jt Comm J Qual Safety.* 2003; 29:329-335.

7. University of Wisconsin–Madison. Office of Human Resource Development. How to Lead Effective Meetings. Available at: www.ohrd.wisc.edu/meetings/howto1.htm. Accessed August 29, 2003.

8. American Hospital Association, Health Research & Education Trust, and the Institute for Safe Medication Practices. Pathways for Medication Safety.SM Leading a Strategic Planning Effort. Section 1.1 Why hospitals need a strategic plan for medication safety. 2002. Available at: www.hospitalconnect.com/medpathways/tools/content/1_1.pdf. Accessed November 8, 2003.

9. Massachusetts Coalition for the Prevention of Medical Errors. MHA Best Practice Recommendations to Reduce Medication Error. 1999. Available at: www.macoalition.org/documents/Best_Practice_Medication_Errors.pdf. Accessed November 8, 2003.

10. National Coordinating Council for Medication Error Reporting and Prevention. Council recommendations. Available at: www.nccmerp.org/councilRecs.html. Accessed September 1, 2003.

11. Institute for Safe Medication Practices. Medication Safety Self-Assessment. 2004. Available at: www.ismp.org/Survey/Hospital/Intro.htm. Accessed October 31, 2004.

12. Health Care Improvement Foundation. Regional Medication Safety Program for Hospitals. 2001. Available at: www.ecri.org/MedicationSafety/mssklink.asp. Accessed September 1, 2003.

13. American Society of Health-System Pharmacists Center on Patient Safety. The Medication-Use-System Safety Strategy. Introduction and Task Analysis. Bethesda, MD: ASHP; 2001. Available at: www.ashp.org/patient-safety/MS3-1.pdf. Accessed November 8, 2003.

14. American Hospital Association, Health Research & Education Trust, and the Institute for Safe Medication Practices. Pathways for Medication Safety.SM Leading a Strategic Planning Effort. Section 1.2 Model strategic plan for medication safety. 2002. Available at: http://www.hospitalconnect.com/medpathways/tools/content/1_2.pdf Accessed November 8, 2003.

15. Joint Commission on Accreditation of Healthcare Organizations. National Patient Safety Goals. Available at: www.jcaho.org/accredited+organizations/patient+safety/npsg.htm/ Accessed September 1, 2003.

16. Joint Commission on Accreditation of Healthcare Organizations. *2004 Hospital Accreditation Standards.* Oak Brook Terrace, IL: JCAHO; 2003.

17. American Hospital Association, Health Research & Education Trust, and the Institute for Safe Medication Practices. Pathways for Medication Safety.SM Leading a Strategic Planning Effort. Section 1.3 Creating an organization-specific strategic plan for medication safety. 2002. Available at: www.hospitalconnect.com/medpathways/tools/content/1_3.pdf. Accessed November 8, 2003.

18. Center of Excellence for Patient Safety Research and Practice. Safety climate survey. University of Texas, Austin. Available at: www.qualityhealth care.org/QHC/Topics/PatientSafety/MedicationSystems/Tools/Safety%20Climate%20Survey%20(IHI%20Tool).htm. Accessed September 12, 2003.

19. Frankel A, Graydon-Baker E, Neppl C, et al. Patient safety leadership WalkRounds™. *Jt Comm J Qual Safety*. 2003;29(1):16-26.

20. American Hospital Association, Health Research & Education Trust, and the Institute for Safe Medication Practices. Pathways for Medication Safety.SM Leading a Strategic Planning Effort. Attachment 1.K Prioritization criteria for selecting medication safety change projects. 2002. Available at: www.hospitalconnect.com/medpathways/tools/content/1_K.pdf. Accessed November 8, 2003.

21. University of Michigan Health System. Patient Safety Toolkit. Improving Patient Safety in Hospitals: Turning Ideas into Actions. 2002. Available at: www.med.umich.edu/patientsafetytoolkit/culture.htm. Accessed September 15, 2003.

22. Beardsley D, Woods K, eds. Performing a root-cause analysis. In: *First Do No Harm—A Practical Guide to Medication Safety and JCAHO Compliance*. Marblehead, MA: Opus Communications;1999:57-109.

23. Bates DW, Pepper GA, Schneider PJ. Measuring medication safety in hospitals. Paper presented at: Conference on Measuring Medication Safety in Hospitals; April 8-9, 2002; Tucson, AZ.

24. Institute for Health Care Improvement and BMJ Publishing Group. Medication Systems—Measures. Available at: www.quality healthcare.org/QHC/Topics/PatientSafety/MedicationSystems/Measures. Accessed September 15, 2003.

25. Beardsley D, Woods K, eds. Designing and implementing improvement proposals. In: *First Do No Harm—A Practical Guide to Medication Safety and JCAHO Compliance*. Marblehead, MA: Opus Communications;1999:111-153.

26. Cohen MR. Prescription for safety in health care. *Am J Health-Syst Pharm*. 2002;59:1511-1517.

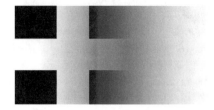

CHAPTER 8

The Practice-Change System Applied to Medication Safety

Christine M. Nimmo and
Ross W. Holland

Introduction

A glance at the titles and themes of the other chapters in this book confirms the centrality of practice change in achieving medication safety. For example, Turnbull calls for a change in culture. Culture does not simply involve mouthing words or tacking a credo on a bulletin board; rather, it is the adoption by the entire staff of a health care system of a philosophy that manifests itself in pervasive change in their daily actions. Pane describes the role of the pharmacist in a safe system. In such a system, the majority of pharmacists view models of patient care as the paramount guides to their work. As a consequence, significant numbers of current practitioners may need to change their current practice models. For example, Lesar emphasizes that pharmacists must change their decision-making processes in order to consistently employ best evidence in the care of patients.

Were there any doubt that change is central to achieving medication safety, the reader need only refer to the chapter by May, which details the job responsibilities and associated tasks of a health system team charged with effecting a safe medication-use system. Among the tasks are 10 different situations in which the medication-use safety coordinator must facilitate a change in the practices not only of pharmacists but also of nurses, physicians, and other health care professionals. For example, prescribers may be required to adopt the use of standardized medication orders, nurses to use different procedures to operate pumps, and pharmacists to rearrange medications in the picking area.

Almost every strategy one can devise for improving medication safety is ultimately attached to a change in what individual practitioners do or in the way in which they do it. Thus, once the path to safety is established, whether it is standardization, informatics, clinical involvement, or another tool or process, the change leader must focus on getting each affected practitioner to make the changes in his or her practice that are consistent with the goals of the safety plan. The realization of safety hinges on the decision of each individual to make changes in his or her practice. This chapter focuses on strategies for maximizing the possibility that practitioners will choose to change and will follow through on that decision.

Toward Facilitating Change

If facilitating individual change among practitioners is central to achieving medication safety, there is a need to ensure that leaders, including pharmacy department managers, have a systematic, effective, and efficient method for maximizing the possibility that the desired changes, once defined, will be made. Where should one look for this sort of guidance?

Well before the emergence of the current nationwide focus on medication safety, the authors of this chapter were engaged in activities at the national level to promote pharmacist adoption of clinical and pharmaceutical care practice models in both health-system and community practices. The goal of these activities was to switch the pharmacist's focus from product to patient. The change methodology described in this chapter evolved from the authors' desire to identify and implement an effective way to make that change happen.

Our first step was to search the change literature for a model that was prescriptive rather than descriptive and that took into account the idiosyncrasies of the pharmacy environment. We did not identify a model that exactly met the need. Most of the models focused on helping a leader understand the type of change needed, and why, but did not give clear direction on what to do in order to move forward to effect it. Many of the models relied on extrinsic rewards, such as promotions and salary increases, which were not available in most pharmacies at a time when cost cutting was widespread. No model seemed to account for the magnitude of change being asked of an individual who had made the decision to enter a technical profession that was transforming itself into one centered on caring.

Having found nothing that adequately addressed this change situation, we created something that we hoped would. The resulting practice-change system (PCS), the theoretical basis for which is described in the Transitions in Pharmacy Practice series in the *American Journal of Health-System Pharmacy*,[1-5] takes into account the profound effect on the practitioner of a change in practice model and the realities of the pharmacy environment in which such change was to take place.

The PCS has now been in use for five years. Evidence shows that when pharmacy managers apply the principles of the PCS they are able not only to facilitate desired changes between different models of practice but also to change pharmacist performance within the context of a single practice model.[6-9] These are the types of practitioner change that safety-enhancement efforts require. Consequently, we believe that the PCS approach to facilitating individual change can be employed to achieve the individual practice changes needed to attain a safe medication system.

This chapter focuses on how pharmacy can apply the PCS to help achieve organizational medication-safety goals. Those in charge of this process, whether members of a medication-safety team or individual pharmacy managers, are referred to as "change leaders."

Overview of the Practice-Change System

Before using the PCS, the change leader must be able to clearly articulate the change desired and how current practices differ from those that will be required under the changed system. The leader must articulate these key ideas not only to those who will be directly involved but also to those who will be affected by it. This simple, but often overlooked, prerequisite is the foundation on which communication and critical decision making for all parties will be based. It makes clear to the practitioner the degree of change that he or she will be expected to make as well as the goal of the new behavior. It helps administrators understand what the desired change can contribute to safety and, at the same time, lays the groundwork for requests for necessary resources. For the change leader, the statement is the reference point for identifying barriers to and facilitators of change, training that must be provided, or the need for a motivational strategy. The statement needs to be written and reviewed for accuracy and clarity. General references to the delivery of "clinical services" or "pharmaceutical care" are not sufficient. The change statement must describe specific tasks.

The PCS is unique among change models in that it is

- prescriptive, i.e., it states clearly what to do;

- efficient, i.e., the prescription for what to do is comprehensive and systematic; and

- effective, i.e., it accounts for the change environment and the impact of required change in professional values on the individual.

The PCS comprises three components: practice environment, learning resources, and motivational strategies (see **Figure 8-1**). All three components are critical in a practitioner's decision to make a major change in practice, and only when all three are concurrently in place is it likely that change will occur.

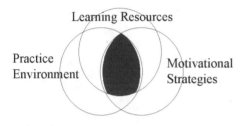

The Holland-Nimmo Practice Change System

Learning Resources

Practice Environment

Motivational Strategies

Figure 8-1. The Holland-Nimmo Practice-Change System

- The practice environment is conducive to performance of the desired practice.

- The practitioner has the knowledge, skills, attitudes, and abilities required for competence in the desired practice.

- The practitioner not only wants to perform the desired practice but also feels capable of doing so.

The PCS guides the change leader through the systematic process of addressing the tasks associated with each component. In the discussion that follows we consider the tasks of each component separately and then tie together the components into an integrated system.

THE PRACTICE-ENVIRONMENT COMPONENT

Approaching the practice-environment component, the change leader's responsibility is to do everything necessary to make it possible and plausible for the practitioner to engage in a changed practice. Where the change for safety is a simple change in procedure, there may be little, perhaps even no, environmental change needed to clear the way for the practitioner to perform in new ways. On the other hand, many safety changes will require changes in staffing, workflow, scheduling, job descriptions, and more before the environment is set aright. The PCS advocates full consideration of the barriers to large and small changes, remembering that it is the little things that can trip us up.

As shown in **Figure 8-2**, the pharmacy practice environment in which change takes place has three levels—society, health system, and practice site. Barriers to making a major change in practice can exist at any of these three levels. Removing these barriers—the small ones that make change difficult as well as the large ones that make change impossible—is the responsibility of the change leader. With the statement of change in hand, the change leader should pose each of the PCS's 20 environmental questions, which are listed in the following paragraphs, working from the societal level down to the practice-site level. If this is done effectively, all barriers will be identified, their significance analyzed, and strategies for overcoming or minimizing them developed.

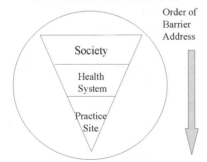

The Practice Environment

Order of Barrier Address

Society

Health System

Practice Site

Figure 8-2. The Practice-Environment Component

Societal-Level Questions

Although it might be tempting to slip past a routine check of the three questions at the societal level, such action would most likely not be wise. Lack of legality or public or professional nonacceptance of a desired practice activity can quickly derail a change process.

Suppose, for example that the desired change is greater pharmacist involvement in direct patient care. One barrier is lack of time, and the identified strategy to create that time is to switch to "tech check tech" for medication preparation. State regulations, however, might not permit this procedure. In this example, the change itself is not prohibited at the societal level, but the mechanism for barrier removal is. This will require either a change in regulations or a switch to another barrier-removal strategy.

The questions posed in each of the components are framed using the term *desired practice* to describe the change to be analyzed. This term can refer to either large or small changes in practice. To better understand the applicability of these questions to the desired change, the reader might think of a specific change in practice of a pharmacist, nurse, physician, or other health professional and substitute a description of that change for the generic term used in these questions.

- Do federal, state, and local laws and regulations permit the desired practice?
- Do the patients to be served accept pharmacists providing the service they would receive in the desired practice?
- At the national level, do the other health care professions accept the desired practice as part of the role of the pharmacist?

Removing barriers at the societal level is the responsibility of local, state, and national associations that lobby or advocate changing laws and regulations.

Health System–Level Questions

Removing barriers at the health-system level is generally the work of the pharmacy department director, working through the customary organizational chain of command or an empowered medication-use safety coordination team, again working through the chain of command and the political structure of the health system. Questions at this level center on availability of resources, administrator support, technology infrastructure, access to information, and other issues beyond the scope of a department to resolve independently. In many ways, the change leader is leading those above him or her to a shared vision for safety that produces the actions they must take to ensure it happens.

As with societal-level questions, the health system–level questions are framed using the generic term *desired practice*. Readers may want to continue to substitute one of their own change goals to increase the perceived relevance of the barrier issues raised.

- Are there health-system administrators whose support for the change in practice will be necessary but who are not convinced of the desirability of the change?
- Are there health-system reporting relationships that may hinder adoption of the desired practice?
- Are there inadequacies in the pharmacy's physical facilities that would hinder establishment of the desired practice?
- Will financial resources be required to establish the desired practice?
- Will additions to staff or changes in staffing patterns be required to establish the desired practice?
- Are there other health care professionals in the health system whose support will be necessary for approval but who have not been convinced of the need for the desired practice?

- Are there limitations in the health system's use of technology (e.g., information systems, robotics) that will hinder establishment of the desired practice?

- Is any unachieved union support required for approval of the desired practice?

- Are there human resources–management restrictions that might hinder establishment of the desired practice?

- Are there limitations in access by the department to information pertinent to the desired practice (e.g., data on medication errors, patient profiles, adverse drug reactions, length of stay)?

- Are there health-system policy constraints on pharmacist practice activities that may hinder the establishment of the desired practice (e.g., writing in the chart, ordering laboratory tests)?

Practice Site–Level Questions

At this level, teams of practitioners may serve as rich sources of information on barrier identification and resolution. These questions drill down to the specifics of how things are done, on interpersonal relationships, on communication patterns, and on other variables that make a department run in a particular way.

- Are there patterns in the pharmacy's workflow that would hinder establishment of the desired practice?

- Are the department's current policies and procedures consistent with any change in processes required when pharmacists begin to engage in the desired practice?

- Are there discrepancies in the existing relationships between the pharmacist and each member of the health care team that will affected by the pharmacist's change in practice and the relationships required for successful establishment of the desired practice?

- Are there financial, staffing, and time implications of staff training needs that must be met to establish the desired practice?

- Are there differences between existing pharmacist job descriptions and job descriptions that accurately describe the pharmacist's desired practice?

- Are there differences in the present pharmacy department staff's (including managers and supervisors) norms, values, and expectations about practice and those that are required to support the desired practice?

The change leader's tasks in this component are complete when all significant barriers to establishment of the desired change have been identified and minimized or removed. At this point, the managerial tasks associated with implementing the change can begin to take place.

THE MOTIVATIONAL-STRATEGIES COMPONENT

Creating a motivational strategy entails persuading practitioners to acquire any knowledge and skills required for competence in the changed practice and to desire to make that mode of practice their own.

Motivation often occurs almost effortlessly. The change leader states that this is an important thing to do, conditions are right for doing it the new way, and practitioners move forward to effect a sustained change. Sometimes, a little more "oomph" is required, maybe because the practitioner must first work hard to learn how to do what is desired. Simple incentives, such as offering scheduling preference or establishing a career ladder that rewards the desired practice, may be effective.

But what of the puzzling situation where training and opportunity are offered, but the practitioner does not grab hold? Why don't standard approaches to workplace motivation consistently work? It may be that trying to change the practice of professionals presents some unique barriers that are not encountered in other groups. Or it may be that change becomes increasingly difficult as the magnitude of change being asked of the individual comes close to being a virtual change in profession. The PCS seeks to deal with these potentials by presenting a systematic strategy for managing these possible barriers to motivation to change (see Figure 8-3).

The Motivation Strategies Component

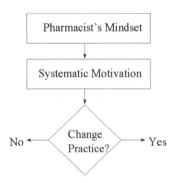

Figure 8-3. The Motivational-Strategies Component

Some members of a profession are members in name only. They think of their work as simply a "job." For them, extrinsic motivation or rewards are the most effective means to produce change.

For others, the situation is different. Individuals who truly embrace their profession are socialized to its values. But what if an individual is strongly professionalized, and the values and attitudes associated with the new desired practice are at odds with those that the practitioner currently holds? Professional socialization determines such things as to whom the practitioner feels ultimately responsible, what tasks are and are not appropriate to perform, the appropriate relationship with other health care professionals, and the appropriate relationship with patients.

When the desired change is an alteration in workflow or in the way in which a particular task is performed, major value differences are unlikely. But what if the desired change is to move from distributive practice to direct involvement in patient care? What if the practitioner will now be expected to interview or counsel the patient, assume responsibility for medication-use outcomes, and work with prescribers on a collegial basis? In this case, the values and attitudes concerning practice emerge as distinctly different. One values applying technical skill to solve well-defined problems and regards the pharmacist's role as supporting the physician's patient-outcome goals. The other sees the pharmacist as part of a team that shares responsibility for achieving optimal medication-use outcomes and for helping solve ill-defined problems.

One cannot assume that all pharmacists, nurses, or physicians share identical values for their respective professions. Despite efforts to standardize the outcomes of professional education, there will always be variance in the values inculcated by different schools and universities. Probably even more significant than differentiated values within a profession, however, is the inevitability of practice evolution: Persons educated in one era may have different notions of the appropriate tasks and responsibilities of the profession than those educated in another era do. Practice experience further complicates the picture. Values acquired in training may be altered by the realities of practice. A final debunker of the assumption of uniform values and beliefs about professional practice is the influence of active participation in professional associations by some, but not all members of the profession. For any one change process, the change leader can be confronted with as many different sets of professional values and beliefs as there are individuals to be changed.

When the change leader compares the individual practitioner's current values with those of the desired practice and sees no significant discrepancies, it would be overkill to engage in a systematic motivational process. On the other hand, when values collide, failing to address the differences through resocialization to the values and beliefs of the desired practice mode is likely to doom the change effort to failure. To help change leaders move professionally socialized practitioners to adoption of practice modes drawing on different assumptions about the profession the PCS advocates the development of a motivational strategy based on professional resocialization.

The Nimmo-Holland Motivational Guide for Practice Change

The change leader's task is to employ motivational strategies that (1) generate an intense desire in the practitioner to adopt the safety-enhancing practice change, (2) make the practitioner believe that he or she is capable of doing so, and (3) encourage the practitioner to resolve to attain any necessary knowledge or skill needed to engage in the practice change. One motivational strategy that can be used to achieve these three objectives is professional resocialization. It is based on Festinger's Theory of Cognitive Dissonance,[10] which asserts that when an individual's belief system is out of sync with his or her actions, it produces such emotional discomfort that the person will change behavior in order to restore internal harmony.

The systematic strategy to produce intrinsic motivation for practice change must be accomplished before the change leader introduces the training identified in the PCS learning-resources component. The purpose of the strategy is to produce a learner with a high degree of motivation to learn and thereby to enable him or her to engage in the new practice. Until this is achieved, the effects of a training program are likely to be disappointing. Put simply, the unmotivated learner is a poor learner.

Teaching the values and attitudes associated with the safety-enhancing practice tasks or model is the change leader's chief task under the motivation component. The educational community's guide for teaching values and attitudes is Krathwohl's Taxonomy for the Affective Domain.[11] The Nimmo-Holland Motivational Guide for Practice Change (see **Table 8-1**) is based on this taxonomy. It adapts Krathwohl's generic model to the current change situation in pharmacy. The change leader's responsibility is to move the practitioner through four learning stages to professionally resocialize him or her to resolute commitment to the values and attitudes of the safety-enhancing practice. The stages may be briefly characterized as follows:

Table 8-1. Nimmo-Holland Motivational Guide for Practice Change

STAGE	MOTIVATIONAL ACTIVITIES	STAGE INDICATORS
1. Finding Out about It	o Interactive lecture/guided discussion o Informal discussions with colleagues o Articles o On-site near-peer role models o Site visits to near-peers o Discuss WIIFM (What's in it for me?) o Brainstorm barriers to adoption	1.1 "I'm aware that some pharmacists do those things, but couldn't care less about it." 1.2. "Well, I guess it's possible for pharmacists to do that." 1.3. "This idea about practice intrigues me." 1.4. "I've been told I must learn more about this new kind of practice. I do what I'm told."
2. Testing the Water	o Provide access to near-peers in this type of practice. o Try practice out on a partial basis. o Make the practitioner feel competent. o Provide feedback.	2.1. "I'm interested in learning more about this new kind of practice." 2.2 "I'm enjoying the idea of playing around with this new kind of practice."

cont'd

Table 8-1. Nimmo-Holland Motivational Guide for Practice Change (cont'd)

STAGE	MOTIVATIONAL ACTIVITIES	STAGE INDICATORS
3. Gaining Commitment	o Continue to provide access to near-peers in this type of practice o Provide opportunities to publicly identify with this practice	3.1 "This type of practice has a place in the role of the pharmacist." 3.2 "If you gave me a choice, I believe I'd choose this type of practice." 3.3 "I am firmly convinced this kind of practice is what I should be doing."
4. Making Sure It Sticks	o Encourage verbalization of practice concept to others. o Provide access to near-peers who have been retrained for this practice.	4.1 "Let me tell you how when a pharmacist practices this way, all the bases for a pharmacist's contribution to patient care are covered." 4.2 "I have a plan for learning the new skills I need to do this kind of practice, and I'm committed to using some of my personal time to do it."

- At stage 1, Finding Out about It, the practitioner acquires a solid comprehension of what the practice change is about.

- In stage 2, Testing the Water, the practitioner begins to understand the emotional response he or she would experience by engaging in the new practice and to see what new learning would be required to adopt the desired practice.

- At stage 3, Gaining Commitment, the practitioner forms the values and attitudes of the desired practice tasks or model and begins to believe that this is what he or she should do.

- During stage 4, Making Sure It Sticks, the practitioner reshuffles his or her existing value system to make room for all that is involved in becoming a practitioner grounded in the safety-enhancing practice.

The motivational guide outlines the teaching tasks of the change leader in helping the practitioner acquire a new set of professional values and attitudes. The stage indicators are responses that the change leader might get from practitioners as they advance through the hierarchical learning process.

The "near-peer" concept is critical to understanding the guide and achieving success in the teaching effort. The literature of the diffusion of innovations reveals the powerful positive influence on the adoption of change when the advocate is a person perceived to be similar to oneself.[12] Thus, a village woman is most likely to adopt birth control practices when encouraged to do so by another woman in the same village, and a physician is most likely to change treatment of a disease when a respected fellow practitioner says he's tried the new way and achieved good outcomes. For this reason, the PCS encourages the use of near-peers, when possible, in attempting to revise the professional values and attitudes of any health care professional. Details on how to carry out the teaching tasks for each of the four stages are published elsewhere.[5,13]

The Influence of Personality

Each practitioner is a unique individual. On the other hand, there are definite shared traits that even the layperson recognizes as predominant in the group known as pharmacists. Research conducted between 1976 and 1997 revealed that the dominant personality type in the profession of pharmacy at that time was characterized by a strong sense of responsibility, conscientiousness, practicality, logic, and, in about one practitioner in five, a fear of interpersonal communication.[14-18] Were similar studies run on today's new practitioners, chances are the effects of pharmacy schools' current emphasis on the ability to communicate might show an upswing in willingness to communicate. Nonetheless, it is reasonable to assume that the majority of today's pharmacists do not feel that communications is their forte.

We can account for the predominance of a particular set of personality characteristics within those who have chosen a given profession by turning to research on vocational choice. This literature has established that individuals select their life work on the basis of a perceived match between their own personalities and the personality characteristics drawn upon by the job. Personality is relatively fixed, but the choice of job is not. The drive to match one's personality with the job is so strong that 74.6 percent of men and 72.3 percent of women between ages 21 and 25 achieve a match.[19] The percentage, moreover, increases with time. Ninety-one percent of men and 90 percent of women between the ages 61 and 65 achieve a job-personality match.[19] Holland states that when there is a mismatch between personality and work environment, one can expect "gross dissatisfaction, ineffective coping behavior, and probably leaving the environment."[20]

Holland also writes about what occurs when the practitioner self-selects into a profession with whom he or she has a match (e.g., distributive pharmacy) but is then required to engage in work that is incompatible with his or her personality (e.g., clinical or pharmaceutical care practice). Perhaps predictably, they may resign or become major managerial problems as they manifest coping behavior such as avoidance, feigned helplessness, subterfuge, or even sabotage.[9]

When practice changes promise to be significant, the PCS advises that change leaders pay attention to the personality of the practitioner and to the personality characteristics that will be drawn on by the safety-enhancing practice role. It is unrealistic to assume that all practitioners will change their personalities to suit new job expectations: Some will be unable to make the required change. At the same time, as the adoption of automated dispensing devices and reliance on pharmacy technicians increase, relegating those distributive pharmacists who cannot make significant changes in practice to distributive roles becomes increasingly impractical. The change leader's obligation is to understand the practitioner's mindset, which is a combination of personality and professional socialization; to weigh that mindset against the expected change; devise a motivational strategy that matches the need; and to follow through on its implementation. If a practitioner cannot make the change in practice, the responsible leader may assist that practitioner in finding a more personally appropriate position in another organization.

THE LEARNING-RESOURCES COMPONENT

The learning resources component (see **Figure 8-4**) comprises those leadership tasks that must be fulfilled to ensure that the practitioner asked to make change has opportunities to gain competence in the new tasks he or she is being asked to perform. Some safety-enhancing changes are as simple as asking the practitioner to make small modifications in an existing procedure; others may require the complexity of training for a new practice model.

The Learning Resources Component

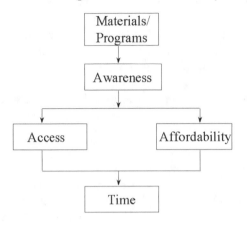

Figure 8-4. *The Learning-Resources Component*

Whatever the extent of learning required to perform the changed practice successfully, the same five baseline principles apply, as described in the following paragraphs.

Materials and Programs
The training materials must be effective resources for learning the tasks to be performed. The training objectives must be directly linked to what the practitioner will be expected to be able to do on the job. Thus, if the revised practice requires the practitioner to interview patients to obtain information for the departmental database, then the training objectives need to state that the learner will be able to *demonstrate* pharmacist-patient communication in that context, not that the learner will simply be able to *describe* effective pharmacist-patient communication techniques. Such a training would need to include practice doing interviews using techniques such as role plays. The trainee must be evaluated on the basis of the behavior stated in the objective, i.e., doing an interview, rather than answering questions about what one would do "if."

Additional information on this issue has been published elsewhere.[21,22]

Awareness
The change leader should make efforts to be well informed of existing programs that would meet the criteria for a specific training need. Developing a training program from scratch is both time- and labor intensive. On the other hand, it is often hard to find a commercially available product that exactly matches an organization's needs. The quality of the program must also be assessed. A program that is poorly designed is unlikely to yield the desired performance results.

Access
The best program in the world is of no value if it is not accessible or not offered at a time when the practitioner can use it.

Affordability
In some instances, the cost of training can be shared by the organizaiton and the practitioner. This is particularly true when the training needs are great. When budgets are tight, departments frequently elect to design and develop their own training. One has to be wary of the cost of staff time in this undertaking.

Time
Time to train will always be a critical element in a busy workplace. Thought must be given to delegation of regular work time and to expectations that the practitioner will spend time of his or her own.

Table 8-2 is a tool that may be used to systematically address the five learning-resources leadership tasks.

Table 8-2. Guiding Questions for the Learning-Resources Component

RESOURCES EXIST THAT MATCH LEARNING NEEDS

- Has there been an analysis of the knowledge, skills, and abilities required to perform each of the proposed practice activity(ies)?

- Has there been an assessment of each practitioner to determine missing knowledge, skills, and abilities required for performance of the proposed practice activity(ies)?

- Has the practitioner been informed of the results of the learning assessment?

- Have the identified learning needs been worded as educational objectives according to a learning taxonomy in order to facilitate the development of effective learning resources or the evaluation of existing resources to determine that they will produce the required learning outcomes?

- Do instructional resources exist that match with the desired learning outcomes to include selection of teaching method that will achieve the desired level of learning?

AWARENESS

- If the practitioner is charged with meeting all or part of the learning needs, is he or she knowledgeable of alternative resources that will fulfill those needs?

ACCESSIBILITY

- Of those existing learning resources that would fulfill the learning need, which are accessible with respect to location and timing?

AFFORDABILITY

- What is the total cost of training to complete the required learning?

- Are any funds allocated by the health system for the change in practice currently available?

- Is there a well-designed plan for the use of health-system funds for training for the practice change?

- Will the practitioner be required to fund all or part of his or her training?

- Has the practitioner committed to his or her portion of the cost of training?

TIME

- If the employer is committed to providing time for study of the required learning, have issues related to making that time available been resolved?

- If the pharmacist is committed to providing time for study of the required learning, has he or she resolved issues related to making that time available?

Creating the Synergy of Systems

To this point, the leadership tasks specified by the PCS have been discussed as separate entities. This has been done to enable the reader to gain a clear understanding of each component. However, in order to achieve the synergy of the use of a system, the PCS user must integrate the three component's leadership activities so that the right things are happening at the right time and, at the critical moment, the tasks of all three components are simultaneously fulfilled, making it likely that the practitioner will make the required practice change.

The first question is, "Where do I start?" The process starts, as noted at the beginning of this chapter, with a clearly written definition of the desired change. The change leader should blend this in-depth understanding of the change with his or her understanding of the environment in which it is to take place and of the individuals to be changed to thoughtfully answer the 20 questions posed by the PCS for each of the components. This exercise will reveal the scope and depth of what must be accomplished to increase the possibility of a successful change process.

When analysis suggests that the practitioners are motivated and able, but practice circumstances are not welcoming to the changed practice, most of the leader's work should be focused on shaping up the environment. If the analysis was accurate and the site has been readied, the staff should dig in and start doing as hoped. If that does not occur, motivation, competence, or both, may have been overestimated.

It is possible to have staff members who are totally competent to perform in desired ways and an environment that seemingly invites them to do so, and yet nothing of consequence changes. This should drive the change leader back into the analysis phase of the PCS. The question to ask is, "What has been overlooked?" It may be that the individuals in question are not sufficiently motivated. It may be that something subtle in the environment component, such as a departmental culture that squashes attempts to change through ostracism from the group, is derailing change. The point is that those who would orchestrate change among individual practitioners in the name of medication safety are most likely to succeed when all three components of the PCS are in place—environment, motivation, and learning resources. A weakness in any one component can negate the best of efforts in the other two.

Manager or Leader?

Throughout this chapter, the reader has no doubt noted the consistent references to "leadership" tasks that sometimes sound more like those of management. We have observed that those who use PCS well often move back and forth as necessary between the role of leader and that of manager. The leadership part of self sets the vision and sets the strategy. The managerial self evaluates the quality of training materials, reframes position descriptions, and writes a proposal for new technology. The successful change leader will cultivate both sets of skills—articulating a vision, persuading others to share that vision, and creating the circumstances that translate that vision into practice reality.

Conclusion

Achieving a safe medication system requires that health care professionals make changes in their day-to-day practice activities. This may entail simply modifying the way in which certain tasks are performed or adopting a totally new practice model. Regardless of the scope of change to be implemented, leaders can benefit by approaching the change process using a systematic strategy. The PCS provides systematic guidance for leaders desiring to maximize the possibility that an individual practitioner will choose to make the desired change in practice. All three components—environment, motivation, and learning resources—must be in place to achieve the synergy of the system effect. Applying the PCS successfully requires both leadership and managerial skills.

References

1. Holland RW, Nimmo CM. Transitions in pharmacy practice, part 1: beyond pharmaceutical care. *Am J Health-Syst Pharm.* 1999;56:1758-1764.

2. Nimmo CM, Holland RW. Transitions in pharmacy practice, part 2: who does what and why. *Am J Health-Syst Pharm.* 1999;56:1981-1987.

3. Holland RW, Nimmo CM. Transitions in pharmacy practice, part 3: effecting change—the three-ring circus. *Am J Health-Syst Pharm.* 1999;56:2235-2241.

4. Nimmo CM, Holland RW. Transitions in pharmacy practice, part 4: can a leopard change its spots? *Am J Health-Syst Pharm.* 1999;56:2458-2462.

5. Nimmo CM, Holland RW. Transitions in pharmacy practice, part 5: walking the tightrope of change. *Am J Health-Syst Pharm.* 2000;57:64-72.

6. Salverson SM, Murante LJ. Clinical training program based on a practice change model. *Am J Health-Syst Pharm.* 2002;59:862-866.

7. Karbowicz SH. Measuring pharmacists' levels of performance. Poster presented at: American Society of Health-System Pharmacists Midyear Clinical Meeting; New Orleans, LA; December 5, 2001.

8. Henry JS, Ober ML. I tried it, I like it: two takes of the practice change model applications for establishing safe medication use practices and transitioning a distributive staff to clinical roles. Paper presented at: American Society of Health-System Pharmacists Midyear Clinical Meeting; Las Vegas, NV; December 5, 2000.

9. Farthing K, Conrad GE, Jordan JE. Motivating pharmacists for a practice change through application of the Holland-Nimmo Practice Change Model. Paper presented at: American Society of Health-System Pharmacists Midyear Clinical Meeting; Orlando, FL; December 8, 1999.

10. Festinger LA. *Theory of Cognitive Dissonance.* Evanston, IL: Row, Peterson, and Co; 1957.

11. Krathwohl DR, Bloom BS, Masia BB. *Taxonomy of Educational Objectives; The Classification of Educational Goals, Handbook II: Affective Domain.* White Plains, NY: Longman Inc; 1964.

12. Rogers EM. *Diffusion of Innovations.* 4th ed. New York: Free Press; 1995.

13. Nimmo CM, Holland RW. Motivating staff for patient care. In: Hagel HP, Rovers JP, eds. *Patient-Centered Pharmacy Management.* Washington, DC: American Pharmaceutical Association; 2002.

14. Manasse HR Jr, Kabat HF, Wertheimer AI. Professional socialization in pharmacy I: a cross-sectional analysis of personality characteristics of agents and objects of socialization. *Drugs Health Care.* 1976;3(winter):3-18.

15. Lowenthal W. Myers-Briggs type inventory preferences of pharmacy students and practitioners. *Eval Health Prof.* 1994;17:22-42.

16. Karmel B. The hospital pharmacist: master or victim of the environment? *Am J Hosp Pharm.* 1978;35:151-154.

17. Cocolas GH, Sleath B, Hanson-Divers EC. Use of the Gordon Personal Profile-Inventory of pharmacists and pharmacy students. *Am J Pharm Educ.* 1997;61:257-265.

18. Anderson-Harper HM, Berger BA, Noel R. Pharmacists' predisposition to communicate, desire to counsel and job satisfaction. *Am J Pharm Educ.* 1992;56:252-258.

19. Gottfredson GD. Career stability and redirection in adulthood. *J Appl Psychol.* 1977;62:436-445.

20. Holland JL. *Making Vocational Choices: A Theory of Vocational Personalities and Work Environments.* 3rd ed. Odessa, FL: Psychological Assessment Resources Inc; 1997.

21. Nimmo CM, Greene SA, Guerrero RM, Taylor JT, eds. *Staff Development for Pharmacy Practice.* Bethesda, MD: American Society of Health-System Pharmacists; 2000.

22. Nimmo CM, Holland RW, Rovers J. Education and training for patient care. In: Hagel HP, Rovers JP, eds. *Patient-Centered Pharmacy Management.* Washington, DC: American Pharmaceutical Association; 2002.

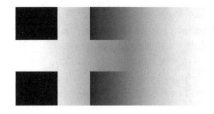

CHAPTER 9

Federal Government, State Government, and Private-Sector Roles in Improving Medication Safety

Jerry Phillips

Introduction

The need for joint involvement of the federal government, state governments, and the private sector in improving medication safety stems from the complexity of the issues related to this activity. In a complex health care environment, every individual medication error has multiple causes and solutions.

As a pharmacist who retired from the U.S. Public Health Service (PHS) with 30 years of service, I have worked in both clinical and regulatory settings. I have experienced my share of close calls and actual medication errors. When I moved from the clinical setting in the Indian Health Service into a regulatory role at the Food and Drug Administration (FDA), I assumed that my days of being involved in medication errors were over. Nothing could have been further from the truth. The following case study highlights this complexity and the role that a federal government agency can play in improving patient safety. The incident occurred when I was a reviewer in FDA's Office of Generic Drugs.

The problem began early in 1993, when Burroughs Wellcome (now GlaxoSmithKline), Abbott Laboratories, and the FDA began to receive reports of problems arising from confusion between the packaging and labeling of the intravenous (i.v.) muscle-relaxant mivacurium chloride and ranitidine. On June 4, 1993, Burroughs Wellcome issued a "statgram" to hospital pharmacists bringing to their attention the possibility of such a mix-up and informed them of new labeling to be forthcoming for the products. In addition, the firm provided stickers to be applied to the current stock of mivacurium in the hospitals.

On July 8, 1993, far away from FDA headquarters in Rockville, Maryland, four patients in one hospital inadvertently received that same product, mivacurium i.v., instead of the anti-infective agent metronidazole. All four patients experienced severe side effects, and two of them died as a result of this medication error.

Following these events, both the hospital and the FDA conducted investigations. Two problems that became apparent immediately were the look-alike packaging and the lack of adequate labeling. Manufactured by Abbott pharmaceuticals, both products were packaged and labeled similarly and had a foil overwrap (see **Figure 9-1**). Both packages had the same dimensions, and both were wrapped with an aluminum-laminated sleeve with a window for the label. The sleeve design allowed the product inside to slide down, thus obscuring the label. Abbott was manufacturing 11 different drug products with this foil overwrap.

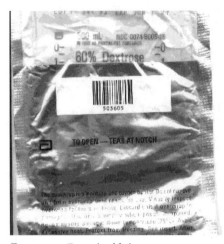

Figure 9-1. Example of foil overwrap.

Even though the problem was due in large part to look-alike packaging, in doing a root-cause analysis of this event, the hospital team found that procedures in the pharmacy and nursing also contributed to the error. First, the team noted that mivacurium had just been added to the formulary. When the pharmacy received the first mivacurium shipment, a pharmacy technician assumed that it was metronidazole injection, the only foil-wrapped product that had formerly existed on the formulary. The technician did not know that mivacurium had just been added to the formulary. Believing the new product to be metronidazole, the technician placed it in the i.v bin intended for that product. Then, when preparing the pharmacy order for the four patients for whom metronidazole had been ordered, the pharmacist stapled the pharmacy label (identifying the correct patient and the intended drug) onto the outside window of the foil overwrap. This was done so that the item could easily be returned to stock if the metronidazole order was not given. The pharmacy label now covered the window, which otherwise could have clearly shown that mivacurium, not metronidazole, was the product inside the foil overwrap. When the nursing department received the product, the nurses concluded that it must be light-sensitive, since it was packaged in a foil overwrap. In an effort to preserve the product's integrity by not exposing it to light, the nurse connected the administration set to the i.v. solution by cutting an opening at the bottom of the foil overwrap. It was then administered to the four patients.

After realizing that the packaging and labeling of the products contributed to the error, the FDA began discussions with Abbott concerning remedial actions. Abbott agreed to issue an alert to all hospital pharmacies concerning all 11 of the similarly packaged products and to place complete labeling on the foil overwrap (see **Figure 9-2**) that would clearly identify each product. Following these changes in labeling and packaging, the FDA received no further reports of errors caused by mix-ups between these products.

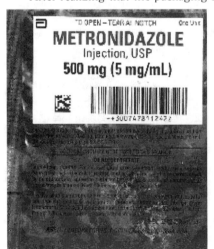

Figure 9-2. Picture of revised labeling.

As is the case with virtually all medication errors, the error described in this case study could be traced to multiple systemic faults. In response, the FDA and the manufacturer worked together to implement changes in the labeling of the products that minimized future errors. In so doing, the FDA continued a tradition of government involvement in the safety of the U.S. population that has its roots in the century of our country's founding. Many other federal agencies, as well as state agencies and private organizations, also have active roles in ensuring the safety of medications, as described in the sections that follow.

Historical Perspective: The Federal Government's Role in Improving Patient Care

Efforts at improving patient care and safety by the U.S. federal government can be traced to July 1798, when the Public Health Service was created to provide for the care and relief of sick and injured merchant seamen.[1,2] This was an era in which the United States depended on maritime trade for economic and national security. The earliest marine hospitals established to care for seamen were located along the East Coast. Boston was the site of the first such facility; later, hospitals were established along inland waterways, the Great Lakes, and the Gulf and Pacific Coasts.

A reorganization in 1870 converted the loose network of locally controlled hospitals into a centrally controlled Marine Hospital Service, with its headquarters in Washington, D.C. The position of supervising surgeon (later surgeon general) was created to administer the PHS, and in 1871, John Maynard Woodworth, called the father of the Public Health Service, became the first individual to occupy this post. He moved quickly to reform the system and adopted a military model for his medical staff, instituting examinations for applicants and putting physicians in uniforms. Woodworth created a cadre of mobile, career-service physicians who could be assigned as needed to the various marine hospitals. The uniformed services component of the Marine Hospital Service was formalized as the Commissioned Corps by legislation enacted in 1889. At first open only to physicians, the corps expanded to include dentists, sanitary engineers, pharmacists, nurses, sanitarians, scientists, and other health professionals.

In the closing decades of the nineteenth century, the activities of the Marine Hospital Service began to expand beyond the care of merchant seamen. That expansion began with the control of infectious diseases. Responsibility for quarantine was originally a function of the states, but the National Quarantine Act of 1878 conferred quarantine authority on the Marine Hospital Service.

Around this same time, the federal government also took over from the states the responsibility for processing immigrants. The Marine Hospital Service was assigned responsibility for the medical inspection of arriving immigrants at sites such as Ellis Island in New York. Commissioned officers played major roles in fulfilling the PHS commitment to prevent disease from entering the country.

The PHS continued to expand its public health activities as the nation entered the twentieth century. PHS-commissioned officers served their country by controlling the spread of contagious diseases such as smallpox and yellow fever, conducting biomedical research, regulating the food and drug supply, providing health care to underserved groups, and supplying medical assistance in the aftermath of disasters, among other functions.

Current Perspective: The Federal Government's Response *To Err Is Human*

To Err is Human: Building a Safer Health System, *a report released in 1999 by the Institute of Medicine (IOM), shocked the nation by estimating that between 44,000 and 98,000 Americans die each year as a result of preventable medical errors.[3] The report concluded that the majority of these errors are the result of systemic problems rather than of poor performance by individual providers, and it outlined a four-pronged approach to prevent medical mistakes and improve patient safety.[3]*

Although the United States provides some of the best health care in the world, the number of errors in health care is unacceptably high.[4] The IOM report estimates that more than half of the adverse medical events occurring each year are due to preventable errors and that these errors cause tens of thousands of deaths. The annual cost associated with these errors in lost income, disability, and health care is as much as $29 billion.[4] The consequences of medical mistakes are often more severe than are those of mistakes in other industries—that is, they may lead to death or disability rather than to simple inconvenience—underscoring the need for aggressive action.

A wide body of research, including many studies funded by federal Agency for Healthcare Research and Quality (AHRQ), supports the IOM conclusions. Two seminal studies on medical error have shown that adverse events occur in approximately 3 percent to 4 percent of patients.[5,6] Leape[7] has reported that the average intensive-care unit (ICU) patient experiences almost two errors per day. One out of five of these errors is serious or potentially fatal. This translates to a level of proficiency of approximately 99 percent. If performance levels of 99.9 percent—substantially higher than those found in the ICU—were applied to the airline and banking industries, it would equate to two dangerous landings per day at O'Hare International Airport and 32,000 checks deducted from the wrong bank account per hour.[7]

Many adverse drug events (ADEs) are associated with the use of pharmaceuticals. The IOM estimates the number of lives lost to preventable medication errors alone at more than 7,000 annually—a figure that exceeds the number of Americans injured in the workplace each year. A 1995 study estimated that problems related to the use of pharmaceutical drugs account for nearly 10 percent of all hospital admissions and that they contribute significantly to increased morbidity and mortality in the United States.[8] A 1991 study of hospitals in New York State indicated that drug complications represented 19 percent of all adverse events, and that 45 percent of these adverse events were caused by medical errors.[9] In this study, 30 percent of the individuals with drug-related injuries died.[9]

Medication errors also represent a significant economic cost to the United States. An article published in 1995 estimated the direct cost of preventable drug-related mortality and morbidity to be $76.6 billion, with drug-related hospital admissions accounting for much of the cost.[10] The authors suggest that indirect costs, such as those relating to lost productivity, might be two to three times as great as direct costs, making the total cost of all preventable, drug-related mortality and morbidity range from $138 to $182 billion. A study published in 2001 used updated figures and revised the direct cost estimate to $177.4 billion.[11] Another article estimated the cost of preventable ADEs in hospitalized patients to be $5,857 for each such event and that the estimated annual cost for preventable ADEs for a 700-bed hospital would be $2.8 million.[12]

In 1997, President Clinton established the Advisory Commission on Consumer Protection and Quality in the Health Care Industry (Quality Commission). The Quality Commission released two seminal reports focusing on patient protections and quality improvement. Following the commission's second report, President Clinton established an umbrella organization, the Quality Interagency Coordination Task Force (QuIC), and charged it with coordinating administration efforts to improve quality. As he established the QuIC, President Clinton stated, "For all of its strengths, our health care system still is plagued by avoidable errors."[4] The QuIC subsequently evaluated the recommendations in To Err Is Human *and responded with a strategy to identify prevalent threats to patient safety and reduce medical errors.*

Consistent with the Quality Commission's recommendations, Vice President Albert Gore launched the National Forum for Health Care Quality Measurement and Reporting. Known as the Quality Forum, it is a broad-based, widely representative private body that establishes standard quality-measurement tools to help purchasers, providers, and consumers of health care better evaluate and ensure the delivery of quality services.

Other federal agencies have made significant efforts to reduce medical errors and increase attention on patient safety. In 2001, the Department of Health and Human Services (HHS) announced formation of a Patient Safety Task Force to coordinate a joint effort to improve data collection on patient safety. The lead agencies are the FDA, the Centers for Disease Control and Prevention (CDC), the Centers for Medicare & Medicaid Services (CMS), and the AHRQ. The vision of the task force is to be a knowledge system for accumulating, exchanging, and integrating relevant information and resources among private and public stakeholders that support local efforts to protect patients and promote health care safety. Its goals are to improve safety by creating and disseminating knowledge necessary to detect and respond to current and emerging health care safety threats, to protect confidentiality, to reduce reporting burden and ensure local access to relevant health care safety information, and to monitor progress toward achieving local, state, and federal patient-safety goals.

In accordance with its recent reauthorization, the AHRQ is the lead agency for the federal government on quality in health care. It sponsors research examining the frequency and cause of medical errors and tests techniques designed to reduce these mistakes. It also examines issues related to health care quality, including overuse and underuse of services.

The Department of Defense and the Department of Veterans Affairs (VA), which serve more than 11 million persons nationwide, have implemented computerized physician order entry (CPOE) systems, a technology that has been proved effective in reducing medical errors. In addition, the VA has implemented computerized medical records and point-of-care bar coding in all its hospitals. Over the past several years, the VA also created an error-reporting system and established four Centers of Inquiry for Patient Safety.

The CMS, through its peer review organizations (PROs), is working to reduce errors of omission for the nation's 39 million Medicare beneficiaries. Under performance-based contracts, the PROs are working to prevent failures and delays in delivering services for patients with breast cancer, diabetes, heart attack, heart failure, pneumonia, and stroke. These efforts have already decreased mortality rates for heart attack victims.

The CDC and the FDA collect data on ADEs that are the result of treatment, such as hospital-acquired infections and on the unintended effects of drugs and medical devices. CDC's National Nosocomial Infections Surveillance system is a hospital-based reporting system that monitors hospital-acquired infections, which afflict more than two million patients every year. Among participating hospitals, bloodstream-infection rates have decreased by more than 30 percent since 1990, and wound infections following surgery have decreased by 60 percent among high-risk patients.[4]

As described in greater detail later in this chapter, FDA receives approximately 100,000 reports per year of adverse events associated with medical devices and over 300,000 reports associated with pharmaceuticals. FDA estimates that more than one-third of the adverse events associated with medical devices and pharmaceuticals are preventable.

In all these efforts, the federal government works closely with the private sector and the states. Many states and organizations in the private sector are moving ahead with actions to reduce the number of medical errors. Approximately 20 states have implemented mandatory or voluntary reporting systems to improve patient safety and to hold health care organizations responsible for the quality of care they provide. The private sector has also taken strides to address the issue of patient safety, most recently with the creation of the Leapfrog Group by executives of some of the nation's largest companies, including General Motors and General Electric. This group is leading an effort to implement CPOE and encourages all employers to make safe medicine a top priority of the health insurance they provide and to steer their employees to the hospitals that make the fewest mistakes.

Overview of Federal Programs Involved in Improving Medication Safety

The following is an overview of some federal programs involved in improving medication safety by providing direct healthcare or influencing healthcare through their regulatory over-sight or influence. This discussion is not meant to be all-inclusive.

U.S. PUBLIC HEALTH SERVICE

Today a part of the Department of Health and Human Services, the PHS consists of the Office of Public Health and Science (headed by the assistant secretary for health and includ-ing the surgeon general), 10 regional health administrators, and 8 operating divisions.

To accomplish the PHS mission,[13] pharmacists within the agencies and programs of the PHS

- provide health care and related services to medically underserved populations (i.e., American Indians, Alaska Natives, other population groups with special needs;
- prevent and control disease, identify health hazards in the environment and help correct them, and promote healthy lifestyles for the nation's citizens;
- improve the nation's mental health;
- ensure that drugs and medical devices are safe and effective, food is safe and whole-some, cosmetics are harmless, and that electronic products do not expose users to dangerous amounts of radiation;
- conduct and support biomedical, behavioral, and health services research and com-municate research results to health professionals and the public; and
- work with other nations and international agencies on global health problems and their solutions.

AGENCY FOR HEALTHCARE RESEARCH AND QUALITY

The AHRQ supports research to improve the outcomes and quality of health care, reduce its costs, address patient safety and medical errors, and broaden access to effective services.[14] The research sponsored, conducted, and disseminated by AHRQ provides information that helps people make better decisions about health care.

In 2001, AHRQ issued a report titled Reducing and Preventing Adverse Drug Events to Decrease Hospital Costs.[15] *The report states that more than 770,000 people are injured or die each year in hospitals from ADEs and that from 28 percent to 95 percent of ADEs could be prevented by reducing medication errors through the use of computerized monitoring systems, especially computerized medication-ordering systems.*

AHRQ's goals[14] are

- To support improvements in health outcomes.

  The field of health outcomes research examines the end results of the structure and processes of health care on the health and well-being of patients and populations. A unique characteristic of such research is the incorporation of the patient's perspec-tive in the assessment of effectiveness. Public and private-sector policy makers are also concerned with the end results of their investments in health care, whether at the individual, community, or population level.

- To strengthen quality measurement and improvement.

  Achieving this goal requires developing and testing quality measures and investigat-ing the best ways to collect, compare, and communicate these data. AHRQ's re-search emphasizes studies of the most effective ways to implement these measures and strategies in order to improve patient safety and health care quality.

- To identify strategies that improve access, foster appropriate use, and reduce unnecessary expenditures.

  Adequate access to and appropriate use of health care services continues to be a challenge for many Americans, particularly the poor, the uninsured, members of minority groups, rural and inner-city residents, and other priority populations. AHRQ supports studies of access, health care utilization, and expenditures to identify whether particular approaches to health care delivery and payment alter behaviors in ways that promote access or economize on health care resource use.

- To improve the quality of health care.

  AHRQ coordinates, conducts, and supports research, demonstrations, and evaluations related to the measurement and improvement of health care quality. This includes the development of an annual report on national trends in health care quality. AHRQ also disseminates scientific findings about what works best and facilitates public access to information on the quality of, and consumer satisfaction with, health care.

- To promote patient safety and reduce medical errors.

  AHRQ develops research and builds partnerships with health care practitioners and health care systems. It has established a permanent program of Centers for Education and Research on Therapeutics. These initiatives will help address concerns raised in the IOM report *To Err Is Human*.

- To advance the use of information technology for coordinating patient care and conducting quality and outcomes research.

  AHRQ works to

  - promote the use of information systems to develop and disseminate performance measures;

  - create effective linkages between health information sources to enhance health care delivery and coordination of evidence-based health care services; and

  - promote protection of individually identifiable patient information used in health services research and health care quality improvement.

- To establish an Office of Priority Populations.

  AHRQ helps ensure that the needs of priority populations (i.e., low-income groups, minorities, women, children, the elderly, and individuals with special heath care needs) are met throughout its intramural and extramural research portfolio. Beginning in fiscal year 2003, this has included developing an annual report on disparities in health care delivery as they relate to these priority populations.

CENTERS FOR DISEASE CONTROL AND PREVENTION

Headquartered in Atlanta, Georgia, the CDC is the lead federal agency for protecting the health and safety of people at home and abroad, providing credible information to enhance health decisions, and promoting health through strong partnerships. CDC serves as the national focus for developing and applying disease prevention and control, environmental health, and health-promotion and -education activities designed to improve the health of the people of the United States.[16]

CDC has developed many partnerships with public and private entities that improve service to the American people. In fiscal year 2000, the CDC workforce comprised approximately 8,500 full-time workers in 170 disciplines, including pharmacy, with a public health focus. More than 2,000 CDC employees work at locations other than the center's Atlanta office, including 47 state health departments. Approximately 120 are assigned overseas in 45 countries.

Infectious diseases, such as HIV/AIDS and tuberculosis, can destroy lives, strain community resources, and even threaten nations. In today's global environment, new diseases have the potential to spread across the world in days, or even hours, making early detection and action more important than ever. CDC plays a critical role in controlling these diseases, traveling at a moment's notice to investigate outbreaks abroad or at home.

Controlling disease outbreaks is only the beginning of CDC's protective role. By assisting state and local health departments, CDC works to protect the public every day: from using innovative fingerprinting technology to identify a food-borne illness to evaluating a family violence-prevention program in an urban community; from training partners in HIV education to protecting children from vaccine-preventable diseases through immunizations.[15]

FOOD AND DRUG ADMINISTRATION

Overview of Responsibilities

The FDA is responsible for protecting the public health by ensuring the safety, efficacy, and security of human and veterinary drugs, biological products, medical devices, our nation's food supply, cosmetics, and products that emit radiation. The FDA advances the public health by helping speed innovations that make medicines and foods more effective, safer, and more affordable and by helping the public get the accurate, science-based information they need to use medicines and foods to improve their health. FDA employees monitor the manufacture, import, transport, storage, and sale of about $1 trillion worth of products each year.[17] In the FDA's purview today are more products than ever before; it was estimated that pharmacists filled 3.2 billion prescriptions in 2003, a 60 percent increase from a decade ago.[18]

In carrying out its responsibilities, the FDA performs a broad range of functions. For example, in 2002, the FDA

- received and evaluated 320,860 reports of ADEs (see **Figure 9-3**);
- reviewed about 3,000 reports of medication errors;
- issued 688 letters to help ensure that the promotion of drug products presents a fair balance of risks and benefits and is not false or misleading;
- issued warnings for misbranded or fraudulent products and products marketed as "street drug alternatives";
- issued 4,733 export certificates for U.S. drug products;
- developed technology for the rapid identification of counterfeit drug products;

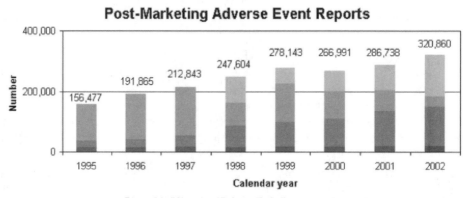

Figure 9-3. Adverse Event Reports Received at FDA, 1995–2002.[17]

- conducted shelf-life extensions for stockpiled drugs;

- proposed a regulation that would require bar coding on all pharmaceutical product labels; and

- proposed a regulation that would require manufacturers to report all medication errors (actual and potential) to the FDA.

In addition, the FDA may require that the manufacturer provide specific written patient information for selected prescription drugs that pose a serious and significant public health concern. This information is called a "Medication Guide." Medication Guides must be distributed to patients with each prescription dispensed. Such guides are required when the information is necessary for patients to use a product safely and effectively or to decide whether to use or to continue to use the product. In 2002, the FDA approved Medication Guides for four innovator products and one generic product:

- alosetron (Lotronex)

- isotretinoin (Amnesteem), generic product; Medication Guide previously approved for Accutane

- ribavirin (Copegus)

- sodium oxybate (Xyrem)

- teriparatide, rDNA origin (Forteo)

Certain FDA controls on 10 prescription drugs include limiting distribution to specific facilities; limiting prescription to physicians with special training or expertise; or requiring certain medical tests with their use. As of April 30, 2003, these drugs were

- alosetron

- bosentan

- clozapine

- dofetilide

- fentanyl citrate

- isotretinoin

- mifepristone

- sodium oxybate

- thalidomide

- trovafloxacin mesylate or alatrofloxacin mesylate injection

Sources of Risk from Drug Products

All drug products, no matter how carefully tested, monitored, and administered, have risks as well as benefits. Even with the best-available data, products sometimes have side effects that were not predictable or detectable in clinical trials and other studies prior to their use in real-world conditions. Major sources of risks associated with drugs are summarized in **Figure 9-4**.

- Product-quality defects. These are controlled through good manufacturing practices, monitoring, and surveillance.

- Known side effects. Predictable adverse events are identified in the drug's labeling. These cause the majority of injuries and deaths from using medicines. Some of these risks are avoidable, and others are unavoidable.

- Avoidable side effects. In many cases drug therapy requires an individualized treatment plan and careful monitoring. Other avoidable side effects are known drug-drug interactions.

- Unavoidable side effects. Side effects occur even a drug is used appropriately. Examples include nausea from antibiotics or bone marrow suppression from chemotherapy.

- Medication errors. Errors occur if, for example, a drug is administered incorrectly or if the wrong drug or dose is administered.

- Remaining uncertainties. These include unexpected side effects, long-term effects, and unstudied uses and populations. For example, a rare event occurring in fewer than 1 in 10,000 persons will not be identified in normal premarket testing.

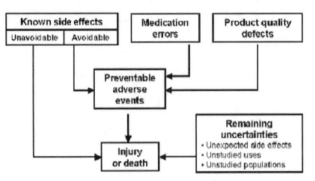

Sources of Risk from Drug Products

Figure 9-4. Sources of Risk from Drug Products.[19]

Virtually all medical therapies have side effects and risks, and it is important that these side effects be well understood so that FDA can be sure that the benefits of the products we approve outweigh their risks. This includes improving the ability to understand particular risks in specific populations, e.g., elderly patients and patients from particular demographic groups or carrying certain genes that may be associated with differences in risks.

FDA monitors these risks and the quality of marketed drugs and their promotional materials through product testing and surveillance. As Americans are increasingly receiving the benefits of important new drugs before they are available to citizens of other countries, FDA is especially vigilant in drug surveillance. In addition, the FDA develops policies, guidance, and standards for drug labeling, current good manufacturing practices, clinical and good laboratory practices, and industry practices to demonstrate the safety and effectiveness of drugs.

FDA has also continued research and evaluation activities in support of private-sector efforts to provide patients with information about prescription drugs. The goal is that by 2006, 95 percent of patients will receive useful information with new prescriptions.

MedWatch

FDA depends on the alertness and responsiveness of pharmacists and other health professionals to learn of ADEs, medication errors, and problems associated with medical products regulated by FDA. Today, these adverse events and product problems can be reported to FDA's MedWatch program.

In 1993, FDA launched MedWatch: The FDA Medical Products Reporting Program.[20] This system consolidated several reporting forms into one and encouraged health care professionals and consumers to report serious adverse events and product problems. FDA regards confidentiality as an important public health issue and protects the identity of the reporter, patient, and institution. Reports can be filed by mail, fax, telephone, or the Internet.

MedWatch is an important tool in identification of drug-safety issues, including preventable medication errors. It helps promote the safe use of drugs by

- providing a mechanism through which health professionals and the public can voluntarily report serious adverse events and problems with FDA-regulated medical products;

- disseminating new safety information on the Internet and providing e-mail notification to health professionals, institutions, the public, and MedWatch partners, which consist of professional societies, health agencies, and patient and consumer groups; and

- educating health professionals and consumers, through Internet outreach, speeches, articles, and exhibits, about the importance of recognizing and reporting serious adverse events and product problems, including medication errors.

In 2002, there were approximately 30,000 subscribers to MedWatch's e-mail notification service, which issues safety alerts for drugs. Notifications were posted on the Internet and e-mailed to individuals and 190 MedWatch partner organizations. In addition, subscribers and partners regularly receive information on safety-related labeling changes for drugs.

Drug Naming and Labeling

In 1991, the FDA began to receive reports of medication errors from a voluntary reporting system operated by the U.S. Pharmacopeia in cooperation with the Institute for Safe Medication Practices. To evaluate those reports, the FDA formed a Medication Errors Committee whose members consisted of a pharmacist, a physician, and a nurse. Every month, this group met to determine whether any of the reported errors were related to the naming, labeling, or packaging of the drug product. If so, the committee referred the report and recommendations to the responsible reviewing division with FDA's Center for Drug Evaluation and Research (CDER). In 1998, this activity was transferred to the Division of Medication Errors and Technical Support within the Office of Drug Safety.

Investigations into error reports frequently reveal that problems are due in part to look-alike labeling or product design or to sound-alike product names. The FDA helps ensure the safe use of newly approved drugs by minimizing the number of proprietary or brand names that look or sound like the names of existing products. Between 1985 and 1999, proprietary names were evaluated by the Labeling and Nomenclature Committee, an expert committee of health professionals within the CDER. In October 1999, primary responsibility for this activity was transferred to the Office of Post-Marketing Drug Risk Assessment. In January 2002, that office was reorganized into the Office of Drug Safety, where medication-error activities are provided by the Division of Medication Errors and Technical Support.

The FDA evaluates every proposed name for look-alike and sound-alike similarity to marketed drug names before it is approved. To simulate the prescription-ordering process, each proposed proprietary name is written within the context of an inpatient and outpatient prescription and recorded as a verbal prescription. These prescriptions are then presented to a group of FDA physicians, pharmacists, and nurses for interpretation. The goal of this activity is to determine whether any of the health care professionals confuse any proposed name with that of a product already on the market. In addition, FDA has developed and implemented a computerized system of evaluating proprietary name similarity. This system is based on an algorithm that determines the orthographic and phonetic similarity of the proposed name to the names in a dictionary of marketed drugs.

Continued Efforts to Improve Drug Safety

As the MedWatch program experience illustrates, the FDA depends on astute health professionals and others to identify problems as soon as they arise in order that appropriate intervention can be made. That intervention may range from revising the product labeling to withdrawing a product that has been deemed too dangerous to be safely used. While these systems are effective in identifying rare and serious adverse events, the need to rely on health care providers and incomplete reporting means that detection of and response to adverse events may be less timely and effective than is desirable.

The FDA recognizes the need to improve its systems for reporting drug-safety problems. One way is by improving the quality and standardization of the adverse event reports that the agency receives through its spontaneous adverse event reporting systems, and the agency is taking steps to do that. Another very promising new way is to have direct and secure access to relevant electronic health information. Increasingly, health care providers are using computerized systems to store patient information. Some of the information in these systems is related to product use and product-related adverse events. Confidential, secure exchange of information with these provider systems could expedite the discovery and reporting of safety problems. At present, however, the use of different technology platforms and applications hampers the flow of information among these systems. The FDA is working with its partners to develop standards to improve the flow of information across systems and to increase the benefits to health care organizations of adopting electronic medical record systems. Through activities such as these, the FDA will identify the most innovative and effective ways to communicate the risks associated with regulated products.

Finally, there are an increasing number of health care databases available to study the use and outcomes associated with medical products. The FDA has the challenge and the opportunity to use the best-available information from the private and public sectors to improve understanding of product safety.

HEALTH RESOURCES AND SERVICES ADMINISTRATION

The Health Resources and Services Administration (HRSA) directs national programs that improve the nation's health by ensuring equitable access to comprehensive, quality care. It works to improve and extend life for people with HIV/AIDS, to provide primary health care to medically underserved people, to serve women and children through state programs, and to train a health workforce that is both diverse and motivated to work in underserved communities.

In 1999, in response to mounting concern regarding a possible shortage of licensed pharmacists in the United States, Congress directed the secretary of HHS, through the appropriate agencies of the PHS, to conduct a study to determine whether and to what extent such a shortage existed. The HRSA study, titled "The Pharmacist Workforce: A Study of the Supply and Demand for Pharmacists," reported that the number of unfilled full- and part-time drugstore pharmacist positions nationally had been rising sharply, from about 2,700 vacancies in February 1998 to nearly 7,000 vacancies in February 2000. HRSA concluded that such vacancies could be expected to continue to grow. The report also warned that "the factors causing the current shortage are of a nature not likely to abate in the near future without fundamental changes in pharmacy practice and education."[21] According to the study, the shortage results in less time for pharmacists to counsel patients, job stress and poor working conditions with reduced professional satisfaction, longer working hours, less scheduling flexibility and greater potential for fatigue-related errors, and fewer pharmacy school faculty because of their recruitment into the workforce.

The HRSA study identified a number of causes for the growing demand for pharmacists, including

- the growing number of prescription medications;
- increased access to health care and more health care providers authorized to prescribe medications;
- expanded health insurance coverage and a resulting increase in prescriptions;
- growing emphasis on the doctor of pharmacy degree, which lengthens the education program and increases the amount of training in clinical practice; and
- strong competition for pharmacists trained at the residency or fellowship level.

As part of the study, HRSA requested comments on possible causes of the shortage and proposals for addressing it. Proposals included using more technicians to perform repetitive manual tasks, which would free pharmacists to focus on tasks that they alone are authorized to do. Other respondents urged greater use of automation to increase efficiency and reduce pharmacists' workloads. Respondents were also concerned that shortages are exacerbated by administrative burdens by health plans and insurers.

INDIAN HEALTH SERVICE

The Indian Health Service (IHS) is the principal federal health care advocate and provider for American Indians and Alaskan Natives who belong to more than 550 federally recognized tribes in 35 states. It provides comprehensive preventive, curative, rehabilitative, and environmental health care services.

Preventive measures involving environmental, educational, and outreach activities are combined with therapeutic measures into a single, national health system. Within these broad categories are special initiatives in traditional medicine, elder care, women's health, pediatric and adolescent care, injury prevention, domestic violence and child abuse, health care financing, state health care, sanitation facilities, and oral health. Most IHS funds are appropriated for American Indians who live on or near reservations, but the Congress has also authorized programs that provide access to care for Indians living in urban areas.

IHS services are provided directly and through tribally contracted and operated health programs. Health services also include health care purchased from more than 9,000 private providers annually. The federal system consists of 36 hospitals, 63 health centers, 44 health stations, and 5 residential treatment centers. In addition, 34 urban Indian health projects provide health and referral services.[22]

IHS pharmacists practice in a true pharmaceutical care environment where they fully use their knowledge and skills. IHS has pioneered many innovative advances over the past 30 years. Pharmacists have access to the patient's entire health record, including laboratory results, immunization status, and medical history. Problems are resolved with providers prior to dispensing medications, and all patients are counseled on their medication therapy. In many locations, pharmacists are credentialed to provide primary care, and they use their prescriptive authority to evaluate and manage the care of certain patients.

In the hospital setting, services provided by IHS pharmacists include unit dose, i.v. admixture, pharmacokinetic consultation, rounding, drug information, and discharge counseling.

DEPARTMENT OF VETERANS AFFAIRS

The Department of Veterans Affairs (VA) was established on 1989, succeeding the Veterans Administration. It provides federal benefits to veterans and their dependents. Headed by the Secretary of Veterans Affairs, VA is the second-largest of the 15 cabinet departments and operates nationwide programs for health care, financial assistance, and burial benefits.

Of the 26 million veterans currently alive, nearly three-quarters served during a war or an official period of conflict. About a quarter of the nation's population, or approximately 70 million people, are potentially eligible for VA benefits and services because they are veterans or family members or survivors of veterans.[23] The responsibility to care for veterans, spouses, survivors and dependents can last a long time; for example, more than 400 children and widows of Spanish-American War veterans still receive VA compensation or pensions, and six descendants of Civil War veterans still draw VA benefits.[23]

The VA health care system includes 163 hospitals, with at least one in each of the 48 contiguous states, Puerto Rico, and the District of Columbia. VA also operates more than 850 ambulatory care and community-based outpatient clinics, 137 nursing homes, 43 domiciliary facilities, and 73 comprehensive home care programs.[23] VA health care facilities provide a broad spectrum of medical, surgical, and rehabilitative care. More than 4.5 million people received care in VA health care facilities in 2002, and 46.5 million visits were recorded in VA's outpatient clinics.[23]

The VA created the National Center for Patient Safety (NCPS) in an effort to reduce and prevent adverse medical events. A unified and cohesive patient-safety program with active participation by all VA hospitals, the NCPS focuses on prevention. The program applies human factor analysis to identify and eliminate system vulnerabilities within the VA. In addition, the VA has implemented an electronic medical record system with CPOE and a point-of-care bar-coding system in all its hospitals, leading to major gains in improving medication safety.

NATIONAL INSTITUTES OF HEALTH

The National Institutes of Health (NIH) has 27 components, mainly institutes and centers. It is one of the world's foremost medical research centers and the focal point for federally supported medical research in this country. Its mission is to uncover new knowledge that will lead to better health for everyone by conducting research in its own laboratories, supporting the research of scientists in universities, medical schools, hospitals, and research institutions throughout the country and abroad, helping in the training of research investigators, and fostering communication of medical information.[24]

The NIH Clinical Center Pharmacy Department provides pharmaceutical care and research support to patients, health care providers, and investigators. Pharmacy staff members conduct and participate in research programs that enhance knowledge regarding optimal dosing and appropriate use of investigational and commercially available agents. The pharmacists provide investigational drug–management services that include protocol development and support, product development and formulation, and investigational drug information development. They also control and hold accountability for investigational agents. Pharmacists at the clinical center manage commercially available and investigational drugs in approximately 1,000 drug protocols.[24] This area is also responsible for preparing customized investigational drug products for clinical center patients, meeting FDA regulatory requirements for the manufacturing of drugs, and assisting investigators in filing investigational new drug applications.

In addition, the NIH pharmacy supports clinical and distributive programs, which include participation in drug selection and experimental protocol design and implementation, monitoring patient response to drug therapy, patient education, provision of drug information, drug use evaluation, and patient counseling.

The center's Clinical Pharmacokinetic Research Laboratory assists clinical investigators in the design, analysis, and interpretation of pharmacokinetic studies. Laboratory staff support NIH scientists in several areas of pharmacokinetic research.

CENTERS FOR MEDICARE & MEDICAID SERVICES (FORMERLY THE HEALTH CARE FINANCING ADMINISTRATION [HCFA])

The Centers for Medicare & Medicaid Services (CMS) administer the Medicare and Medicaid programs, which ensure provision of care to America's aged and indigent populations as well as oversee the State Children's Health Insurance Program. CMS performs a number of quality-focused activities, including regulation of laboratory testing, coverage policies, and quality-of-care improvement. It oversees the survey and certification of nursing homes and continuing-care providers, including home health agencies, intermediate-care facilities for the mentally challenged, and hospitals.

CMS's goals are to[25]

- protect and improve beneficiary health and satisfaction;
- foster appropriate and predictable payments and high-quality care;
- promote understanding of CMS programs among beneficiaries, the health care community, and the public;
- promote the fiscal integrity of CMS programs and be an accountable steward of public funds;
- foster excellence in the design and administration of CMS programs; and
- provide leadership in the broader health care marketplace to improve health.

CMS is an excellent position to have a positive influence on the safe use of medications as a measure of participation for hospitals and nursing homes.

States and Nongovernmental Bodies

The states have critical roles in improving medication safety. They bear the chief responsibility for licensing and monitoring health care providers. Medication safety is influenced by state licensing and regulatory authorities and legislative mandates. Recommendation 5.1 of the IOM report *To Err Is Human* states that a "nationwide system should be established that provides for the collection of standardized information by state governments about adverse events that result in death or serious harm."[3] Thus, states are in the center of federal recommendations to improve patient safety.

In 2000, the National Academy for State Health Policy surveyed state activities in tracking and reducing medical and adverse events.[26] Findings included the following:

- Fifteen states require mandatory reporting of ADEs from general and acute-care hospitals.
- Six states, including the District of Columbia, have voluntary reporting systems for medical errors or adverse events.
- In 10 states, the most frequent use of reported data is to identify trends.
- Underreporting and inadequate resources are the states' two greatest concerns with their reporting systems.

JOINT COMMISSION ON ACCREDITATION OF HEALTHCARE ORGANIZATIONS

Over the past few decades, the states have delegated their hospital-oversight activities to the Joint Commission on Accreditation of Healthcare Organizations (JCAHO). They have done so largely in response to the 1965 Medicare Act, which required hospitals to meet certain minimum health and safety requirements in order to participate in this national program. The act states that Congress will deem a hospital in compliance with Medicare conditions of participation if it is accredited by JCAHO. (As an alternative, hospitals can go through a Medicare certification process.) JCAHO evaluates and accredits more than 16,000 health care organizations and programs in the United States. An independent, not-for-profit organization, it is the nation's predominant standard-setting and accrediting body in health care.

JCAHO National Patient Safety Goals[27] for health care organizations in relationship to improving medication safety are to

- improve the effectiveness of communication among caregivers;
- implement a process for taking verbal or telephone orders or critical test results that require a verification "read back" of the complete order or test result by the person receiving the order or test result;
- standardize the abbreviations, acronyms, and symbols used throughout the organization, including a list of abbreviations, acronyms, and symbols not to use;

- improve the safety of high-alert medications;
- remove concentrated electrolytes (including, but not limited to, potassium chloride, potassium phosphate, and sodium chloride >0.9 percent) from patient care units;
- standardize and limit the number of drug concentrations available in the organization;
- improve the safety of using infusion pumps; and
- ensure free-flow protection on all general-use and patient-controlled analgesia i.v. infusion pumps used in the organization.

INSTITUTE FOR SAFE MEDICATION PRACTICES

The Institute for Safe Medication Practices (ISMP) was established in 1994 as a nonprofit organization that works closely with practitioners, regulatory agencies, health care institutions, professional organizations, and the pharmaceutical industry to provide education about ADEs.[28] ISMP is governed by a board of trustees representing a cross-section of the health care community, academia, pharmaceutical industry, professional health care organizations, managed care, and consumers. ISMP shares information about medication errors and other ADEs through four publications: ISMP Medication Safety Alert for Acute Care, Community/ Ambulatory, Consumer, and Nursing. In addition, ISMP communicates medication safety through columns and articles published in the journals and newsletters of health care associations.

The ISMP cooperates with the United States Pharmacopeia in a voluntary reporting effort called the Medication Errors Reporting (MER) program. This nationwide program, which was established in 1991, makes it possible for health professionals who encounter actual or potential medication errors to report them confidentially and anonymously. By sharing these experiences, pharmacists, nurses, physicians, and other health care practitioners contribute to improved patient safety and to the development of educational services for the prevention of future errors. Reporters can report medication errors by calling 1-800-FAIL-SAFE at ISMP or 1-800-23ERROR at the USP.

UNITED STATES PHARMACOPEIA

The United States Pharmacopeia (USP) is a nonprofit, nongovernmental, standard-setting organization that advances public health by ensuring the quality and consistency of medicines, promoting the safe and proper use of medications, and verifying ingredients in dietary supplements. USP standards are developed by a unique process of public involvement and are accepted worldwide. Other USP programs focus on promoting optimal health care delivery. USP achieves its goals through the contributions of volunteers representing pharmacy, medicine, and other health care professions, as well as science, academia, the U.S. government, the pharmaceutical industry, and consumer organizations.[29]

The USP created the Center for the Advancement of Patient Safety (CAPS) in order to broaden its work in the patient-safety arena. CAPS conducts data analysis and research, seeks grants, develops professional education programs, publishes articles on issues related to medication errors, participates in legislative activities, and proposes standards recommendations and guidelines for the goal of improving patient safety by preventing and reducing medication errors.[29]

As noted above, USP, with the ISMP, supports the MER program, a national voluntary reporting system. To date, this effort has collected more than 7,000 reports of medication errors. In addition, USP operates MEDMARX[SM], an Internet-accessible database on which hospitals can anonymously report and track medication errors.

CENTERS FOR EDUCATION & RESEARCH ON THERAPEUTICS

The Centers for Education & Research on Therapeutics (CERTS) is administered by Agency for Healthcare Research and Quality, in consultation with the FDA. It was established in 1999 and authorized under the FDA Modernization Act of 1997. The CERTS program consists of seven centers, a steering committee, and numerous partnerships. The seven centers are Duke University, the HMO Research Network, the University of Alabama, the University of Arizona, the University of North Carolina, the University of Pennsylvania, and Vanderbilt University Medical Center. The goal of CERTS is to improve the effectiveness and safety of the use of therapeutics by conducting research and educational programs that examine the benefits and risks of new, existing, or combined uses of therapeutics.[30] Developing collaborative relationships with public and private organizations is a key activity. To date, the centers have worked on over 130 projects. Improving the safe use of therapies has been central to the goals of the CERTS, which has more than 70 projects focused on this area.[31]

NATIONAL COORDINATING COUNCIL FOR MEDICATION ERROR REPORTING AND PREVENTION

The National Coordinating Council for Medication Error Reporting and Prevention (NCC MERP) was formed in 1995 and is an independent body consisting of 25 national and international organizations devoted to improving the reporting and minimization of medication errors.[32] The council comprises representatives of health care regulatory groups, the pharmaceutical industry, government agencies, standards-setting organizations, professional organizations, and consumers. The NCC MERP has led the way in improving medication safety by issuing numerous recommendations on how to report and prevent medication errors. It also developed a national taxonomy for classifying the types and causes of medication errors and issued recommendations to the FDA on the need to bar code pharmaceutical products.

INSTITUTE OF MEDICINE

For independent science-based advice about issues of medicine and public health, the government and the nation's leaders often turn to an institution that was created specifically for providing such counsel: the Institute of Medicine (IOM) of The National Academies (formerly the National Academy of Sciences, or NAS). The NAS was created by the federal government to be an adviser on scientific and technological matters. However, the academy and its associated organizations are private organizations and do not receive direct federal appropriations for their work. The IOM's mission is to advance and disseminate scientific knowledge to improve human health.[33] The institute provides objective, timely, authoritative information and advice concerning health and science policy to government, industry, the professions, and the public. Studies undertaken by the academies are usually funded out of appropriations made available to federal agencies and are done at the agencies' request.

The NAS congressional charter places the IOM in a unique role. Beyond that, the IOM process establishes it as an independent body. It relies on unpaid volunteer experts to author most of its reports. Each report must go through the IOM/National Research Council institutional process, ensuring a rigorous and formal peer review, a requirement that findings and recommendations be evidence based whenever possible, and that, when this is not possible, the findings be noted as expert opinion. Because the IOM is an independent entity, its experts and committees have a greater variety of options to conduct their studies than members of government-supported groups would have. In particular, although many meetings are open to the public, IOM committee members may deliberate among themselves and are not obligated to conduct all their work in a public forum.

The IOM has released numerous important reports on improving medication safety and health care quality. They include

- Patient Safety: Achieving a New Standard of Care (2003)
- Leadership by Example: Coordinating Government Roles in Improving Health Care Quality (2002)
- Crossing the Quality Chasm: A New Health System for the 21ˢᵗ Century (2001)
- Ensuring Quality Cancer Care (1999)
- Envisioning the National Health Care Quality Report (2001)
- To Err Is Human: Building a Safer Health System (1999)

Conclusion

Improving medication safety is a collaborative effort that is often spearheaded by an agency of the federal government but that also involves the collaboration of states, private organizations, consumers, and individual health care practitioners. Improved medication safety begins with the initial research, development, and approval of a drug product and extends throughout its commercial life.

While both the public and private sectors have made notable contributions to reducing preventable medical errors, additional and aggressive efforts are needed, both within and outside of the federal government, to further reduce these mistakes.

References

1. http://www.usphs.gov/html/history.html. Accessed November 1, 2003.

2. Department of Health and Human Services. *50 Years of Service*. Rockville, MD: Department of Health and Human Services; 2003;32-39.

3. Kohn LT, Corrigan JM, Donaldson MD, eds. Committee on Quality of Health in America, Institute of Medicine. *To Err Is Human: Building a Safer Health System*. Washington, DC: National Academy Press; 1999.

4. Quality Interagency Coordination Task Force. Report of the Quality Interagency Coordination Task Force to the President. Doing What Counts for Patient Safety: Federal Actions to Reduce Medical Errors and their Impact. February 2000. Available at: www.quic.gov/report/errors6.pdf.

5. Brennan TA, Leape LL, Laird N, et al. Incidence of adverse events and negligence in hospitalized patients: Results of the Harvard Medical Practice Study I. *New Engl J Med*. 1991;324:370-376.

6. Thomas EJ, Studdert DM, Newhouse JP, et al. Costs of medical injuries in Utah and Colorado. Inquiry. 1999;36:255-264.

7. Leape LL. Error in medicine. *JAMA*. 1994;272:1851-1857.

8. Bates DW, Cullen DJ, Laird N, et al. Incidence of adverse drug events and potential adverse drug events: Implications for prevention. ADE Prevention Study Group. *JAMA*. 1995;274:29-34.

9. Leape LL, Brennan TA, Laird N, et al. The nature of adverse events in hospitalized patients: Results of the Harvard Medical Practice Study II. *N Engl J Med*. 1991;324:377-384.

10. Johnson JA, Bootman JL. Drug-related morbidity and mortality: a cost-of-illness model. *Arch Intern Med*. 1995;155:1949-1956.

11. Ernst FR, Grizzle AJ. Drug-related morbidity and mortality: updating the cost-of-illness model. *J Am Pharm Assoc*. 2001;41:192-199.

12. Bates DW, Spell N, Cullen D, et al. The cost of adverse drug events in hospitalized patients. *JAMA*. 1997;277:307-311.

13. www.usphs.gov. Accessed October 15, 2003.

14. www.ahrq.gov. Accessed October 15, 2003.

15. Agency for Healthcare Quality and Research. Reducing and Preventing Adverse Drug Events to Decrease Hospital Costs. Research in Action, Issue 1. March 2001. Rockville, MD: Department of Health and Human Services; March 2001. AHRQ publication 01-0020. Available at: www.ahrq.gov/qual/aderia/aderia.htm.

16. www.cdc.gov. Accessed November 26, 2003.

17. Food and Drug Administration. Center for Drug Evaluation and Research. Improving Public Health through Human Drugs. Report to the Nation. Rockville, MD: Department of Health and Human Services; 2002. Available at: www.fda.gov/cder/reports/rtn/2002/rtn2002-3.HTM#Highlights.

18. www.fda.gov. Accessed October 30, 2003.

19. Food and Drug Administration. Managing the Risks from Medical Product Use—Creating a Risk-Management Framework. Rockville, MD: FDA. 1999. Available at: www.fda.gov/oc/tfrm/executivesummary.html.

20. Kessler DA. Introducing MedWatch: a new approach to reporting medication and device adverse effects and product problems. *JAMA*. 1993:269:2765-2768.

21. http://bhpr.hrsa.gov/healthworkforce/pharmacist.html. Accessed November 26, 2003.

22. www.ihs.gov. Accessed November 1, 2003.

23. www.va.gov. Accessed November 22, 2003.

24. www.nih.gov. Accessed November 26, 2003.

25. www.cms.gov. Accessed October 1, 2003.

26. National Academy for State Health Policy. State Reporting of Medical Errors and Adverse Events: Results of a 50-State Survey. Portland, ME: National Academy for State Health Policy; April 2000.

27. http://www.jcaho.org/about+us/index.htm. Accessed November 14, 2003.

28. www.ismp.org. Accessed November 21, 2003.

29. http://usp.org. Accessed November 21, 2003.

30. Centers for Education & Research on Therapeutics. CERTs Annual Report: Year 3. October 2001–September 2002. Rockville, MD: Department of Health and Human Services; July 2003. AHRQ publication 03-0021.

31. http://www.certs.hhs.gov. Accessed November 26, 2003.

32. http://nccmerp.org. Accessed November 21, 2003.

33. www.iom.edu. Accessed November 22, 2003.

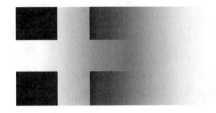

CHAPTER 10

Applying Best Practices and Scientific Evidence to Improving Patient Safety

Timothy S. Lesar

Introduction

Health care providers and organizations face many challenges when implementing patient-safety improvements. Making significant improvements in patient safety is complex, difficult, time-consuming, and, in some cases, costly. Failure to implement improvement aims may result in negative patient outcomes and increased patient care costs. Considering the importance of success, health care providers must approach this undertaking in a data-driven and systematic manner.

Numerous organizations have provided both general and specific recommendations for the safe provision of drug therapy to patients. A large number of resources, tools, products, and technologies exist that individual caregivers and health care organizations can use to improve medication safety. In large part, medication practices to reduce patient risk for error have been defined; the challenge is to ensure these practices are implemented effectively. The value of specific safety strategies will vary from one care setting and organization to another. Moreover, simply changing a policy or process, or implementing a new technology, does not guarantee improved patient safety; indeed, it could increase risk. To successfully and efficiently adopt appropriate safety recommendations, each organization must assess its current culture, structure, and care practices; evaluate the potential benefits of proposed changes for specific care settings; determine whether and how change is to be undertaken; and, finally, decide how to monitor improvement.

This chapter addresses the assessment and implementation of recommended medication-safety practices. Those involved in implementing improvements should understand the basis for commonly used and emerging medication-safety practices. The importance of considering the rationale and evidence for the recommended practices is discussed. A sound knowledge of improvement techniques and of established safety strategies is a necessity when adopting and implementing recommended safety practices in a specific care setting.

Principles of Improving Medication Safety

Recommendations for safe practices spanning much of the medication-use system are available from a number of sources. Most organizations already incorporate many elements of these practices in their medication-use systems, and much of the current efforts to improve medication safety involves ongoing efforts to expand and improve safety systems that are currently in place. Additional efforts may involve major system redesign and adoption of new practices, processes, and technologies.

USE A SYSTEMS-BASED AND HUMAN FACTORS APPROACH

The landmark 1999 Institute of Medicine (IOM) report *To Err Is Human: Building a Safer Health System*[1] and subsequent reports from the IOM's Committee on the Quality of Health Care in America[2-5] established a general framework and broad guidelines for improving the safety and quality of patient care. The IOM reports strongly support a *systems* approach to improving patient safety, a philosophy that has also been generally adopted by the current patient-safety movement. A systems approach to improving safety focuses on the processes, systems, and environment in which people work rather than simply attempting to improve individual skills and performance.[6-14] The systems approach runs counter to the traditional medical model of stressing individual performance as the primary determinant of outcomes. Another major recommendation of the 1999 IOM report was the application of error-prevention and quality-improvement methods widely used outside medicine.[15-17]

On the basis of these approaches, the initial IOM report delineated the following widely accepted set of general strategies and principles for improving patient safety:[1]

- Increase visibility of processes so that users can see what and how things need to be done and what happens if a step is not completed.

- Simplify tasks to reduce reliance on individual performance skills (e.g., planning, memory, vigilance, problem solving).

- Apply design principles with allowances for error, and design processes and equipment that communicate how they work to the user and lead to desired outcomes.

- Use forcing functions (i.e., processes that limit options or force processes to occur as desired) and constraints to guide individuals in the correct performance of functions and reduce the possibility of wrong action. Establish error-recovery processes that make it easy to recover or back out if a wrong action is taken.

- Implement standardization with resultant simplification and consistency of processes. (Standardization will have inherent forcing function effects as well.)

- Respect human limits by applying knowledge about human factors in process design.

- Promote effective team functioning.

- Anticipate the unexpected. Monitor all changes carefully for their effectiveness and unanticipated consequences.

- Create a learning environment in which detection of process deficiencies and failures is seen as an opportunity for improvement.

Despite the emphasis on systems, medication-use processes are also highly dependent on human performance and behavior. Safety improvements will always involve caregivers, patients, and others at some level. Humans are a part of any health care system. To be maximally effective, safety strategies must always consider the role and interactions of humans and their behaviors with the systems of care.

In recognition of the role of individuals, application of human factors is central to the design and implementation of medication-safety strategies. *Human factors* is the study of the interaction between humans and the systems in which they work and of the resulting outcomes. The goal of studying human factors is to design systems, environments, work practices, and equipment that produce improved outcomes. Human factors has been widely used in nonmedical industries to design, implement, and assess systems. Human factors considerations play a large part in medication-safety practices such as medication control, unit dose systems, and medical equipment design.[18-21] Human nature, in sum, must be considered when designing and implementing medication-safety processes.

Anthony Grasha[21] suggested the following three principles of the human factors approach as applied to medication safety:

1. Strong and effective systems make people more effective.
2. Strong and effective people make systems more effective.
3. Medication-safety systems work best when they consider the design and goals of the system and the needs of the humans who interact with it.

These principles stress the importance of developing and choosing staff on the basis of their ability to perform specific high-risk tasks.

Grasha[20] also developed a set of useful principles concerning human nature as it relates to identifying causes of, and preventing, human errors in complex systems such as health care. These principles are as follows:

Optimism encourages and nurtures change.
The manner in which change is sought is often more important than the methods used to achieve it. A positive, collaborative, and cooperative effort will produce benefits well beyond any immediate goals.

Old solutions seldom fix new problems.
The medication-use process has changed dramatically over the past two decades, requiring new approaches to deal with new problems. Improving the medication-use system can be more effective when ideas for change cross traditional boundaries and escape established frameworks.

A system perspective is not enough.
For maximum performance, individuals must be held accountable and feel responsible for their roles within any care system. Not all individuals are equally well suited to perform complex tasks, and task assignments should reflect this fact.

People internalize components of systems in that they work and live.
The systems in an individual's life affect how that individual behaves and reacts. Systems can have positive or negative influences on people's actions and decisions.

Factors producing errors operate at manifest and latent levels.
We commonly make the mistake of placing low priority on fixing latent error-producing conditions, such as understaffing and inadequate technological support. We often rationalize this inaction with statements such as, "There has never been a problem before." One only has to consider the National Aeronautics and Space Administration's two space shuttle disasters to find disturbing illustrations of this principle.

Error in complex systems is both predictable and unpredictable.
Many errors are unpredictable. Although hindsight bias may tell us that an error was predictable, it must not lead us to assume that we can predict most future errors. Error monitoring and learning must be an ongoing process, and the lessons learned must be applied to reduce future patient risk.

These principles of human nature are an important complement to the nonhuman aspects of systems-based safety recommendations of the IOM and others. The success of system-based improvements depends to a great extent on the success of the human-system interface and, as such, must be considered when designing and implementing medication-safety processes. It is widely accepted that a systems-based approach, which applies human factors principles and human behavior considerations, should be used to guide the development and implementation of medication-safety strategies and practices.

Safe Medication-Use Practice Recommendations

The 1999 IOM report[1] provided general recommendations related to improving medication safety (see **Table 10-1**). Many medication-safety experts and organizations have echoed and expanded on the IOM report. More-detailed descriptions of safe medication-use practices have been provided by a number of experts[22-31] and organizations (see **Table 10-2**). These recommendations provide sound guidance for the design of safer medication-use systems.

Table 10-1. Medication-Safety Recommendations from the Institute of Medicine[1]

- Implement standard processes for medication doses, dose timing, and dose scales in a given patient care unit.
- Standardize prescription writing and prescribing rules.
- Limit the number of types of common drug administration equipment.
- Implement physician computerized order entry.
- Use pharmaceutical software.
- Have the central pharmacy supply high-risk intravenous medications.
- Use special procedures and written protocols for the use of high-risk medications.
- Do not store concentrated solutions of hazardous medications on patient care units.
- Ensure the availability of pharmaceutical decision support.
- Include a pharmacist during rounds of patient care units.
- Make relevant patient information available at the point of care.
- Improve patient knowledge about their treatments.

Specific Medication-Safety Recommendations from the Institute of Medicine's *To Err Is Human: Building a Safer Health System* Report.

Table 10-2. Medication-Safety Resources*

- Agency for Healthcare Quality and Research (AHRQ), www.ahrq.gov
- AHRQ Morbidity and Mortality Rounds on the Web, www.webmm.ahrq.gov
- American Hospital Association (AHA), www.aha.org
- Healthcare Research and Education Trust (HRET), www.hospitalconnect.com/hret
- American Pharmacy Association (formerly American Pharmaceutical Association), www.apha.org
- American Society of Consultant Pharmacists (AACP), www.aacp.org
- American Academy of Pediatrics (AAP), www.aap.org
- American Society for Parenteral and Enteral Nutrition (ASPEN), www.aspen.org
- American Society of Health-Systems Pharmacists (ASHP), www.ashp.org
  - Patient Safety Resource Center, www.ashp.org/patient-safety/index.cfm
  - Safe medication.com (consumer patient-safety information), www.safemedication.com
- California Institute for Health Systems Performance (CIHSP), www.cihsp.org
- Food and Drug Administration (FDA), www.fda.gov
  - Center for Drug Evaluation and Research (CDER), www.fda.gov/cder
  - Office of Drug Safety, www.fda.gov/cder/Offices/ODS/default.htm
- Institute for Healthcare Improvement (IHI), www.ihi.org

- Institute for Safe Medication Practices (ISMP), www.ismp.org
- Joint Commission for Accreditation of Healthcare Organizations (JCAHO), www.jcaho.org
- Leapfrog Group, www.leapfroggroup.org
- Massachusetts Coalition for the Prevention of Medical Error, www.macoalition.org
- National Coordinating Council for Medication Error Reporting Programs (NCC MERP), www.nccmerp.org
- National Council on Patient Information and Education, www.talkaboutrx.org
- National Patient Safety Foundation (NPSF), www.npsf.org
- National Quality Forum (NQF), www.qualityforum.org
- Partnership for Patient Safety, www.p4ps.org
- PatientSafety.net, www.patientsafety.net
- Pediatric Pharmacy Advocacy Group (PPAG), www.ppag.org
- United States Pharmacopeia (USP), www.usp.org
- Veterans Administration National Center for Patient Safety, www.patientsafety.gov

*All sites accessed October 15, 2004.

Those participating in implementing safety practices must understand that many current practices and recommendations for improving medication safety are based on experience, logic and common sense, and tradition as well as on human factors–based applications developed in fields other than medicine. Consequently, few recommendations are based on the type of supportive scientific evidence, such as controlled trials, commonly expected for medical interventions. Those practices for which evidence does exist are often narrow in scope or lack evidence of effectiveness when applied broadly in medical care. There are, however, some notable exceptions; for example, the increased safety associated with the use of unit dose systems rather than floor stock systems has been documented for more than 30 years.[24,32] More recently, considerable evidence has been generated regarding the benefits of computerized prescriber order entry (CPOE).[33]

This does not mean processes lacking substantial evidence to support their effectiveness are unlikely to improve safety. Rather, the lack of evidence for common safety practices usually reflects their inherently obvious value, based on other sources of evidence (e.g., noncontrolled trials, nonmedical applications) and experience with common use (e.g., medication-access controls), or the difficulty, limitations, and expense of studying effectiveness of safety practice impact on patient outcomes. The science of patient safety is still in its developing stages, and adequate and widely accepted techniques for measuring the value of safety practices are not yet available.

In order to move the patient safety and quality movement forward despite such limitations, the National Quality Forum has published a set of universal recommendations for safe medical care (see **Table 10-3**). These recommendations are based on available evidence for effectiveness, expert opinion, generalizability across health care settings, and value. The recommendations were partly based on a comprehensive, evidence-based review of patient-safety practices commissioned by the Agency for Health Care Improvement (AHRQ).[33] This report reviewed the available evidence for the effectiveness of a number of practices related to medication safety. The strength-of-evidence ratings for medication-safety practices evaluated in the report are listed in **Table 10-4**. The results of this review reflect the application of a medical care methodology of evidence-based review that places greater weight on controlled trials.[34,35] The report focused on strategies that would produce improved safety over current practice; for this reason, common practices such as unit dose dispensing and pharmacist order review were not rated highly. Because many commonly accepted and recommended medication-safety practices have not specifically undergone substantial scientific evaluation, they were either not included in the final recommendations or were rated as having limited supporting evidence. The many recommendations provided by the Institute for Safe Medication Practices (ISMP) and other organizations (see Table 10-2) are based primarily on the application of well-established safety principles rather than on data from controlled trials. The AHRQ report clearly demonstrates the need for improving methods for assessing safety strategies. While it is critical that practices be based on evidence, it is not sensible, possible, or economically prudent to expect convincing controlled trials for all currently used safety practices.[34, 35]

Table 10-3. Practices Related to Safe Medication Practices Endorsed by the National Quality Forum

- Create a culture of safety.
- Pharmacists should actively participate in the medication-use process:
  - be available for consultation
  - interpret and review medication orders
  - prepare medications
  - dispense medications
  - administer and monitor medications
- Record verbal orders immediately and read them back for verification.
- Use only standardized abbreviations and dose designations.
- Do not prepare patient care summaries and other records (e.g., medication history) from memory.
- Communicate or transfer all care information, such as orders and important information, to all providers who need the information.
- Implement computer prescriber order entry systems.
- Assess each patient undergoing elective surgery and provide prophylactic beta blockers to patients at high risk for cardiac ischemic events.
- Evaluate each patient and provide appropriate venothromboembolism prophylaxis.
- Use dedicated anticoagulation services.
- Provide appropriate antibiotic surgical prophylaxis.
- Evaluate patients for risk of contrast media–induced nephropathy and provide appropriate preventive care.
- Vaccinate health care workers for influenza.
- Ensure that medication storage and work areas are uncluttered, well lit, and clean. Reduce distraction, interruptions, and noise.
- Evaluate for risk of malnutrition and employ strategies to avoid malnutrition.
- Standardize medication labeling, packaging, and storage.
- Identify all high-alert medications.
- Use unit dose and unit-of-use medication-dispensing systems.

Adapted from National Quality Forum–Endorsed Set of Safe Practices. Available at:www.qualityforum.org. Accessed October 20, 2004.

Table 10-4. Practices Related to Medication Safety Included in the Agency for Healthcare Research and Quality Evidence-Based Review of Patient-Safety Practices[33]

Practices rated as having the greatest strength of evidence
- Provision of appropriate venothromboembolism prophylaxis*
- Reduction of cardiac events by use of perioperative beta blockers in select noncardiac surgery patients*
- Provision of appropriate perioperative antibiotic prophylaxis*
- Appropriate nutritional strategies in postoperative patients*
- Self-managed home monitoring of chronic warfarin anticoagulation*

Practices rated as having a high strength of evidence
- Use of computer monitoring or surveillance for adverse drug events
- Selective decontamination of digestive tract to prevent ventilator-associated pneumonia*
- Information transfer between inpatient and outpatient pharmacies

Practices rated as having a medium strength of evidence
- Computerized prescriber order entry and decision support
- Clinical pharmacist consultation services
- Perioperative glucose control*
- Use of H_2 antagonists for stress-ulcer prevention*
- Increased use of pneumococcal vaccination*
- Acute pain services*
- Anticoagulation services and clinics*
- Antibiotic controls to reduce development of resistance*
- Hydration and oral acetylcysteine protocols to prevent contrast media–induced nephropathy
- Use of heparin protocols to guide anticoagulation therapy*
- Use of low osmolar contrast media*

Practices rated as having a lower impact or strength of evidence
- Use of antiseptics to prevent central venous catheter infections*
- Use of heparin to prevent central venous catheter infections*
- Use of analgesics in patients with acute abdomen*
- Use of automated dispensing devices
- Use of bar coding for patient identification
- Unit dose dispensing systems
- Improving team performance through application of aviation-style crew-resource management techniques and other methods+
- Limitation of caregiver work hours+

Practices rated as having lowest impact and/or strength of evidence
- Use of sucralfate to prevent ventilator-associated pneumonia*
- Hydration and theophylline protocols to prevent contrast media–induced nephropathy*

Table 10-4. Practices Related to Medication Safety Included in the Agency for Healthcare Research and Quality Evidence-Based Review of Patient-Safety Practices[33] (cont'd)

- Routine antibiotic to prevent central venous catheter infections

Other medication safety–related practices reviewed but strength of evidence not rated
- Use of structured discharge summaries+
- Promotion of a culture of safety+
- Use of human factors in design and assessment of medical devices+

Key:
    * Patient-outcome benefits related to consistent and effective delivery of specific medical care.
    + General safety strategies applicable to medication-use systems.

The nature of medication safety does not lend itself to the type of scientific assessment typically used to evaluate care and interventions. Wide variations in practice exist from one health care organization to another, and the medication-use system comprises multiple interdependent and interacting individuals, processes, and technologies. Patient outcome is a net result of the entire system, rather than of its individual components. Controlling and accounting for variables when testing the effectiveness of safety strategies is difficult, if not impossible. Measuring effectiveness of safety practices is compounded by the fact that medication errors and their resulting effects on patients are difficult to identify, given the multiple variables involved and the ethical need to correct and ameliorate errors that are detected. Medication errors occur and progress through the system in countless ways and are difficult to study. Medication errors that occur in similar ways are common; errors occurring in *exactly* the same way are rare. Implementing changes to reduce errors in one isolated component of the system may not be measurable in terms of patient outcome because of the low frequency of errors or because the effectiveness of the change was dependent upon other system components.

Many safety practices are based on an understanding of the multiple factors and system deficiencies related to error.[1,6, 9,12,22,28,36-50] Systems-based and human factors–based risk-reduction strategies are developed on the basis of this knowledge. This approach to safety is widely used in industries other than medicine and is a hallmark of high-reliability organizations.[11,14,16] Thus, many medication systems that lack specific scientific evidence for effectiveness are nonetheless based on well-established and evidence-based safety-design principles. The lack of evidence of generalizability of specific safety practices across the health care system does increase the importance of careful assessment, planning, and effective process implementation and of the need to obtain baseline and follow-up measures of safety. However, the difficulty of assessing the potential value and risks of a recommended process change, and its eventual impact once implemented, is compounded by the inability of most organizations to accurately measure medication safety within their organizations.[51,52] Given the urgent need to improve medication safety, it is necessary to carefully move forward with changes without the clear medical-model evidence base to which most caregivers are accustomed. Applying the established principles of safe systems design while recognizing and accounting for the limitations of the available evidence will enable organizations to implement effective changes in their medication-use processes.

While there are numerous recommendations for safe medication practices, there is a notable amount of consistency, and all strategies reflect a systems-based approach to reducing risk. The ISMP Medication Safety Self Assessments[53] contain an excellent compilation of nearly 200 representative characteristics of safe medication-use systems that are reflected in and expanded on by the recommendations of the organizations listed in Table 10-2. The 20 core characteristics of safe medication-use systems recommended by the ISMP are listed in **Table 10-5.** Individual organizations must translate these recommendations and adapt or modify them in order to implement improvements in their own care settings.

Table 10-5. Institute for Safe Medication Practices Medication Safety Self-Assessment: Core Distinguishing Characteristics

1. Essential patient information is obtained, readily available in useful form, and considered when prescribing, dispensing, and administering medications.

2. Essential drug information is readily available in useful form and considered when ordering, dispensing, and administering medications.

3. A closed drug formulary system is established to limit choice to essential drugs, minimize the number of drugs with which practitioners must be familiar, and provide adequate time for designing safe processes for the use of drugs added to the formulary.

4. Methods of communicating drug orders and other information are standardized and automated.

5. Strategies are undertaken to minimize the possibility of errors with drug products that have similar or confusing manufacturer labeling/packaging or names that look or sound alike.

6. Readable labels that identify drugs clearly are on all drug containers, and drugs remain labeled up to the point of administration.

7. IV drug solutions, drug concentrations, doses, and administration times are standardized whenever possible.

8. Medications are delivered to patient care units in a safe and secure manner and available for administration within a time frame that meets essential patient needs.

9. Unit-based floor stock is restricted.

10. Hazardous chemicals are sequestered from patients and not accessible in drug-preparation areas.

11. The potential for human error is mitigated through careful procurement, maintenance, use, and standardization of medication-delivery devices.

12. Medications are prescribed, transcribed, prepared, dispensed, and administered in a physical environment that offers adequate space and lighting and allows practitioners to remain free of distractions.

13. The complement of qualified, well-rested practitioners matches the clinical workload without compromising patient safety.

14. Practitioners receive sufficient orientation to medication use and undergo baseline and annual competency evaluations of knowledge and skills related to safe medication practices.

15. Practitioners involved in medication use undergo ongoing education about medication error prevention and the safe use of drugs that have the greatest potential to cause harm if misused.

16. Patients are active partners in their care through education about their medications and ways to avert errors.

17. A nonpunitive, system-based approach to error reduction is in place and supported by senior administration and the board of trustees/directors.

18. Practitioners are stimulated to detect and report errors, and multidisciplinary teams regularly analyze errors that have occurred within the organization and in other organizations for the purpose of redesigning systems to best support safe practitioner performance.

19. Simple redundancies that support a system of independent double checks or an automated verification process are used for vulnerable parts of the medication system.

20. Proven infection-control practices are followed when storing, preparing, and administering medications.

Adapted from ISMP Medication Safety Self-Assessment.[53] Available at: www.ismp.org. Accessed September 18, 2003.

Most medication-safety practices recommendations, guidelines, and standards can be organized into the following 10 categories. Many recommended safety practices have an impact on a number of these categories.

LEADERSHIP, ORGANIZATIONAL STRUCTURE, AND CULTURE

Organizational culture and leadership play critical roles when implementing improvements in patient safety. Leaders as well as caregivers must consider themselves personally responsible for patient safety.[54,55] Establishing and enhancing a culture of safety and quality among all individuals, and as a core characteristic of the organization as a whole, will promote behaviors necessary for system-based improvements.[11,12,15-17, 53-74] The organization must clearly communicate a vision that patient safety is everyone's primary responsibility and define how it strives to attain this goal. Executive leaders should establish clearly delineated expectations and lines of accountability and responsibility. This includes ensuring the existence of an organizational framework with appropriate authority and resources. All managers and supervisors should be oriented to the systems-based approach to safety and to the importance of supporting and fostering a nonpunitive reporting and learning process in their day-to-day activities.

Four useful tools describing leadership responsibilities and providing a work plan for safety are Pathways for Medication Safety: Leading a Strategic Planning Effort,[54] Pathways for Medication Safety Looking at Risk Collectively,[55] the ISMP Medication Safety Self-Assessments,[53] and the American Society of Health-System Pharmacists (ASHP) Medication System Safety Strategy (MS³).[70] Key leadership groups in improving medication safety in hospitals include the pharmacy, nursing, and medical staff; leadership, risk-management, and quality-improvement staff; and the pharmacy and therapeutics committee. In many settings, other groups may play important roles, including laboratory services, respiratory care, biomedical engineering, patient information services, patient representatives, environmental services, and public relations.[53-55, 70-74] A multidisciplinary team specifically organized to lead and address medication use and safety throughout the organization should be considered if not already in place. Many health care organizations have designated a medication-safety officer to lead and coordinate improvement efforts. The specific characteristics of practice, organizational, or corporate structure will determine the appropriate leadership structure for settings such as long-term care facilities, community pharmacies, home care, and mail-order pharmacies. In all settings, making substantive improvements requires that multiple individuals and groups work in a coordinated fashion.

The individual caregivers and the culture within the workplace will often determine the effectiveness of changes intended to improve safety.[1-4,8,11,12] The evidence supporting the role of a culture of safety was evaluated in the aforementioned AHRQ report.[33] Despite the lack of evidence specifically supporting the effectiveness of improving culture, the rationale and experience in nonmedical settings are compelling. Culture is considered the critical component of the safety processes of nonmedical high-reliability industries.[10,15,16,33] The multifaceted patient-safety initiatives of the Veterans Health Administration provide a model for improving culture for health care organizations to adapt.[67]

INFORMATION AVAILABILITY, TRANSFER, AND USE

Lack of information availability, sharing, or communication and the failure to use important patient and drug information, contribute to a large proportion of preventable adverse drug events (ADEs).[9,24,28,42,43,50,74] Thus, many medication-safety recommendations relate to making information more accessible to, and appropriately applied by, caregivers. Improving the availability and use of information involves many interrelated functions, including technologies, staff training and competency, teamwork, staff deployment, communications, formulary policies, documentation practices, organizational processes and structure, culture, workload, and environmental factors.

COMMUNICATION, TEAMWORK, AND WORKFLOW SIMPLIFICATION

The medication-use process is highly interdisciplinary and therefore highly dependent on teamwork, communication, coordination, and effective interpersonal interactions.[1,9,11,24,53,74] A number of safe medication practices address the communication and teamwork among all involved in this process. These safe practices involve not only the operational but also the interpersonal and behavioral aspects and characteristics of communication and teamwork.

MEDICATION STANDARDIZATION, TASK SIMPLIFICATION, AND CONTROL

Controlling access to medications, standardizing processes, and reducing variability are basic engineering methods of reducing the risk of medication errors.[17,24,53,70,74, Table 2] Commonly used examples of this strategy are unit dose systems, standardized intravenous (i.v.) drug solutions, limitations on floor stocks, and limitations on access to automated dispensing cabinets prior to pharmacist order review. While simple in concept, comprehensive implementation of such practices is challenging because of competing priorities and the culture and complexity of health care organizations. Medication standardization and control involves all components and individuals involved in the process. Reduction of error risk through medication-control processes often involves limiting caregiver access to medications and making efforts to restrict variability in practice. These limitations may inherently produce delays and less efficient (albeit safer) workflow processes that potentially produce work-arounds to circumvent the safety practice.[33] Working to limit the potential workflow inefficiencies and engaging affected staff will improve the possibility of effective implementation and compliance.

IMPROVING IDENTIFICATION, VERIFICATION, CHECKING, RECONCILIATION, WARNINGS, AND ALERTS

Many important safety processes involve verification of the patient and medication, along with the use of warnings and alerts.[1,6-9,11,28,53,74] This strategy is particularly important in association with high-alert medications. Examples include pharmacist order review, independent double checks, medication reconciliation, smart IV pump limits and warnings or use of precalculated tables for setting i.v. pumps, pharmacy and prescriber computer flags and warnings, dispensing systems that use bar-code drug identification, and machine-readable patient identification. These safety practices are often intended to support caregivers as they work.

STAFFING AND COMPETENCY

The effectiveness and safety of the medication-use system depend highly on individual performance. Adequate numbers of competent staff are critical. Effective orientation and ongoing training, combined with constructive performance assessments, should address competency in drug therapy and in the ability to function safely within the medication-use system. Education of caregivers is a necessary component of any medication-use system improvement[1-4,20,21,50,74]

ENVIRONMENT AND EQUIPMENT

Environmental factors such as space and lighting, clutter, temperature, noise levels, and distractions and interruptions can be modified to support staff performance and reduce errors.

Assessing, controlling, distributing, and maintaining all medical equipment should be an organizational priority.[24,50,53,70,Table 2]

TECHNOLOGIES TO IMPROVE MEDICATION SAFETY

A number of technologies have been designed or adapted to improve medication safety.[75-81] These include pharmacy computers, automated dispensing and drug-preparation technologies, smart IV pumps, CPOE, computer-generated medication administration records, complete electronic medical records, and medication-safety surveillance software. Currently available and emerging technologies have the potential to be extremely useful tools to improve medication safety on many levels. Technologies can improve information availability, transfer, and use. They can enhance communication, teamwork, and decision-support systems. They can also improve work efficiency, identification and verification processes, and monitoring. Despite increasing use of technologies, only limited evidence supporting a positive impact of widespread use on patient safety is available.[31,33,75,79]

The implementation of technologies can be difficult, time-consuming, and, in many cases, costly. Failures in implementation have occurred. As such, the effectiveness of implementation and appropriate ongoing use of any technology will determine the impact on patient safety.[75,80,81] Much of the effort in implementing technologies will involve managing the human-technology interface.

PATIENT INVOLVEMENT

Routine education and continued engagement of patients in their care results in improved medication use, fewer errors, and earlier detection of problems.[24,42,53,70, Table 2] Patients should be educated regarding medication safety and instructed to actively participate in their care and in error-prevention activities. Teaching and encouraging patients and families to communicate issues and concerns with their drug therapy is an effective risk-reduction strategy. Simple patient counseling and education throughout the process often detects and averts errors.

MONITORING SAFETY AND LEARNING FROM ERRORS

Implementing and enhancing medication-safety monitoring and measurement serve a number of functions. On an immediate basis, monitoring and reporting provide an opportunity to improve care, reduce imminent risk to others, and provide a more accurate record of events. In the longer term, robust detection and reporting processes provide an opportunity to learn about medication-safety deficiencies within the organization, identify their causes, and develop prevention strategies and error defenses. Obtaining and assessing information from an effective medication-safety monitoring process will help guide and promote improvements. Data from safety-monitoring and error-reporting programs helps create a culture of safety. Common methods of error analysis include critical incident analysis, root-cause analysis (RCA), theory of constraints, and failure mode and effects analysis (FMEA).[1,24,39,40,53,54,70,82-85]

Implementing Best Medication-Safety Recommendations in Specific Patient Care Settings

The nature and causes of common safety deficiencies in medication-use systems have been well defined. General strategies and specific practices for improving medication safety have been developed and widely recommended (Table 10-2). The goal of many attempting to improve safety is to maximize the safety of current processes. Other improvements may involve system redesign and implementation of new practices, process, and technologies; improving safety reporting and monitoring of systems; or improving the culture of safety and quality within the organization. The Institute for Healthcare Improvement (IHI)[74] recommends that organizations prioritize implementing change in the following areas:

- Develop a culture of safety.

- Decrease risk for harm from high-alert medications.

- Improve the core processes of the medication-use system (prescribing, dispensing, administration).

- Reconcile medication information at multiple points in the care process.

The major challenge to those implementing improvements is to effectively and efficiently change internal processes and hold the gains made. Applying the fundamental aspects of a systems-based, blamefree, collaborative approach to improvement is critical to success.

Implementing specific medication-safety practices begins with identifying a team or group to be responsible for overseeing and leading overall organizational improvements, assessing needs and determining opportunities, establishing priorities, and then choosing specific target processes for improvement.[38] The targets may focus on prevention of medication-use process errors,[39] on preventing injuries from errors,[40] or on both. Different types of targets (i.e., error versus injury focus) may result in similar or very different prevention strategies.

Once a target is chosen, a team with membership chosen specifically to address that target should be formed. This team should start by conducting a systematic and well-informed assessment of the targeted process. This assessment should lead to the development of potential strategies, methods, and plans for improvement. The team should set clear and measurable aims for the proposed changes. The statement should include a quantifiable goal and set time frame for accomplishing the aim (e.g., "We will achieve a 90 percent reduction in use of prohibited abbreviations in three months."). Process stakeholders from a number of perspectives should critically evaluate these plans. The evaluation should include all costs related to the change. Potential for unintended consequences and introduction of new types of errors are then systematically evaluated through methods such as FMEA.[24,84-86] A plan for implementing, communicating, and monitoring the changes is developed and the new processes are implemented. Monitoring of changes allows assessment of impact on safety and identification of problems, issues, and further opportunities for improvement. Once a change has been successfully implemented, follow-up assessment should be performed to monitor continuation of improvements made.

ORGANIZATIONAL NEEDS ASSESSMENT AND IDENTIFICATION OF OPPORTUNITIES FOR IMPROVEMENT

Opportunities for improving the safety of medication use exist in all health care organizations and care settings. Prioritizing improvement efforts is often necessary because of resource constraints, the complexity of most health care systems, and the difficulty and expense of making many large-scale changes at once. The team or individual responsible for medication safety should undertake organizational assessments and set priorities. The areas of focus vary but are usually chosen on the basis of identification of areas with known safety problems or high risk for problems, areas with opportunities for major improvement, or the need for compliance with regulatory, accreditation, or professional standards and guidelines. Internal medication-error reporting and safety-monitoring programs can provide important information regarding the frequency and nature of existing problems. Establishing a culture of safety and promoting error and ADE reporting provide extremely useful information to guide safety efforts.[24,70,82,83] Simple discussions with patients and caregivers often reveal safety-related issues that can be addressed through the process-improvement program.

Systematically assessing an organization's medication-use system in terms of adherence to regulatory requirements, accreditation, and professional standards often identifies areas of noncompliance. The ISMP Medication Safety Self-Assessments[74] and ASHP Practice Standards Self-Assessment [87] are excellent tools for comprehensive evaluation of an organization and identification of opportunities for improvement. The Joint Commission on Accreditation of Healthcare Organizations provides standards, Sentinel Event Alerts, and Patient Safety Goals as recommended or required safety practices.[88,89] A consistent and collective view of the medication-use process and its deficiencies is critical to establish focus, teamwork, and common goals.[55] Many organizations and publications provide recommendations for safe medication practice that can be used to assess an individual care setting or organization. Many organizations participate in collaboratives focusing on medication safety. Such collaboratives provide focus, direction, training, information sharing, and support to those involved in implementing change.[90-93] Organizational self-assessments should occur continuously at all levels of the organization. Effective leadership and coordination at all levels of an organization are necessary to manage the effort and to identify priority targets for improvement. No matter what process-improvement target is chosen, the task needs to be undertaken by an appropriate team, driven by data, and instituted in a well-planned and communicated process.

ESTABLISHING A QUALITY-IMPROVEMENT TEAM FOR SPECIFIC IMPROVEMENTS

Once a specific target medication-use process is identified, a team should be formed to undertake the task of implementing improvements. In all care settings, the medication-use system involves numerous individuals and groups. Collectively, team members should have extensive knowledge about the specific care processes being targeted for improvement. It is also necessary that the team have members who are part of, or have close working relationships with, the caregivers to be affected by any changes implemented. Team members should have appropriate levels of authority and autonomy to serve effectively. Individuals willing to collaborate and who have good communication skills are critical. A mix of members who are broad systems thinkers and those with more narrow patient care delivery perspectives, but with detailed understanding of the specific process targeted, provide creative group dynamics. Including thought leaders, advocates, and champions will vastly improve the chance of success. Individuals with expertise and experience in risk management and quality improvement can help the team stay focused. All team members should be committed to the process. Work teams with responsibility for implementing medication-safety practices typically include pharmacists, nurses, physicians, quality specialists and risk managers, and patient-safety officers. Physicians should be included in the process whenever changes to be implemented will affect their practice or patients. When appropriate, it is critical to include other stakeholders, such as staff from management, finance, human resources, respiratory care, laboratory, information services, medical records, and imaging, as well as patient-care-unit clerks, transporters, and pharmacy technicians. Lines of communication and reporting to management and stakeholders should be clearly established.

STRUCTURED PROCESS-IMPROVEMENT METHODS

When addressing an opportunity for improvement, using an established process-improvement method may be helpful. A number of process-improvement methodologies have been applied to medication safety. Those new to process improvement will find these methods useful in guiding them to reach goals. Such methodologies are also particularly useful when complex or major projects are undertaken. Common improvement methods have many similarities, often approaching the task from slightly different perspectives and with different priorities. Two outcome-focused and data-driven methods are the FOCUS-PDCA Model for Improvement method[94] (also called the Deming method) and the Design for Six Sigma (DFSS) methodology developed at the Motorola Corporation.[95] The Model for Improvement [94] has been used by the Institute for Healthcare Improvement and others.

The FOCUS-PDCA method involves the following steps:

- Finding an opportunity for improvement;
- Organizing to improve–form a team and develop an overall plan;
- Clarifying and understanding the problem;
- Understanding the sources of error and variation; and
- Selecting solutions.

Changes are then implemented and tested in small, incremental steps using multiple Plan-Do-Check-Act (PDCA) cycles.

The DFSS method[95-97] approaches improvement in a highly structured and data-driven way by

- defining what process outcomes need to be addressed and what outcomes should be expected;
- measuring the performance of the current system;
- analyzing the most important factors that drive results and what changes will improve those processes;
- improving and remeasuring each of the important processes; and
- controlling and sustaining the improvement through ongoing measurement and support.

Both methodologies have many common elements. Six sigma methodologies are highly structured and have numerous established tools and defined methods and processes.[96]

Including a team member who has training and experience with structured process-improvement methods may increase the effectiveness of changes made. Developing all team members' knowledge of process-improvement methodologies may be similarly beneficial.[54] Use of process-improvement methodologies will help teams avoid mistakes due to inadequate problem assessment (e.g., jumping to conclusions) and implementing ineffective or even potentially harmful changes. However, to the inexperienced, the application of these methodologies will appear to be time-consuming and overly process-driven. To avoid frustration and avoid unnecessary delay, team members must understand the link between processes and intended outcomes.

UNDERSTANDING THE PROBLEM AND DETERMINING CHANGE STRATEGIES FOR THE TARGETED PROCESS

The first step in evaluating potential medication-use system safety practices is to establish a thorough understanding of the process itself, all the subprocesses, the process context, associated processes, known problems and failures, effective process components, confounding factors, and any other useful considerations. This process should always include discussion with individuals involved in the process. Using standardized approaches, process assessment such as RCA, FMEA,[24,85] DFSS, [95-97] and hazard analysis and critical control point (HACCP) methods[98] will assist in organization and provide a consistently thorough evaluation. Combining knowledge of the process with knowledge of potential change strategies, such as standardization, simplification, constraints, application of technologies, improving communication, and enhancing staff coordination, will identify a set of potential change strategies. For most medication-use processes, a number of potentially effective safety-improvement strategies will be identified. One or more strategies may be chosen. Teams may determine that implementation of a number of simultaneously or sequentially initiated strategies is necessary for aims to be achieved.

Once a change strategy is chosen, it is useful to create a step-by-step description or workflow diagram. Necessary policies and procedures should be drafted. Once the new or revised processes have been delineated, they should be submitted for review by individuals involved with all aspects of the process. These users' input should be evaluated and, when appropriate, incorporated into a revised plan. The revised plan should then again be distributed for review. A number of comment-and-revision cycles may be necessary. The proposed process change may be evaluated using FMEA, DFSS,[97] HACCP,[98] or similar techniques to supplement and enhance other evaluation processes.

Once a final draft is complete, the proposed plan should be presented to all appropriate leadership and staff for comments. Draft policies should be sent to appropriate groups and individuals within the organizations for approval. The product of this team process is a detailed plan for improvement that is ready to be tested through implementation.

ESTABLISHING MEASURES

Measuring the impact of implemented change is a necessary component of any improvement process. Optimally, measurements of outcome, such as a reduction in ADEs or the number of medication errors that reach the patient, are preferred. Because of the many variables involved in preventable ADEs, and the narrow scope of most medication-use improvements, it is unlikely (but not impossible[45,99,100]) that general measures of successful change, such as decreased mortality, length of stay, and overall ADE rates, will provide meaningful information. Measures chosen to monitor changes should reflect the expected specific impact of the process changes and have as few confounding factors as possible. Teams should understand the limitations of most methods for monitoring medication safety. Some steps in the medication process are more easily and accurately measurable than others, and available measurement techniques vary in their utility.[51,52] For example, observational[32,36-38] measurement methods for evaluating drug-administration discrepancies are likely to produce accurate and reproducible results. Medical record reviews that rely on documentation of ADEs or errors are much less reproducible measures.[101, 102]

Because of the nature of medication errors, errors may occur in one step of the process at a high rate but few of them might actually have an impact on the patient. An example would be a team working on reducing dose errors in pediatrics that is measuring the change in the number of detected errors after introduction of a new policy that requires pharmacists to recalculate all doses as a double check. Measures of change may also involve monitoring of processes rather than outcomes. For example, the impact of a policy restricting the use of certain abbreviations can be measured by monitoring the change in the frequency of use of the prohibited abbreviations. A third factor to measure is the creation of unintended consequences and introduction of new errors into the system as changes are made. Such negative consequences of change are often difficult to predict, and as such the monitoring process should be designed to evaluate a wide variety of operational, human factors, and organizational issues that could occur as a result of a change. Monitoring changes should always involve discussion and feedback from all involved in the process.

IMPLEMENTING AND TESTING MEDICATION-SAFETY IMPROVEMENTS

The plan for implementing and testing changes is as important as designing the plan itself. Communication and obtaining cooperation of all involved are critical to success.

The FOCUS-PDCA model stresses the use of small-scale changes prior to wider implementation, with the use of multiple, concurrent, and sequential change-evaluate-revise cycles. When the option exists, partial and small-scale implementation of a planned improvement process is usually preferable to full-scale implementation for a number of reasons. Small-scale implementation allows an opportunity for evaluation of effectiveness and detection of any major problems prior to widespread use and allows careful coordination with those first implementing the change. Revisions can be quickly made. Small-scale success will provide justification for widespread application. Using the PDCA approach, proposed changes (Plan) are implemented on a small scale (Do), assessed (Check), with subsequent changes made based on findings (Act). Small changes in processes implemented using the PDCA model may occur sequentially or concurrently. By performing repeated PDCA cycles, considerable improvements in the medication-use process can be implemented. The PDCA process is particularly applicable to the medication-use process because of its multiple interdependent subcomponents and involvement of multiple individuals. The PDCA method may also reduce risk of any unintended negative consequences of changes. Following successful small-scale PDCA cycles, the process can be adapted in additional medication-use processes or in other parts of the organization. The established measurements of change should be monitored to assess results versus stated aims.

MAINTAINING AND EXPANDING THE GAINS IN SAFETY

The dynamic environment of health systems necessitates the ongoing care and nurturing of medication-system processes. Without such active intervention, many safety processes erode in effectiveness as lessons are forgotten, attention is diverted, bad habits emerge, staff change, competing priorities develop, and new factors emerge. Seldom is a patient-safety problem completely fixed or "solved for good." Practice-improvement initiatives often provide excellent learning opportunities and identify opportunities for additional progress. Further safety improvements should be built on previous successes. Those involved will learn and develop new ways to improve safety.

Expanding successful existing practices or applying successful strategies to new areas and processes is often easier than the initial change. Multiple successful changes teach the staff important lessons in safety and help drive improvements in the culture, further propelling forward the system. Ongoing safety-improvement activities and the communication of successfully implemented initiatives keep patient safety in the minds of the staff. Those responsible for managing the medication-use system should maintain up-to-date knowledge of medication safety and continually apply this knowledge through the organization's established system-based assessment and improvement processes.

Summary

Comprehensive and widely accepted safe medication-use practices are recommended for implementation in all appropriate care settings. Organizational leadership and culture play critical roles in achieving substantive improvements in patient safety. Present safety efforts involve improving the safety of medication-use practices, system redesign, and implementation of new practices and technologies. The ability to measure safety using current medical models of evidence is limited, difficult, and costly, and only a limited number of safety practices have been demonstrated to be effective in controlled clinical trials. Safety practices are primarily based on well-established models of risk reduction rather than on traditional medical standards of evidence. Medication-safety recommendations apply a systems and human factors–based approach to improvement rather than the traditional person approach used in medical care. To be successful, the process by which improvements are introduced should be systematic and data driven. Established process-improvement methodologies are applicable to instituting medication safety in health care organizations. Substantial improvements in medication safety are possible through successful application of available knowledge and tools.

References

1. Kohn L, Corrigan J, Donaldson M, eds. Committee on Quality of Health Care in America. Institute of Medicine. *To Err Is Human Building a Safer Health System* Washington, DC: National Academy Press; 1999.

2. Committee on Quality of Health Care in America, Institute of Medicine. *Crossing the Quality Chasm: A New Health System for the 21st Century.* Washington, DC: National Academy Press; 2001.

3. Board on Health Care Services, Institute of Medicine. Priority Areas for National Action. Transforming Health Care Quality. Washington, DC: National Academy Press; 2003.

4. Committee on Health Professions Education Summit, Institute of Medicine. *Health Profession Education: A Bridge to Quality.* Greiner AC, Knebel E, eds. Washington, DC: National Academy Press; 2003.

5. Knapp KK, Ray MD. A pharmacy response to the Institute of Medicine's 2001 initiative on quality health care. *Am J Health-Syst Pharm.* 2002;59:2443-2450.

6. Leape LL. Error in medicine. *JAMA.* 1994;272:1851-1857.

7. Nolan TW. System change to improve patient safety. *Br Med J.* 2000;320:771-773.

8. Berwick, DM. Not again! Preventing errors lies in redesign—not exhortation. *Br Med J.* 2001;322:247-248.

9. Leape LL, Bates DW, Cullen DJ, et al. Systems analysis of adverse drug events. *JAMA.* 995;274:35-43.

10. Reason JT. *Human Error.* Cambridge, England: Cambridge University Press; 1990.

11. Reason JT. Human error. Models and management. *Br Med J.* 2000;320:768-770.

12. Manasse HR. Not too perfect. Hard lessons and small victories in patient safety. *Am J Health-Syst Pharm.* 2003;60:78-88.

13. Lesar TS. Recommendations for Reducing Medication Errors Medscape Pharmacists Available at: www.medscape.com/Medscape/pharmacists/journal/2000/v01.n04/mph7175.lesa/mph7175.lesa-01.html. Accessed October 21, 2004.

14. National Patient Safety Partnership. Healthcare leaders urge adoption of methods to reduce adverse drug events. Washington, DC: Veterans Administration. May 1, 1999.

15. Barach P, Small SD. Reporting and preventing medical mishaps: lessons from non-medical near miss reporting systems. *Br Med J.* 2000;320:759-763.

16. Helmreich RL. On error management: lessons from aviation. *Br Med J.* 2000;320:781-785.

17. Gaba DM. Structural and organizational issues in patient safety: a comparison of health care with other high-hazard industries. *Calif Manage Rev.* 2000;43:1-20.

18. Schneider PJ. Applying human factors in improving medication-use safety. *Am J Health-Syst Pharm.* 2002;59:1155-1159.

19. Gosbee JW, Anderson T. Human factors engineering design demonstrations can enlighten your RCA team. *Qual Safety Health Care.* 2003;12:119-121.

20. Grasha AT. Into the abyss: seven principles for identifying the causes of and preventing human errors in complex systems *Am J Health-Syst Pharm.* 2000;57:554-564.

21. Grasha AT. Human factors annotated checklist/Version3. Available at: www.pharmsafety.net/articles.htm. Accessed September 10, 2003.

22. Allard J, Carthey J, Pitt M, Woodward S. Medication errors: causes, prevention and reduction. *Brit J Hematol.* 2002;116:755-765.

23. Brushwood DB. Pharmacy practice guidelines for medication error prevention. Available at: www.cop.ufl.edu/safezone/root/programs/ce/MedErr-2hr/Introduction-1.htm Accessed September 18, 2003.

24. Cohen MR, ed. *Medication Errors.* Washington, DC: American Pharmaceutical Association; 1999.

25. Summerfield MR, Lawrence T. Rethinking approaches to reducing medication errors: an examination of 10 core processes. *Formulary.* 2002;37:462-472.

26. Cipolle RJ, Strand LM, Morley PC. *Pharmaceutical Care Practice.* New York: McGraw Hill; 1998.

27. Cohen M. Prescription for safety in health care. *Am J Health-Syst Pharm.* 2002;59:1311-1317.

28. Fortescue EB, Kaushal R, Androgen CP, et al. Prioritizing strategies for preventing medication errors and adverse events in pediatric inpatients. *Pediatrics.* 2003;111:722-729.

29. Beckwith M, Tyler L. Preventing medication errors with antineoplastic agents. *Hosp Pharm*

(parts 1 and 2) 2002;35:511-525 and 732-749.

30. Schiff GD, Klass D, Peterson J, et al. Linking laboratory and pharmacy. Opportunities for reducing errors and improving care. *Arch Intern Med.* 2003;163:893-900.

31. Bates DW, Gawanda AA. Improving patient safety with information technology. *N Engl J Med.* 2003;348:2526-2534.

32. Allan EL, Barker KN. Fundamentals of medication error research. *Am J Hosp Pharm.* 1990;47:555-571.

33. Shojania KC, Duncan BW, McDonald KM, Watcher R, eds. Making Health Safer: A Critical Analysis of Patient Safety Practices. Evidence Report/ Technology Assessment No. 43. Rockville, MD: Agency for Healthcare Research and Quality. 2001. AHRQ publication 01-E058.

34. Shojania KC. Duncan BW, McDonald KM, Wachter RM. Safe but sound. Patient safety meets evidence-based medicine. *JAMA.* 2002;288:508-513.

35. Leape LL, Berwick DM, Bates DW. What practices will most improve safety? Patient safety meets evidence-based medicine. *JAMA.* 2002;288:501-507.

36. Taxis K, Barber N. Ethnographic study of incidence and severity of intravenous drug errors. *Br Med J.* 2003;226:684-687.

37. Allen-Flynn E, Barker KN, Carnahan BJ. National observation study of prescription dispensing accuracy and safety in 50 pharmacies. *J Am Pharm Assoc.* 2003;43:191-200.

38. Allan-Flynn E, Pearson RE, Barker K. Observational study of accuracy in compounding IV admixtures at five hospitals. *Am J Health-Syst Pharm.* 1997;54:904-912.

39. McNutt RA, Abrams R, Aron DC. Patient safety efforts should focus on medical errors. *JAMA.* 2002;287:1997-2001.

40. Layde PM, Maas LA, Teret SP, et al. Patient safety efforts should focus on medical injuries. *JAMA.* 2002;287:1993-1997.

41. Barker KN, Flynn EA, Pepper G, et al. Medication errors observed in 36 health care facilities. *Arch Intern Med.* 2002;162:1897-1903.

42. Ghandi TK, Weingart SN, Borus J, et al. Adverse drug events in ambulatory care. *N Engl J Med.* 2003;348:1556-1564.

43. Bates DW, Cullen DJ, Laird N, et al. Incidence of adverse drug events and potential adverse drug events. Implications for prevention. *JAMA.* 1995;274:29-34.

44. Bates DW, Miller EB, Cullen DJ, et al. Patient risk factors for ADEs in hospitalized patients. *Arch Intern Med.* 1999;159:253-260.

45. Leape LL, Cullen DJ, Clapp MD, et al. Pharmacist participation on physician rounds and adverse drug events in the intensive care unit. *JAMA.* 1999;282:267-270.

46. Forster AJ, Murff HJ, Peterson JF, Gandhi TK, Bates DW. The incidence and severity of adverse events affecting patients after discharge from the hospital. *Ann Intern Med.* 2003;138:161-167.

47. Gurwitz G, Field TS, Harrold HR, et al. Incidence and preventability of adverse drug events among older persons in the ambulatory setting. *JAMA.* 2003;289:1107-1116.

48. Gurwitz JH, Field TS, Avorn J, et. al. Incidence and preventability of adverse drug events in nursing homes. *Am J Med.* 2000;109:87-94.

49. Kaushal R, Bates DW, Landrigan R, et al. Medication errors and adverse drug events pediatric inpatients. *JAMA.* 2001;285:2114-2120.

50. Dean B, Schachter M, Vincent D, Barber B. Causes of prescribing error in hospital inpatients: a prospective study. *Lancet.* 2002;359:373-378.

51. Measuring medication safety in hospitals. *Am J Health-Syst Pharm.* 2002;59:2313-2336.

52. Measuring Medication Safety in Hospitals. Report of an Invitational Conference on Measuring Medication Safety in Hospitals; April 5-9, 2002; Tucson, AZ, Available at www.latiolais.org. Accessed December 9, 2004.

53. Institute for Safe Medication Practices. Medication Safety Self-Assessment. Huntingdon, PA: Institute for Safe Medication Practices; 2004. Available at: www.ismp.org. Accessed October 10, 2004.

54. Pathways for Medication Safety. Leading a strategic planning effort. Available at: www.hospitalconnect.com/medpathways/tools/content/Section_1.pdf. Accessed September 18, 2003.

55. Pathways for Medication Safety. Looking at risk collectively. Available at: www.hospital connect.com/medpathways/tools/content/Section_2.pdf. Accessed September 18, 2003.

56. Lamb RM, Studdert DM, Bohmer RM, Berwick DM, Brennan TA. Hospital disclosure practices. Results of a national survey.

Health Affairs. 2003;22:243-254.

57. Marx D. Safety and the "just culture": A primer for health care executives. 2001. Available at: www.mers-tm.net/support/marxxprimer.pdf. Accessed July 2003.

58. Ryan KD. Driving fear out of the medication-use process so that improvement can occur. *Am J Heath-Syst Pharm.* 1999;56:1765-1769.

59. Runciman WB, Merry AF, Tito F. Error, blame, and the law in health care—an antipodean perspective. *Ann Intern Med.* 2003;138:974-979.

60. Rosner FR, Berger JT, Kark P, Bennett AJ. Disclosure and prevention of medical errors. *Arch Intern Med.* 2002;160;2089-2092.

61. Robinson AR, Hohmann KB, Rifkin JL. Physician and public opinions on the quality of healthcare and the problem of medical errors. *Arch Intern Med.* 2002;162;2186-2190.

62. Gallagher TH, Waterman AD, Ebers AC, Fraser VJ, Levinson W. Patients' and physicians' attitudes regarding the disclosure of medical errors. *JAMA.* 2003;289:1001-1007.

63. Blendon RJ, DesRoches CM, Brodie M, et al. Views of practicing physicians and the public on medical errors. *N Engl J Med.* 2002;347:1933-1940.

64. Hibbard JH, Stockard J, Tusler M. Does publicizing hospital performance stimulate quality improvement efforts? *Health Affairs.* 2003;22:84-94.

65. Shaller D, Sofaer S, Findlay SD, Hibbard JH, Lansky D, Delbanco S. Consumer and quality driven health care: a call to action. *Health Affairs.* 2003;22:95-100.

66. Bates DW, Gawande AA, Error in medicine: what have we learned? *Ann Intern Med.* 2000;132:763-766.

67. Weeks WB, Bagian JP. Developing a culture of safety in the Veterans Health Administration. *Eff Clin Pract.* 2000;3:270-276.

68. Reinertsen JI. Let's talk about error. *Br Med J.* 2000;320:730.

69. Bagian J, Lee C, Gosbee J, et al. Developing and deploying a patient safety program in a large health delivery system: you can't fix what you don't know about. *Jt Comm J Qual Improve.* 2001;27:527-532.

70. American Society of Health Systems Pharmacists. Medication-Use System Safety Strategy (MS³). Available at: www.ashp.org. Accessed September 10, 2003.

71. Rozich JD, Resar RK. Medication safety: one organization's approach to the challenge. *J Clin Outcome Manage.* 2001;8:27-34.

72. Goldmann D, Kaushal R. Time to tackle tough issues in patient safety. *Pediatrics.* 2002;110:823-826.

73. Silverman JB, Stapinski CD, Churchill WW, Neppl C, Bates DW, Gandhi TK. Multifaceted approach to reducing preventable adverse drug events. *Am J Health-Syst Pharm.* 2003;60:582-586.

74. The Institute for Healthcare Improvement. Available at:www.ihi.org/IHI/Topics/Patient Safety/MedicationSystems. Accessed September 10, 2003.

75. Oren E, Shaffer ER, Guglielmo J. Impact of technology on medication errors and adverse events. *Am J Health-Syst Pharm.* 2003;60:1447-1458.

76. Neuenschwander M, Cohen MR, Vaida AJ, Patchett JA, Kelly J, Trohimovich B. Practical guide to bar coding for patient medication safety. *Am J Health-Syst Pharm.* 2003;60:768-779.

77. Schiff GD. Computerized prescriber order entry: models and hurdles. *Am J Health-Syst Pharm.* 2002;59:1456-1460.

78. First Consulting Group. Computerized physician order entry: costs, benefits and challenges. A case study approach. Prepared for the American Hospital Association and the Federation of American Hospitals. January 2003. Available at: www.aha.org. Accessed September 30, 2003.

79. Kuperman GJ, Gibson R. Computer physician order entry: Benefits, costs, and issues. *Ann Intern Med.* 2003;139:31-39.

80. Kelly K, Cohen M. Smetzer J. Optimizing computer systems for medication safety. *ISMP Medication Safety Alert.* Community/Ambulatory Care. 2003;2(7):1-2.

81. American Society of Health-System Pharmacists. CPOE, bedside technology, and patient safety: A roundtable discussion. *Am J Health-Syst Pharm.* 2003;60:1219-1928.

82. Vincent C. Analysis of critical events. *N Engl J Med.* 2003;348:1051-1056.

83. Leape LL. Reporting of adverse events. *N Engl J Med.* 2002;347:1633-1838.

84. DeRosier , Stalhandske E, Bagian JP, Nudell T. Using health care failure mode and effects analysis: a VA National Center for Patient Safety's prospective risk analysis system. *Joint Comm J Qual Improve.* 2002;28:248-267.

85. Cohen MR, Senders J, Davis NM. Failure mode and effects analysis: a novel approach to avoiding dangerous medication errors and accidents. *Hosp Pharm.* 1994;29:319-330.

86. Hieb B, Stumpf J. Improving patient safety through expert knowledge and critical knowledge and critical healthcare decision support. Available at: www.misys.com. Accessed July 15, 2003.

87. American Society of Health-System Pharmacists. Best Practices Self-Assessment Tool. Available at:www.ashp.org/practicemanager/self-assessment.cfm. Accessed September 10, 2003.

88. Joint Commission on Accreditation of Healthcare Organizations. 2004 Patient Safety Goals. Oak Brook, IL: JCAHO. Available at: www.jcaho.org. Accessed September 10, 2003.

89. Joint Commission on Accreditation of Healthcare Organizations. 2004 Medication Management Standards.Oak Brook, IL: JCAHO. Available at: www. jcaho.org. Accessed September 10, 2003.

90. Leape LL, Kabcenell AI, Gandhi TK, Carver P, Nolan TW, Berwick DM. Reducing adverse drug events: lessons from a breakthrough series collaborative. *Joint Comm J Qual Improve.* 2000;26:321-331.

91. Farbstein K,, Clough J. Improving medication safety across a multihospital system. *Jt Comm J Qual Improve.* 2001;27:123-137.

92. Lesar T, Mattis A, Anderson E, Avery J, Fields J, Gregoire J, Vaida A.Using the ISMP Medication Safety Self-Assessment to improve medication use processes. *Jt Comm J Qual Safety.* 2003;29:211-226.

93. Voelker R. Hospital collaborative creates tools to help reduce medication errors. *JAMA.* 2001;286:3067-3070.

94. The Institute for Healthcare Improvement. How to improve. Available at: www.ihi.org/IHI/Topics/PatientSafety/Medication Systems/HowToImprove. Accessed July 15, 2003.

95. Hicks, J. Six sigma—PDCA on steroids? Available at: healthcare.isixsigma.com/library/content/c030624a.asp. Accessed September 14, 2003.

96. Kooy MV, Edell L, Melchiorre Sceckner H. Use of six sigma to improve safety and efficacy of acute anticoagulation with heparin. *J Clin Outcome Manage.* 2002;9:445-453.

97. Simon K. What is DFSS? And how does design for six sigma compare to DMAIC? Available at: healthcare.isixsigma.com/library/content/c020722a.asp. Accessed September 15, 2003.

98. Food and Drug Administration, Hazard Analysis and Critical Control Point (HACCP). Available at:vm.cfsan.fda.gov/~lrd/haccp.html. Accessed September 10, 2003.

99. Raschke RA, Gollihare B, Wunderlich TA, Guidry JR, Leibowitz AI, Peirce JC et al. A computer alert system to prevent injury from adverse drug events. *JAMA.* 1998;280:1317-1320.

100. Kucukarslan SN, Peters M, Mlynarek M, Nafziger DA. Pharmacists on rounding teams reduce preventable adverse drug events in hospital general medicine units. *Arch Intern Med.* 2003;163:2014-2018.

101. Voluntary Hospitals of America. Monitoring ADE: Finding the needle in the haystack. Irving, TX: VHA Inc; 2002.

102. The Institute for Healthcare Improvement. Trigger Tool for measuring ADE. Available at: www.ihi.org/qhc/workspace/tools/trigger. Accessed September 10, 2003.

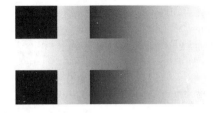

CHAPTER 11

The Role of Effective Communication in Health Care Delivery Systems

C. J. Biddle

Introduction

Today's health care delivery system may be the most complex integrated system imaginable, and it likely poses greater safety challenges than does any other human activity on the planet. The reasons for this are wide-ranging and are discussed in detail elsewhere in this book. Fundamental to the success (efficiency, efficacy, safety) of any complex system involving humans is communication, which is the focus of this chapter.

Although I had worked in clinical anesthesia since 1980, my own epiphany relating to patient safety did not occur until 1991, when I read a Harvard study reporting that 4 percent of hospital admissions in New York State resulted in iatrogenesis.[1] Of those admissions, 70 percent resulted in minor or temporary disability, but in 7 percent of the patients, the resultant disability was permanent and in 14 percent, the iatrogenesis either caused or contributed to patient death. This was but the first of numerous subsequent reports,[2-4] capped by an Institute of Medicine text,[5] that fueled my interest in patient safety and helped form my current clinical, teaching, and research pursuits.

Traditional and modern approaches to system design have relied on requiring individuals to engage in errorfree performance. When that level of performance is not achieved, punishment in some form or another usually results, and a feedback loop evolves that actively, or passively, discourages undesirable or unsafe practice. Although still in widespread use in medicine, this approach is no longer employed by industries such as nuclear power and commercial aviation, whose business is to do business safely.

Fundamental to making patient care safer is rethinking and redesigning the component systems within health care delivery so that errors are harder to make and that errors that do occur are buffered so that they have the least-possible impact on the patient. Creating a culture of safety, as Turnbull notes elsewhere in this volume, is essential to this process: The goal is to create a climate in which risk reduction and medication-misadventure prevention are recognized as everyone's responsibility. Central to this is an understanding of the importance of open, respectful communication among patients and providers within the system.

Connecting the Silos of Health Care

In its April 2, 2004 issue, *U.S. News & World Report* ranked the department in which I work as the

163

number-one graduate program in the nation in its discipline. We have highly active research, clinical, and teaching programs in place, yet intradepartmental collaboration and communication are virtually nonexistent. I often feel that I am in a silo akin to those that house underground ballistic missiles or that store grain or feed for farm animals. One might assume that a respected program such as ours would be characterized by a lot of collaboration and communication with other successful (or even less-successful) programs. In reality, such communication rarely occurs.

The medical center of which we are a part is a complex system of departments and divisions, of clinics and treatment areas, of laboratories and specialty diagnostic centers, of drug-processing and drug-distribution complexes, of administration offices, and of legions of support offices and facilities. More often than not, this complex takes on the appearance of a mass of silos, where integration or connections among the different areas are tenuous, sporadic, or even absent (see **Figure 11-1**).

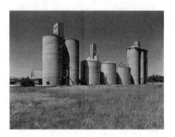 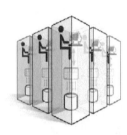

Like the silos seen in agriculture or industry, health care systems are plagued with numerous "silos" where vertical information sharing occurs (within a department or unit) but where horizontal exchange among different departments or units does not.

Figure 11-1. The "silos" of health care.

There is little doubt to the educated mind that pitfalls in communication are major players in medical errors and misadventures. Systems designed to facilitate effective and timely communication among the stakeholders within the health care delivery process are crucial to reducing error. Such systems must promote communication among physicians, nurses, administrators, and staff of labs, pharmacies, and other components of the delivery universe.

In the wake of the 2003 Columbia space shuttle catastrophe, National Aeronautics and Space Administration officials, scientists, technicians, and other "insiders" were noteworthy in their willingness to share information. The resultant flushing out of details of what took place enabled the agency to quickly orchestrate an investigation and, it is hoped, to help ensure that future missions would not experience the same fate. Remarkably absent from this process was any finger-pointing, guilt-assigning behavior. This most certainly contributed to the rapid detection of the source of the problem, which was insulating-foam fragments that broke off from the external fuel tank and struck and compromised the integrity of the shuttle wing surface.

A recent example of an active campaign to facilitate intradepartmental communication— and connecting those silos in an efficient and timely manner within a complex health care environment—is the DocLink™ system, which was installed at Barnes-Jewish Hospital in St. Louis.[6] DocLink is a Web, Internet, or institutional communication tool that electronically manages scheduling, physicians' orders, and medical and nursing interventions by automating communication between physicians, staff, and hospitals. Such a system, by prompting communication-based interactions among patients, medical, nursing, laboratory, and pharmacy personnel, facilitates patient interventions and enhances outcomes. This system has great relevance to the clinical pharmacist; for example, it has been shown to produce a substantial reduction in cycle time (time from drug-order start to drug-order stop) and significant improvement in pharmacists' response time. The authors of this report note that use of simplified, effective information-dissemination processes could save thousands of lives annually.[6]

Systems designed to enhance the routing, sharing, and dissemination of patient care–related communication are critical to any effort to improve patient safety and health outcomes. The domain of communication is sufficiently important that it is a specified research and funding objective for the Agency for Healthcare Research and Quality in its effort to promote and improve patient safety.[5]

Individual Leadership Responsibility

Early in their studies, physics and chemistry students learn that diffusion occurs down a concentration gradient. In examining a material that exists at two concentrations, separated only by a diffusible biological membrane, students discover that molecular diffusion occurs from the area of greater concentration to that of lower concentration. Eventually, equilibrium is achieved, and the concentration of the material exists in a balanced fashion on both sides of the membrane. Until equilibrium is reached, flow is unidirectional.

This experience can serve as a metaphor for the health care system. In this metaphor, let the word *power* (of the individuals within the system) replace the word *concentration* (of the chemical or material). In systems where there are few obstacles to the flow of information, regardless of the power gradient, information freely disseminates in all directions.

Open communication, like any other domain of knowledge or set of skills, is not something that one should presume to be present. Likewise, if it is not present, one should not presume that it is impossible to achieve. Individuals within an organization can be taught to communicate more effectively. The concept of "stakeholder" comes to mind, that is, one who has an interest, or stake, in the outcome. Stakeholders in a health care organization include patients, providers, administrators, and technicians—in fact, everyone within the system is a stakeholder. By virtue of that designation, everyone within the organization has a stake in the communication domain.

Case in point: We generally think of aircraft pilots (whether civilian or military) as being "take charge," "no nonsense," "rule by fiat" types. Yet senior pilots, whether flying an F-15 Eagle over Iraq or a Boeing 737 over Missouri, are taught to invite others to communicate safety concerns to them. Junior members of flight teams in both the civilian and military sectors are assigned the responsibility of communicating information about performance and safety concerns to their superiors; they are not forced to adhere to any preconceived or preexistent "power/concentration" gradient. Senior pilots are obliged to respond to concerns that are raised. If a senior pilot is challenged twice about a safety concern without providing a satisfactory reply, the junior team member is empowered to take over the controls of the craft.

Transferring that philosophical orientation to the health care environment is not an easy task. Regardless of whether the environment is academic, private, community, for-profit, or not for-profit, there are historical and cultural roots that ground the power and communication pathways in a somewhat turgid and inflexible manner.

Intimidation

Intimidation is a pervasive phenomenon in the workplace. It is not at all uncommon for physicians to make errors in prescribing drugs. The errors may occur because they have misinterpreted published materials or because of misprints in otherwise highly reliable references. A recent case illustrates the point.

A new pharmacist received an order for "Fluorouracil 4,100 mg to be administered over 12 hours for 8 doses covering 4 days." Recognizing the overdose, she contacted the physician. His response was hostile, and he refused to change the order. He cited the article that he had used as a reference and became verbally abusive to the pharmacist.

This pharmacist encountered a physician whose ego and anger overwhelmed both his judgment and communication. Only through the intervention of the pharmacist's manager and the institution's chief of staff was a potentially fatal dose of fluorouracil avoided. Later, when the reference cited by the physician was checked, it was determined that it had incorrectly listed the four-day cumulative dose as the recommended daily dose.

Most of us can attest to the role of intimidation as a barrier to patient safety. An atmosphere of intimidation restricts the ability of the system to detect, acknowledge, and correct mistakes before they reach the patient. There is no place for intimidating behaviors in this domain. Those who justify abusive behaviors as a form of punishment for those who err are seriously misguided. Intimidating or abusive behaviors promote stress and job dissatisfaction and lead to employee resentment and turnover. Such behavior promotes miscommunication of its own, which may further jeopardize patient outcomes. Workplace intimidation is so serious and so pervasive a problem that it should be proactively dealt with in institutional and departmental policies and procedures. It should be discussed at staff orientation and be on the agenda at ongoing departmental meetings.

The example just cited illustrates the essential role of effective communication in health care. Interestingly, in other complex industries, such as aviation, nuclear power, and assembly line manufacturing, expressing concerns about safety does not put the individual or individuals who raise the issue on the defensive. Once voiced, a safety concern is considered real until proved otherwise. The "two-challenge rule" is a reasonable and effective methodology to employ in assessing safety risks. Under this rule, if a concern (and the basis for the concern) is voiced twice without being resolved, then the matter is automatically referred to a third party. This avoids ego-dominated situations in which a "win/lose" attitude drives the equation and ensures an objective review before any decision is made.

The Art and Science of Getting the Right Medication to the Right Patient

While medication errors are often preventable, reducing error rates in a meaningful and sustained way involves a number of interventions directed at the many layers of the process. The often-quoted study of Lesar et al.[7] revealed that failure in the knowledge of drug therapy, knowledge of patient factors, calculation factors, and nomenclature accounted for the majority of medication errors. Poor transfer of information within and among places where care is provided is an important and correctable contributor to adverse events.

The problem is compounded by the communication chasm that exists in many settings. Emergency department (ED) care is fertile ground for medication-related errors because of many factors described elsewhere in this text. Among these are care providers who routinely encounter patients in a random, happenstance manner, limitations in accessing background information in a comprehensive fashion, and dealing simultaneously with acute, life-threatening problems, such as a gunshot wound, as well myriad preexisting issues, such as asthma, hypertension, or diabetes.

In the ED, screening for drug interactions is rarely routine. In one study, 47 percent of visits to an ED resulted in adding at least one medication to the patient's drug regimen, and 10 percent of these changes resulted in an order for a drug that had a significant potential for an adverse drug interaction.[8]

It is clear that the complexities and potential problems associated with decision making in health care are enhanced by poor communication. The patient record is one readily available, relevant information source. Informatics has evolved to the extent that comprehensive, user-friendly patient information in an electronic, computerized system is accessible. Traditional manual systems are often sloppy, do not promote information sharing, and are time-intensive; information is often lost, illegible, or misfiled. Patient-centered, computerized clinical information systems linking all relevant health care providers and domains are practical, economical, and effective.

Getting It Right—Good Communication as a Goal

Quality communication is essential to the delivery of quality health care, but it would be naïve to view communication in this setting as anything but highly complex. Communication is determined by the coordinated perceptions of two or more individuals; as such, it appears seductively easy to achieve. When we experience a communication failure, we are often surprised, and finger-pointing or blame shedding often results. Poor transfer and application of knowledge between and among the players responsible for delivering health care is a contributor to adverse events.

Because communication is a human enterprise, simple solutions rarely do justice to its complexities. One approach to improving communications would be to recruit only individuals with manifest communication skills. This is rarely considered in candidates applying for medical, nursing, pharmacy, laboratory, or administrative educational programs in our country. In Australia, however, concern about improving communication among health care workers is such that a national task force has recommended that incentives be instituted to ensure that educators assess students' communication skills at the same level as they do their cognitive skills.[9]

Building an Effective Team Environment

Even the modest sports enthusiast recognizes that a group of athletes playing football or basketball is much different from a team of players. Even when its members have shared objectives, a group is much less effective than a team, whose members make a collective effort to focus on decisions and interventions that will optimize the possibility for the desired outcome.

Several principles have emerged from recent research in teamwork theory that have direct application to health care.[10-13] Among the most important principles are the following:

- Teamwork skills are highly identifiable and can be taught, learned, and assessed.
- Although there are common attributes across disciplines, specific teamwork interventions must be tailored to the environment in which the work is to be accomplished.
- Communication and monitoring are essential team actions that enable the generation as well as the efficient exchange of information.
- A team setting is the ideal context within which to detect, minimize, and manage human- and technology-related error.

The delivery of health care involves large numbers of individuals making complicated decisions and engaging in complex, and often dangerous, interventions, all with the common objective of enhancing patient outcome. Achieving this objective requires teamwork, yet the involved individuals are unlikely to have had any training in effective team dynamics.

An excellent template for such teaching comes from my own discipline of anesthesia care. It is a model that has borrowed heavily from lessons learned in the aviation industry. The process of crew resource management training, used in the airline industry, is the foundation for anesthesia crisis management training that is employed extensively in training programs nationwide, including our program at Virginia Commonwealth University.[14] This approach employs simulations that reenact real-world events and allows for a follow-up debriefing dialogue with experienced clinicians in which everyone can reflect on what took place.

While difficult to study as an independent risk-management approach, this training has contributed meaningfully to the patient-safety advances that have been observed in the delivery of surgical anesthesia care. A similar program, designed specifically for ED workers, is the MedTeams approach, which focuses on educating providers and support staff working in that setting.[11]

Our patients have the right to expect that all known information relevant to their care is immediately accessible to everyone involved in decisions concerning that care. This necessitates the coordination of communication among the stakeholders involved in the patient's care. If this is to occur, incentives must be built into our system that encourage, rather than impede or distort, information flow. The best approach to this is through enhancement of communication skills through active team training. Furthermore, attention must be given to promoting thoughtful human collaboration with electronic, computerized technology that not only enhances but also safeguards information exchange.

References

1. Brennan TA, Leape LL, Laird NM, Hebert L, Localio AR, Lawthers AG, et al. Incidence of adverse events and negligence in hospitalized patients. *N Engl J Med.* 1991;324:370-376.

2. Kahn KL. Above all, "Do no harm." How shall we avoid errors in medicine? *JAMA.* 1995;274:75-76.

3. Leape LL. Error in medicine. *JAMA.* 1994;272:1851-1857.

4. Bogner MS, ed. *Human Error in Medicine.* Hillsdale, NJ: Lawrence Erlbaum Assoc; 1998.

5. Kohn LT, Corrigan JM, Donaldson MD, eds. Committee on Quality of Health in America, Institute of Medicine. *To Err Is Human: Building a Safer Health System.* Washington, DC: National Academy Press; 1999.

6. Balas EA, Weingarten S, Garb CT, Blumenthal D, Boren SA, Brown GD. Improving preventive care by prompting physicians. *Arch Intern Med.* 2000;160:301-308.

7. Lesar TS, Briceland L, Stein DS. Factors related to errors in medication prescribing. *JAMA.* 1997;277:312-317.

8. Beers MH, Storrie M, Lee G. Potential adverse drug interactions in the emergency room. *Ann Intern Med.* 1990;112:61-64.

9. Department of Health and Ageing. Government of Australia. Improving communication. Available at: www.health.gov.au/pubs/hlthcare/ch4/improv.htm. Accessed October 14, 2004.

10. Katzenbach JR, Roberts DK. The discipline of teams. *Harvard Business Review.* 1993;71:111-120.

11. Risser DT, Simon R, Rice MM, et al. A structured teamwork system to reduce clinical errors. In: Spath PL, ed. *Error Reduction in Healthcare.* San Francisco: Jossey-Bass; 1999:234-278.

12. Risser DT, Rice MM, Salisbury ML, et al. The potential to improved teamwork to reduce medical errors in the emergency department. *Ann Emerg Med.* 1999;34:373-383.

13. Sexton JB, Thomas EJ, Helmreich RL. Error, stress and teamwork in medicine and aviation: cross-sectional surveys. *Br Med J.* 2000;320:745-749.

14. Gaba DM, Fish KJ, Howard SK. *Crisis Management in Anesthesiology.* Philadelphia: Churchill Livingstone; 1994.

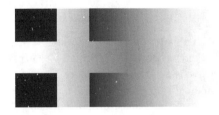

Designing an Internal Reporting and Learning System

David N. Gragg

Introduction

The fundamental purpose of medical-error reporting systems is to prevent future errors. The primary goal of voluntary reporting of medical errors should be to learn how to improve the health quality and enhance patient safety. Reports of errors and near misses by frontline practitioners may be seen as strengths of such programs when report analysis and communication lead to prevention of similar occurrences. Reporting, in other words, is a learning process. The public interest will be served if protection is granted to individuals who submit reports to voluntary reporting programs.[1]

Why take time to document a mistake for which *we* may have been at fault? Health professionals face this question every day. The purpose of this chapter is to help answer it. The chapter reviews the voluntary reporting of medication-related errors, the barriers to compliance with voluntary reporting, the goals of voluntary reporting, and the attributes of functional error-reporting systems. As will be seen, capturing valuable information in a nonpunitive atmosphere and ensuring the appropriate use of that information are the goals of a voluntary reporting system. The chapter concludes with a discussion of the current system and the reasons and rationale for its current operation.

So why report? To begin with, patient and medication safety is front-page news. Recommendation 5.2 of the Institute of Medicine (IOM) report *To Err Is Human: Building a Safer Health System* states that "the development of voluntary reporting efforts should be encouraged."[2] The IOM's best-practice recommendations suggest the need to "improve voluntary reporting of adverse drug events and near misses." The report outlines two important functions served by reporting systems. First, they hold providers accountable for performance; second, they can provide information that leads to improved safety.[2]

This chapter, although not inclusive, describes the basic challenges, thought processes, and decisions that are among my responsibilities as medication-safety officer at The Cleveland Clinic Foundation (CCF). CCF is a 1,000+-bed, multidisciplinary academic medical center and a national referral center. The Cleveland Clinic (CC) has more than 1,400 physicians, representing 120 specialties and subspecialties, on staff. The CCF has a partnership affiliation with nine community hospitals through the Cleveland Clinic Health System (CCHS). The procedures and issues described here are based mainly on experiences and reporting methods observed at the CCF.

Goals of a Voluntary Reporting System

Voluntary reporting systems can be designed to accomplish a variety of functions. They can be designed to capture only errors or events that are defined as "potential" errors, i.e., near misses or errors that do not cause harm. Systems exclusively designed to capture nursing medical administration record (MAR) and pharmacy medication profile discrepancies are largely of this type. Systems can also be designed to capture only those errors that cause harm.

Thus, institutions must first determine what they expect to accomplish with their systems. Is the objective to capture every event happening within the institution or only events that may affect inpatients? Is it acceptable to exclude certain patient groups, such as those in the emergency department, surgery, or radiology?

Regardless of the type of reporting system an institution elects to design and implement, there are several common goals that any reporting system must address in order to be of value. While this list is not exclusive, these goals helped define our system road map at CCF. Four of the most important goals are discussed in the paragraphs that follow.

TO CREATE REAL-TIME REPORTING, I.E., TO CAPTURE EVENTS AND ALLOW THEM TO BE REPORTED IN A TIMELY MANNER

Before we implemented our reporting system, one of the biggest roadblocks to effective error-event analysis was timing. Suppose, for example, that an error occurred on the first of the month. The involved unit would then generate a paper report, which would eventually end up on the unit manager's desk. From there, the report would be mailed to the risk management or quality office (most likely for categorization purposes). Only then would the report reach my attention.

This process took at least three weeks; often it could take four or five weeks. By that time, the facts surrounding the event were no longer fresh in the reporter's mind, and finding the employees involved was a task in itself. Two of the most important goals of analyzing any error report are to identify steps to correct the error and to report this information to the affected staff members promptly. Timely reporting involves the identification of roadblocks that may facilitate the timely transfer of information to the appropriate people.

TO MAXIMIZE THE QUALITY OF DATA IN EACH REPORT

A report is only as good as the data that it contains. Voluntary reports often suffer because the information reported is limited; only the easiest data fields have been completed. As a result, essential information may be missing. For example, a report may include only the name of the patient and perhaps the medical record number, unit, and bed space, which are required fields in any report. The medication name and class, as well as a description of the event, are missing. Monthly discussions by the medication-systems committee in the nine hospitals in our system have revealed that this is one of the biggest roadblocks to effective voluntary reporting.

To remedy this problem, voluntary reporting systems must be designed to allow an individual to report all requested and needed data easily and in a timely fashion. An advanced degree in computer processing should not be required. Going hand in hand with receiving timely error information is receiving as much information as possible.

TO MINIMIZE THE ROLE OF THE INDIVIDUAL INVOLVED AND TO EMPHASIZE THE IMPORTANCE OF SYSTEM-RELATED CAUSES

Providers will be reluctant to report if they fear retribution. Reporters must feel that they are providing needed information and that reporting an event is not synonymous with being linked with having caused it. Only if reporting the event and responsibility for causing it are separated will a complete exchange of information be possible. Tips for creating a nonpunitive atmosphere are discussed below.

TO IDENTIFY DEFICIENCIES IN MEDICATION-USE SYSTEMS AND ALLOW SAFER SYSTEMS TO BE DESIGNED

Manasse[3] has written, "One cannot argue with the fact that reporting provides data, and that data—not merely stored, but applied, data—drive discovery, understanding, and improvement. Deficiencies in medication-use systems cause medication-related errors. Safer systems result from planning and analysis. To build a safer system one needs to know what the current problems are and where they exist. To reiterate . . . data—not merely stored, but applied, data—drive discovery, understanding, and improvement."

What good is collecting information if it is not going to be used in a constructive method to prevent other errors or events? Too many times, we create reports for reports' sake. With no offense to, and in complete support of, my colleagues at the Joint Commission on Accreditation of Healthcare Organizations (JCAHO), I have heard a colleague say, "We're collecting this information for JCAHO," with no mention of its relevance to patient care, far too many times. I would have liked to have seen an equal amount of time dedicated to preventing medication errors as there was devoted to recording and graphing the temperature of our institution's refrigerators.

If data are not going to be reviewed, analyzed, and constructively used, there is no reason to collect it. Even monthly medication-error reports, detailing only when and where events occur, are underused if not evaluated.

Institutions must make a commitment to identify resources in every department involved in the medication-use system to analyze all reported events and to force issues to the next level. One department's (for our purposes, pharmacy's) report of a weakness in the system must be followed by implementation of a system-improvement effort that may be institution-wide in scope. The solution to a problem identified in one nursing unit must be implemented by staff of all the hospital's nursing units. The pharmacy-designated safety-resource officer works the issue through pharmacy work groups, committees, and red tape; having a dedicated point person in nursing facilitates the same constructive action flow from one unit to the entire facility. The issue must then be shared with other relevant departments and gradually be moved upward in the organizational hierarchy until it reaches the group that holds authority to act on the data analyzed. The process has to come full circle—error occurrence, data capture, review of data for further applicability, identification of action steps, institution of preventive action, and reporting of outcomes to the individuals and staff affected by the error. Only when this cycle is complete will reporters know that their efforts were not in vain. And only then will medication-related events be prevented from recurring.

Components of an Effective Reporting System

COMMITMENT AND STRUCTURE

These fundamental organizational objectives can originate from only one place: the top. Executive officers and governing boards must demonstrate a commitment to high-reliability precepts that is not only clear to all employees but also contagious. Rarely will a rank-and-file staff member—or a pharmacy director, for that matter—take a stand for safety or encourage error reporting if he or she is not confident that superiors will support and reward safety-related undertakings.[3] Promoting a "culture of safety" is foremost among the National Quality Forum's core safe practices.[2] This requires that managers encourage all employees to focus on risk reduction. Along with removing the climate of fear, an institution's leaders should demonstrate timely, highly visible, corrective responses to problems. Management needs to understand that more reporting leads to more reports, which in turn leads to a safer organization.[4] An effective reporting and learning system, in summary, has to involve the decision-making bodies of that institution. All the good intentions of individual staff or committees can get stonewalled if leadership is not on the same page.

Schneider,[5] in a series of commentaries on Building a Safer Health System, writes, "In my opinion, the best institutional administrative structure for improving medication safety is a physician-led committee composed of prescribers, nurses, pharmacists, and risk-management personnel." At CCHC, we found that a physician-led committee has been the most effective by far. Strong physician and pharmacy champions, either within the committee or aligned with its goals, help ensure that action will be taken and safety advances implemented.

Politics are inherent to all institutions. The questions facing pharmacies are many. They include, for example, physician preference for the medications they customarily prescribe versus those on the formulary, or an institution's buying preferences for automated devices (e.g., do we purchase several different intravenous (i.v.) pumps or one pump for all uses?). Another difficult issue is whether to sacrifice the proven safety net of unit dose packaging of all medications in favor of a more convenient method under which pharmacists dispense multiple doses or multiple days' supplies in one container. A strong physician champion can cut through medical staff red tape.

At CCF, we have been fortunate to have this strong physician champion in the position of medical director in the Office of Quality Management. This individual was instrumental in securing the support of the chair of the medical staff for our pharmacy-led effort to eliminate use of potentially confusing abbreviations. Pharmacy's physician champion helped us achieve our purpose, starting with the top medical staff chairs and administrators and then ensuring that the needed actions would be taken by the entire medical staff. The department chairs of medicine approached their staff physicians concerning the importance of eliminating dangerous medical abbreviations. Staff physicians, in turn, approached their fellows, residents, and medical students.

This was only one of several physician interventions at our institution that have been aided by our physician safety advocate. Just as important, if not more so, is a strong pharmacy advocate. We have also had the complete support from pharmacy leadership in assuming responsibility for implementation of safety initiatives, even when the methods and changes may have not been the most popular for all involved. The patient had to remain the most important part of all plans.

A NONPUNITIVE ENVIRONMENT

Medicine, pharmacy, and nursing management must assure their staffs that error reports will not be used for evaluative or disciplinary purposes. Reports must be evaluated and investigated for their system-related causes to promote a nonpunitive, cooperative atmosphere surrounding reporting. The practicality of this method may be limited by the culture of the organization, particularly if staff are not comfortable voluntarily reporting errors and events.[6]

Voluntary and nonpunitive reporting go hand in hand. To be effective, voluntary reporting has to be nonpunitive for all respondents and individuals involved in reporting.

COMPLETING THE LOOP: THE IMPORTANCE OF FEEDBACK

Consider the following scenarios:

I am a nurse. I recently caused a medication error involving one of my patients. I reported this error. What followed was despair over the event, concern for my patient, and a building uncertainty over what would happen to me and my professional life as a result of the occurrence.

I am a nurse manager. A nurse on my unit reported an error in which she was involved. The error involved use of an i.v. pump. This error has happened before and probably will happen again. I know that other nursing units use the same i.v. pump and the same medications. I might be able to take the initiative and discuss this event with my staff, in the hope that it doesn't happen again, with us and on our unit. This event may occur on their units too. I hope someone at the top will address the situation.

Webster's dictionary defines the feedback as "the return to the input of a part of the output of a machine, system, or process as for producing changes that improve performance that provide self-corrective action."[7]

In response to the situation described in the two preceding paragraphs, feedback might include the following.

Key Points of Feedback to the Reporting Nurse
- The reported event was analyzed for its system cause.

- The incident was one of several events of the same type that were reported, which will alleviate the reporting nurse's apprehension that she was the only person ever to have caused such an error.

- A plan had been developed to prevent recurrence of the error.

- The report and review will prevent similar events of this type from recurring. A negative event will have a positive outcome.

Key Points of Feedback to the Nurse Manager
- The event has been evaluated from a systems perspective.

- The event has occurred several times before.

- As a result of the information your nurse provided and your prompt follow-up, we have been able to implement changes in process or procedure that will reduce the likelihood that this will happen again—on your unit or on others.

With the provision of this feedback, the loop was complete. All involved in this incident received feedback that helped them understand that safe patient care is of utmost importance. The bottom line is that, "We found a problem, we identified the cause, and we corrected the situation." The next time a medication error occurs, the employees will be in a position to help facilitate change.

A SHARED DEFINITION OF MEDICATION ERROR

Having a complete and shared definition of what constitutes a medication error is essential to the review and reporting of data and analysis. Reporting requires a definition of medication error that is concise, precise, and exact. The definition must also be unambiguous; that is, it must mean the same thing for everyone. The National Coordinating Council on Medication Error Reporting and Prevention (NCC MERP) defines a medication error as any preventable event that may cause or lead to inappropriate medication use or patient harm while the medication is in the control of the health care professional, patient, or consumer. Such events may be related to professional practice, health care products, procedures, and systems, including prescribing; order communication; product labeling, packaging, and nomenclature; compounding; dispensing; distribution; administration; education; monitoring; and use.[8]

The definition covers the entire medication-use process and includes actual and potential errors. It goes beyond the administration of the drug and addresses errors that occur when medications are in the hands of the patient. Severity of consequences is rated using an index ranging from no error (category A) to errors leading nearly to death or to death (categories H and I).

The taxonomy for error reports provides a means of dissecting and coding the information that has been reported. It includes such information as the step, or "node," in the process where the error occurred, the type of error, causes, contributing factors, personnel categories involved, product information, and patient outcomes. While institutions can develop their own reporting taxonomies, we chose the NCC MERP Taxonomy of Medication Errors as our guide.[8]

Issues to Consider in Developing a Shared Reporting System

CCHC is a nine-hospital group that analyzes and shares data. We needed to develop guidelines to follow in an effort to be productive as a group. We needed to identify what we wanted reported and by whom. The initial cornerstone of our efforts was to adopt the NCC MERP definition as our shared definition of a medication error.

When participating in a multi-institution effort, it is also important to agree at the outset to define your institution's reporting parameters, i.e., just exactly what reports you want reported into your system. Voluntary reporting of events can come to include events not usually associated with such reporting. Events occur daily that can be overlooked by the usual medication-error reporting systems. Recent overtures by JCAHO have encouraged institutions to include medication events occurring in such areas as respiratory therapy into their regularly scheduled review of all medication events. These events, such as respiratory treatment omissions, which previously might have been tallied or recorded, now must be evaluated just as any other medication-related event for cause, patient effect, system-related influence, and similar factors.

Thus, it is incumbent on institutions to determine what constitutes a medication error, what data they will collect, where the data will reside, and what the scope of evaluation and analysis will be. Will your institution collect the data? Yes. Will the data be included into the institutions medication error database? Maybe. The answer to this question may be complex.

For example, at the CCF, we share and analyze our medication error data with nine other hospitals. When JCAHO raised the issue of respiratory therapy–related medication errors, one of our member institutions decided to include these data in its single medication-error database. Respiratory therapy omissions accounted for around 100 to 200 events each month. When comparing these data with the remainder of all reported medication-error events, the respiratory figures dwarfed the other causes and types, skewing considerably the data for all reported events.

Our own hospital took a different approach. We coordinated efforts with the respiratory therapy department to agree on what data we needed to collect to allow effective analysis and review. Respiratory therapy collects its medication-related event data and reports to our multidisciplinary medication-safety committee. Just as we would review any of the other medication-error categories, causes, or types, we routinely review all the respiratory therapy data. The committee can then develop recommendations and submit them to the multidisciplinary body for further review and analysis as well as proposed corrective measures. The respiratory therapy department maintains these cumulative data in its own database, whish is separate from the institution's medication-error database. In keeping with the intent of the JCAHO, this information is collected, evaluated, and acted upon to enhance and improve patient safety where needed.

A second area where medication-related events occur and the error reports may or may not appear in an individual institution's database is conscious sedation. Conscious sedation may involve the use of reversal agents, such as naloxone (Narcan®) and flumazenil (Romazicon®), as well as medical intervention to reverse effects of agents used during conscious-sedation procedures. In many institutions, the fact that reversal agents were used requires the reporting of a medication error. Institutions must decide whether these events will continue to be reported to internal departments, such as anesthesia and quality improvement, or included in their voluntary reporting networks.

Finally, voluntary reporting numbers may be inadvertently influenced by special projects or initiatives undertaken to target certain identified problem. Later in this chapter I discuss one such project, which involved a nursing unit and which resulted in an increase in order transcription errors in the magnitude of 30 to 40 reports per month. Institutions must be aware of individual projects and initiative undertaken that may have an unanticipated effect on their total numbers of reported events.

Barriers to Effective Voluntary Reporting

DELAYS IN REPORT PROCESSING

Ideally, the investigator or those analyzing an event will be notified immediately upon discovery of the error. Immediate notification makes it possible to contact those involved for additional information. Receiving reports after the data trail has vanished hinders analysis. The best-case scenario for retrieving data related to error reports is to discover that data within the first 24 hours. The longer the period of time from reporting to analysis, the lower the likelihood for retrieval of additional reliable data.

INCOMPLETE DATA FIELDS

It is important to use data fields that will capture specific facts that will be useful in error analysis and lead to medication-use improvement. Reports should be designed to prevent incomplete or missing data fields, such as drug name, that will hamper the analysis. Other reports may have a drug name, but no information on route of administration. In others, the narrative of what happened may be missing. Any incomplete fields greatly impede the proper analysis of the report. Prior to the implementation of our current system, specific data related to the drug product were not found in our reports. Reports that lacked information on such matters as the drug packaging, labeling, or appearance, all of which might have contributed to the cause of the error, were prone to faulty analysis.

One important barrier to proper analysis of reports, we discovered, was how our voluntary reports were set up. We wanted to be able to compare data among several hospitals. Initially, each hospital in our system had its own reporting template. No two of these reporting forms or templates matched with regard to data fields. We realized that all institutions that are being compared within our group needed to capture the same definitions and data fields. Different fields or choices influence the way errors are identified and classified. All reporting departments and patient-care areas must capture the identical information if they are to be compared. This is also true for different hospitals within the same health system or comparative group.

INSUFFICIENT VOLUME OF REPORTING

The IOM report states that two challenges that confront reporting systems are getting sufficient participation in the programs and building an adequate response system. All reporting programs, whether mandatory or voluntary, are perceived to suffer from underreporting.[2]

The numbers of reports received can be influenced by whether the reporting system is voluntary or mandatory. If reporting is not mandatory, there are a number of major deterrents. Confidentiality and fear of reprisal are high on the list of reasons for failure to report medication errors. They are, in fact, perhaps the main reasons I might not share information on what has been happening at our institution with those outside our doors. Even today, years after the progress of Annenbergs I, II, and III[b] in promoting the free exchange of information, we still find ourselves reluctant to claim ownership of documented errors; instead, we speak hypothetically in national forums. Honestly, when asked to work on this chapter, my first thought was, "What a great opportunity!" and second, "I'd better be careful what I say!"

Health care workers have been raised in a punitive environment. Just as health care practitioners are reluctant to report sentinel events to JCAHO, they are reluctant to report medication errors internally within institutions.[2] In discussions with nurses and pharmacists at our institution, the number-one reason given for not reporting is that they "don't want to get into trouble." In the past, under a punitive environment, employees' errors were tabulated and held as points against them. After a certain number of points, an employee was subjected to disciplinary action, including suspension and even termination. An employee could be terminated for just one infraction if it was deemed serious enough. For example, one institution where I worked terminated a pharmacist who dispensed a penicillin derivative to a patient without determining whether the patient was allergic to penicillin. The patient had a severe reaction, and the pharmacist was held responsible. What was not determined, or even considered, was whether the allergy information was accessible by the pharmacist or was even documented in the patient's chart. The backlash from this event made many pharmacists and nurses reluctant to report errors and perhaps even to cover their mistakes to some extent.

LACK OF CLARITY CONCERNING HOW DATA WILL BE USED

Staff are reluctant to report for a variety of reasons. Topping the list are fear of blame or reprisal and uncertainty about how the information reported will be used. Fear that their association with this event, as a reporter or a perpetrator, will become a factor used in performance evaluations is another fear.

Managers who must prepare performance evaluations like data. Data are clean; data remove the need for subjective determinations. The number of medication errors in which an employee has been involved are quantifiable, just like days absent, meetings attended, or educational modules completed. Whether the employee or the system was at fault rarely enters into the equation. If an employee was involved in any way with a reported medication error, the information, and perhaps even a disciplinary write-up, will be included in his or her annual performance review.

Thus, a key factor in the quest for safer patient care is broader immunity for error reports and a nonpunitive culture that places a higher value on resolving system-based problems than on punishing practitioners for errors.[9] Managers must make clear to all employees how the data used in error reporting will be used. Employees must know that data will be used constructively and related to patient-safety improvements.

Applying the Approach to Design and Implementation of an Effective Voluntary Reporting System

The following discussion describes how the principles just described were applied in the course of implementing a voluntary reporting system, called the Patient Incident Reporting System (PIRS), at the main campus of the Cleveland Clinic Foundation. Although we now use the online reporting system only on our main campus, we plan to implement it throughout the CCHS.

TO CAPTURE EVENTS AND ALLOW THEM TO BE REPORTED IN A TIMELY MANNER

When we designed the PIRS intranet version of our reporting system, we made real-time reporting one of our "musts." We'd previously used a paper system that asked reporters to fill in blanks. Without a selection of choice answers, many of the blanks went unfilled. Our goal was to design a system that allowed the reporter to report an incident in the fewest possible keystrokes but that would capture the maximum amount of information. At the time of our system design we were realizing many of these desired features with the MEDMARX, the medication-error database system of the United States Pharmacopeia (USP).

We originally planned to design an in-house system that would interface with the MEDMARX system to allow timely transfer of information into the MEDMARX database and save time in report analysis. About this same time, PIRS work group was redesigning the internal institution-wide reporting system for all events (e.g., falls, blood administration events, anesthesia, treatment delay, skin analysis, and medication errors). We ultimately incorporated all types of events into a single, reporter-friendly system. (MEDMARX has since released its own, institution-specific interface for customers that accomplishes data transfer between their institutions and USP.)

To facilitate efficiency in report filing and review, we found the institution-wide intranet vehicle to be the best option. The intranet was available to all employees. Printed medication-error reports, by contrast, were available only in certain hospital areas, and they had to be filled out manually. With paper reports, we found that nurses were making virtually all the reports; occasionally, a pharmacist or physician would do so. With the intranet available to all, reporter options would no longer be so limited.

Employees reported using a secure and individual sign-in procedure that required the use of their employee identification number and a password. Passwords are updated every six months. All our nursing and pharmacy personnel had been using the same sign-on approach with the Pyxis automated dispensing cabinets (ADCs) for several years. Getting the data into report format in a relatively timely fashion was accomplished by the institution-wide intranet system. When an event happened, the reporter signed in, accessed the intranet site, and filed the report.

The next major roadblock was crossed when we incorporated a manager-notification function into the PIRS. We designed the system so that it would trigger an e-mail that is sent to the supervisor of the employee reporting the event. Notification is also sent to the pharmacy medication-safety officer or the nursing quality officer. The pharmacy and nursing officers are the gatekeepers for data and event review.

Thus, as the pharmacy medication-safety officer, I would be notified immediately of a medication-related error report being filed. I found it crucial to have the ability to contact those involved in the event as soon as possible, while the event was still fresh in their minds. The timely notification also allowed me to access printed records and patient medical records immediately. Under the other system, after receiving a report that might have been days old, more often than not I found that the patient's medical record had been returned to medical records because the patient had been discharged.

Upon receiving notification that an event occurred, I would access the documented report, where I would find the recorded data, including the name and phone or pager number of the reporter as well as his or her manager. With several mouse clicks I could send an e-mail to the reporter or manager and request further information. The nursing quality gatekeeper would frequently do the same, and we shared information each step of the way.

Reporters had a maximum of 72 hours in which they could update records and augment the original report. The reporter's managers had the option to approve the report anytime before the 72-hour limit.

With the implementation of these systems, we fulfilled of one of our greatest needs—the timely reporting and notification of reports. We now had the report, initial data reported, the names of the reporting individuals, and the ability to augment that data with several prompt and directed questions.

TO DEVELOP DATA FIELDS THAT EASILY ALLOW THE CAPTURE OF DATA

To capture the maximum amount of data elements related to the event and allow the reporter to report this information in as few steps as possible, we designed the following into our system.

First, whenever possible, we provided drop-down screens that listed data elements from which the user could select. Knowing that we needed to be able to transfer these data into MEDMARX, we designed the drop-down screens to mimic MEDMARX drop-downs. We found the MEDMARX report template to be the most efficient for capturing the most data needed for report analysis. MEDMARX has consistently revised, refined, and updated its data fields to capture information even more efficiently, and we continue to revise our own reporting system accordingly. Whenever possible, we linked data elements to existing internal, hospital-wide databases for easy drop-down selection. By linking to our own online formulary system, reporters had at their fingertips an alphabetical (brand/generic) list of all formulary medications. When the reporter selected the medication related to the event, several report fields were populated with the single selection (generic and brand names, medication form, strength and route of administration). Names of medications not listed could be entered manually.

Our initial plans also included linking the report to the hospital ADT (admission/discharge/transfer) database. Under this system, the reporter had access to an alphabetical list of all current inpatients. By scrolling and selecting a patient, the user could populate the report form with the patient's name, medical record number, current bed space and unit, and admitting physician name. This system was linked to our employee database; thus, when a reporter scrolled and selected his or her own name as the reporter, the incident report would automatically generate not only the reporter's name but also his or her employee number, unit, and phone or pager number. We found this to be invaluable in times where follow-up was required. The process of selecting patient names from a rolling list was a function with which all employees were familiar because they had done the same for years with our Pyxis ADCs. Keeping aspects of our new system identical to those already used reduced training time and increased employee acceptance.

By linking to existing databases, such as formulary, ADT, and employee rosters, and by providing drop-down screens, we greatly increased the accuracy of the data we received on each report. Reporters were still required to complete manually the event-description field, which details what happened during the event. Once data entry of the other fields had been streamlined, the reporting of the event-description field greatly improved.

TO EMPHASIZE THE IMPORTANCE OF SYSTEM-RELATED CAUSES RATHER THAN OF INDIVIDUAL ACTION

Over time, our commitment to nonpunitive reporting has resulted in increased reporting of events. One particular project might be seen as a turning point in this respect. As a result of monthly feedback provided to nursing units, we determined that one particular unit experienced several transcription-related events each month. Upon review, the entire process, which involved transcription of medication orders into the MAR by a unit secretary, verification of those transcriptions by a nurse, and the administration of medications to the patients using the MAR, was found to have several weak points that might have led to the commission of errors.

Collaboration between the nursing unit and the medication-safety officer resulted in a project under which all nurses and secretaries of this unit would take part in reviewing order transcription and error identification for a selected period of time. The goal of this project was defined as error identification and process review, not identification of responsible individuals. Each error or potential error identified was viewed as an opportunity for improvement. All these opportunities were reported into the error-reporting system and tabulated along with other errors reported throughout the month.

Within the short period that this project encompassed, the reporting of transcription-related events for this nursing unit rose from around 6 reports per month to more than 30. Weekly analysis of the reports by the entire staff identified several process deficiencies that were easily corrected. The nurses found themselves concentrating their efforts as a unit, reporting findings as a unit, and ultimately celebrating their efforts, not as individuals at fault but as an entire unit. The outcome of their efforts was the identification of several weak points in the process, process improvement, and a reduction in transcription-related events.

We wanted to find a way to reward reporters and to place a positive spin on their reporting. Thus, as an incentive to participation in the project, reporters of all events, as a matter of policy, received a coupon for a free pizza. In addition, we mailed each reporter a note with the following message:

> This card is being sent in appreciation for your diligence and attention to detail in reporting a recent medication-related incident. With the understanding, and within the framework, of our nonpunitive approach to medication-error reporting, we extend a sincere appreciation for your efforts. Statistics have shown that a fair majority of reported errors are in fact "problems with the system," as opposed to individual negligence. It is very important that we be able to correlate as many errors and as much data as possible to get at and correct the proximate causes of errors.
>
> Thank you once again for your efforts. They are greatly appreciated
>
> David N. Gragg
> Medication-Safety Officer

The project received great acclaim within the institution. It was subsequently presented to the nursing leadership and showcased to the entire hospital. The most important impact of this program was that, in addition to the documented decrease in the transcription errors, it promoted the concept that the system and its processes, not individuals, were at the cause of these events.

About a year and a half after we began the pizza coupon for medication-error report program, I was asked whether I felt that it had an impact on our reporting or employee attitudes, and whether its cost could be justified. I responded that while we could definitely show a positive increase in the numbers of reports received (when we started the program we were receiving an average of 35 reports monthly and we currently receive an average of 80 reports), the greatest victory was that if, from the data gleaned from these reports and the following analyses, we prevented one repeated medication error requiring one additional inpatient day, our $6,000 investment in pizza coupons was well worthwhile.

Final Thoughts

In dealing with voluntary reporting, we must never forget that we are dealing with people—fellow health care workers, patients, and their family members. We don't start out our day thinking that we will harm one another. We approach our professions with the willingness to care for the sick above all. If we can keep that thought in front of us at all times, i.e., that our actions and reactions are what will drive good patient care, then we will do just that. On the contrary, if our actions and inactions lead to poor-quality care, then we have failed. Keeping the patient safe is our goal. Acknowledging that errors do occur and then facilitating the action steps to prevent their occurrence is movement in the right direction. In final reference to the value of voluntary and nonpunitive reporting, I am reminded of an ancient Chinese proverb that states, "Love truth, but pardon error."

Footnotes

[a] The National Quality Forum (NQF) is a private, not-for-profit membership organization created to develop and implement a national strategy for measuring and reporting health care quality. The mission of NQF is to improve American health care through endorsement of consensus-based national standards for measurement and public reporting of health care performance data that provide meaningful information about whether care is safe, timely, beneficial, patient centered, equitable, and efficient.

[b] The Annenberg Conferences were a series of patient-safety conferences sponsored by the Annenberg Center for the Health Sciences. Annenberg I, held in 1996, was entitled "Examining Errors in Health Care: Developing a Prevention, Education, and Research Agenda." Annenberg II, held in November 1998, took the next step with "Enhancing Patient Safety and Reducing Errors in Health Care." The third conference, held in May 2004, moved the patient-safety emphasis toward communication issues with the theme "Let's Talk: Communicating Risk and Safety in Health Care."

References

1. American Society of Health-System Pharmacists. ASHP Statement on Reporting Medical Errors. *Am J Health-Syst Pharm.* 2000;57:1531-1532.

2. Kohn LT, Corrigan JM, Donaldson MD, eds. Committee on Quality of Health in America, Institute of Medicine. *To Err Is Human: Building a Safer Health System.* Washington, DC: National Academy Press; 1999.

3. Manasse H. Not too perfect: hard lessons and small victories in patient safety. *Am J Health-Syst Pharm.* 2003;60:780-787.

4. Phillips M. Voluntary reporting of medication errors. *Am J Health-Syst Pharm.* 2002; 59:2326-2328.

5. Schneider P. Commentaries on building a safer health system. *Am J Health-Syst Pharm.* 2002;58:66-68.

6. Schneider P. Workshop summaries. Workshop 5: Voluntary Reporting Method. *Am J Health-Syst Pharm.* 2002;59:2333-2336.

7. *Merriam-Webster's Collegiate Dictionary.* 9th ed. Springfield, MA: Merriam-Webster Inc; 1984.

8. National Coordinating Council for Medication Error Reporting and Prevention Web site. Available at: www.nccmerp.org/ aboutMedError.html. Accessed December 7, 2004.

9. Cohen M. Why error reporting systems should be voluntary [editorial]. *Br Med J.* 2000;320:728-729.

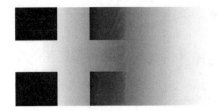

CHAPTER 13

The Safe Use of Technology in Hospitals and Health Systems

Kevin Marvin

Overview

This chapter presents a conceptual framework for the safe and effective use of information technology to improve patient safety. Strategies for the integration of automated systems and clinical workflows and for the optimization of interactions between health practitioners and patients are outlined, and the importance of these functions to patient safety is described. Also included is a review of current and future information technologies.

Role of Technology in Safe Medication Use

Technology is a tool that can support safer medication processes. Information and automation technology can be used to

- perform repetitive tasks with consistency and accuracy;
- provide fast access to information from multiple locations;
- monitor information to identify conditions requiring intervention;
- assist with communication between caregivers;
- assist with the accurate and efficient capture of clinical data; and
- support safe and efficient workflows.

Much has been done in pharmacy to automate the preparation and distribution components of the medication process. Replacement of repetitive human tasks with automation can enhance accuracy and efficiency. Unit-based cabinets and the use of robotics for cart filling, preparation of intravenous (i.v.) solutions, and product delivery have become common. Investments in these systems are justified primarily on the basis of labor savings or revenue enhancement. Additional benefits of preparation and distribution technology are the support and automation of safe practices. Though studies have shown that information technologies can reduce errors in the medication process, more studies are needed to better quantify these reductions and to identify the appropriate use of these technologies.[1,2]

Although automation has done a great deal to support medication-distribution processes, more patient-safety benefits can be effected by supporting other parts of the medication-use process. Research has shown that most of the errors in the medication process occur during activities other than preparation and distribution. For example, one study reported that only 4 percent of medication errors occur in dispensing (i.e., preparation and distribution) while 56 percent occur in ordering (i.e., prescribing and monitoring), 34 percent in administration, and 6 percent in transcribing.[3] Findings such as these indicate the existence of a significant potential for safety increases in the prescribing, administration, and monitoring components of the medication process.

Safety Issues Created by Technology and Automation

New technologies in medical devices and medications require thorough design, testing, education, and monitoring to ensure their safe and efficient use. Information and automation technology require the same care. New information technologies are often implemented to address a specific need within the medication process. It is important to consider the side effects of the technology and to develop procedures to ensure that the safety of the overall process is not compromised by such changes.

Safety may also be compromised if an automated system does not adequately support the user's work. When this happens, users often find shortcuts in the system processes. Such shortcuts can compromise safety. The same problems may occur if the user is not appropriately trained on how to use the system and does not understand why certain procedures are in place.

The term *back-end operations* refers to the maintenance, stocking, and monitoring required to keep a technology tool operating efficiently and safely. Back-end operations are important to the safe use of information technology. If not properly managed, these operations can result in errors. Common errors in back-end operations occur in the maintenance of medication data tables and in how these tables affect system operations and interfaces to other systems, such as electronic charting, robotic dispensing, and billing. A common problem with back-end robotic-system operations is improper stocking, which results in stock outages. Stock outages necessitate increased manual effort and create a potential for unsafe shortcuts as nursing and pharmacy staff try to meet patient needs.

UNSAFE WORKFLOWS AND FORCING FUNCTIONS

As they carry out their assigned functions, nurses, pharmacists, and technicians develop specific sequences for performing repetitive tasks that will help ensure completeness and accuracy. Technology tools and work sequences need to match in order to create a safe and comfortable work environment. The introduction of new technologies requires careful workflow design,[4] as discussed elsewhere in this volume.

Forcing functions are useful tools to enforce proper workflows and prevent medication errors.[5] Forcing functions require the user to complete specific tasks before they continue their workflow process. Information and automation systems can use forcing functions to maintain safe workflows. Examples of such functions include

- requiring documentation of patient allergies prior to entering medication orders;
- requiring the scanning of a patient wristband prior to electronically charting medication administration;
- preventing a medication from being removed from a unit-based cabinet until pharmacy has verified the order; and
- requiring a second person's verification prior to electronically charting a high-alert medication.

When forcing functions are not possible, other mechanisms, such as monitoring, can be used to manage safe medication practices. When the capture of necessary monitoring information becomes part of the workflows, accurate process monitoring is the result. When a nurse withdraws a medication from a unit-based cabinet as an override, the system can require that the nurse enter a reason for requesting the override. Data captured in this way can be used to generate reports to identify areas of improvement that will eventually reduce the number of overrides. Data capture and analysis are possible for management of unit-based cabinet stock outages, pharmacist order interventions, orders for products that are not on the formulary, computerized physician order entry (CPOE), clinical alerts, verbal orders, and other functions.

CORRECT AND INCORRECT ASSUMPTIONS ABOUT SAFETY IN AN AUTOMATED SYSTEM

When designing and implementing an automated system, planners make many assumptions about how the technology works and how best to meld it into human processes. Because technology and health care are always changing, it is important to continually verify that the original assumptions still apply to current medication processes. If those prior assumptions are no longer valid, the processes or automated systems may need to be adjusted.

It is human nature to resist change. Simple changes, such as the reordering of data elements on a data-entry screen, the relocation of a computer workstation, or the implementation of a new clinical computer application, force users to change their work processes. If the change decision is not correct, the user may resort to unsafe workflows. For example, mismatched workflows in a bar-code charting application may lead nurses to omit the scan of the patient's wristband or to skip the charting altogether.[4] A decision to display all levels of clinical warnings may need to be changed if the number of warnings displayed is so great that physicians and pharmacists ignore them.[6]

In some cases, it may be necessary to implement extra efforts to be sure old processes do not continue to be used after new, automated systems have been implemented. This may involve eliminating the ability to perform functions on an old system that has been replaced. For example, when paper processes are replaced with automated processes, a careful search may be needed to find and destroy all the paper forms.

IMPLEMENTATION METHODS AND EFFECTS ON SAFETY

Automation of the medication process puts significant stresses on pharmacists, nurses, and other health care providers. For this reason, the way in which the new technology is introduced must be carefully planned.

There are several common methods to introduce or implement new processes and technologies. Pilot testing is a method under which a change is introduced in a small area in order to determine how well it is suited to a new and broader application. It enables the user to identify and correct issues prior to full-scale implementation.

A pilot test may be run for a short time or for an extended time. The length of the test is important. It must be long enough to achieve its intended purpose; however, an extended pilot run may compromise safety by creating a more complicated work environment. Upon completion, successful pilot tests may be slowly extended into additional areas or quickly expanded, depending on the circumstances. Decisions concerning methods of pilot testing and the pace of expansion need to consider the needs of all departments. A pilot test should never replace a detailed design of workflows and the technology support that they require.

The sequence and timing of the implementation of technologies are important. Examples of sequencing decisions include

- implementing electronic charting applications prior to CPOE;
- implementing automated distribution systems prior to bar-code charting; and
- delaying the implementation of significant order-entry decision support until after CPOE implementation.

Rushing to implementation without adequate process design and training is a common phenomenon, and it can have a serious effect on safety. Nursing and pharmacy need to allocate resources to this effort and to insist that the design team have adequate time to design workflows.

Once a new technology is implemented, time must be allowed to resolve any issues that have arisen before resources are removed from the project. Implementation is an iterative process; we seldom get it right the first time. Resources need to be available after implementation to make any necessary adjustments in the technology and procedures.

DOWNTIME

Downtime is inevitable with automation and information technology. Reducing downtime requires investments in equipment, software, and personnel. Studies have determined the operational costs for downtime but have not quantified its effects on patient safety.[7] Few if any systems can guarantee 100 percent uptime. Health organizations need to develop downtime processes as part of the implementation of clinical systems. Part of this process should include developing estimates of operational costs and assessing the impact of downtime on patient safety. Leaders can use these estimates to justify an investment in more-reliable hardware and software.[8]

Even though an automated system is running, other areas of downtime may have significant impacts. Examples of such impacts are as follows:

- A bar-code charting application does not work because a patient's bar code is not readable or the medication bar code is not recognized in the application's database.

- A pharmacy technician's absence delays restocking of unit-based cabinets. As a result, several patients do not receive their medications at the scheduled times.

- The hospital registration system is undergoing maintenance, and all admissions must temporarily be handled manually.

Downtimes may be of short or long duration. Long-duration downtimes are those that span more than one shift of caregivers. Procedures may be different for each type of downtime.

Processes to support the recovery from downtime are also important. Once a system again becomes available, it is important to switch safely and efficiently from the manual procedures to the automated procedures.

The Computer-Based Patient Record

The computer-based patient record (CPR) is commonly called the electronic medical record (EMR). The Institute of Medicine (IOM) has defined the CPR as to tool to provide universal access to patient and other clinical information.[9] Although this definition focuses on the storage and viewing of medical data, it includes access to reference material and decision-support rules to augment the data.

In two subsequent landmark reports relating to medication safety, the IOM stated, "Information technology solutions, access to clinical guidelines at the point of care and support and redesign of clinical workflows are key to improving patient safety.[10,11] Further definitions of CPR by Gartner and others have added that the CPR must support the care-delivery process across the continuum of care.[12] This expanded definition is important because it recognizes that a CPR and its technology tools can do more than simply replace the paper medical record: They can support processes and workflows in a way that paper records never could. This expanded definition brings support of the medication-use process into the CPR's domain.

CLINICAL WORKFLOWS

Clinical workflows place heavy demands on computing devices and equipment. These devices need to support the display and capture of many types of data. They need to meet hospital electrical-safety requirements. Mobile devices need to be washable, to withstand drops to hard floors, be lightweight, to have long battery lives, and to require minimal training for efficient use.

Clinical workflows have complexities that are difficult to define, much less automate. In a hospital, many tasks take place concurrently against multiple workflows. All these tasks must be coordinated around the condition, location, and needs of the patient.

Why is the support of workflows important in a CPR? In the medication process, a substantial amount of the workflow consists of communication between caregivers and of scheduling and documentation of activities. These workflows must be designed to maximize efficiency and safe practices. Each step in the workflow must be logical, and each step needs to be completed before the next one begins.

To support workflows, the information technology system must be process oriented. This means that it should offer the right tasks at the right time to the right person, as well as supply the information needed to perform those tasks.[13]

The medication-use process has been well described, and best practices are being identified through research. Process-oriented information technologies can be used to support medication-process workflows in many ways.

With manual processes, workflows are designed around paperwork associated with documentation and communication. Many technology systems are implemented to replace components of these manual processes without modifying other process components. In many cases, process changes are needed to take full advantage of the efficiency and safety that technology can provide (see section entitled Integration of Workflows).

OWNERSHIP AND INTEGRITY OF CLINICAL DATA

A CPR stores and displays medical data gathered from multiple sources. In some cases, the data are directly captured by the CPR; in others, data are entered into it from other systems. The latter data could include patient registration data coming from a hospital system, test results coming from a laboratory computer, medication-dispensing data from unit-based cabinets, and information from an electronic medication charting system or other source. The source, or master, of the data is the system in which the data originate. In most cases, the source of the specific data stored in a CPR is well understood. Health Level Seven (HL7) is one of several American National Standards Institute–accredited standards-development organizations operating in the health care arena.[14] HL7 standards for interfacing of medical data allow for a significant amount of data sharing among applications.

A major issue with clinical information systems is how to handle maintenance of data when the ownership, or master, is shared by multiple systems. For example, responsibility for the maintenance of allergy lists is often shared by pharmacy, nursing, and medicine. Separate computer systems are often used for CPOE, pharmacy operations, and nurse documentation. Each system may require access to view, enter, and modify information on a patient's allergies. In such a situation, it becomes difficult to keep data consistent between the systems. Two-way interfaces between systems can be used to address this problem, but they are complex and seldom work well. This complexity increases substantially if each system has a different method of allergy coding. If patient-allergy data are maintained in multiple systems, it is highly likely that inconsistencies will develop and that the integrity of the data will be compromised. In most cases, a decision needs to be made as to which system is the master for the shared data, and all users must then use that system to modify the shared data. If the processes to maintain allergies on this other system do not fit well into workflows, users may take shortcuts and safety issues may develop.

These problems exist whenever separate clinical systems are interfaced and share ownership of data. Patient-order profiles produce similar problems when maintained on multiple systems. Maintaining this complete data is difficult when the pharmacist and physician medication profiles are kept on separate systems. The complexity grows when medication charting is implemented on a third system.

Many hospitals are implementing enterprise CPR systems to avoid the complexities associated with interfaced systems. Standardization of data between systems will reduce these complexities but may not eliminate them.

Computerized Prescriber Order Entry

CPOE has been identified as a tool to reduce medication-related errors when used in combination with clinical decision-support systems.[15] The Leapfrog Group has identified CPOE as one of the three practices that have tremendous potential to save lives by reducing preventable mistakes in hospitals.[16] Despite the attention applied to CPOE, only 4.3 percent of hospitals had implemented CPOE at the time of a survey conducted by the American Society of Health-System Pharmacists (ASHP) in 2001.[17] Many reasons for the slow adoption of this technology into health systems have been proposed. The following discussion focuses on the technology barriers.

DIFFERING NEEDS OF PHYSICIANS, PHARMACISTS, AND NURSES

The ordering process involves many health care workers. Implementation of CPOE has an impact on workflows in all areas of the medication-use process, and each group of providers has different needs.

Physician

The physician is interested in efficiently documenting the order and supporting timely therapy for the patient. The physician trusts that pharmacy and nursing will satisfactorily complete their roles in the medication process. The physician wants the order workflow to have no interruptions unless absolutely necessary. Doctors have little interest in entering or reviewing order information on such matters as product choice, availability, or specific administration times.

Pharmacist

The pharmacist is interested in verifying that the order is clinically appropriate for the patient. The pharmacist expects this check to be done efficiently and with maximum use of automation. If the pharmacist intervenes on an order, the system needs to support the communication and documentation needs of this intervention. Finally, the pharmacist needs to ensure that the medication is correctly dispensed or prepared and is available to nursing when needed. The pharmacist has minimal interest in specific medication administration times, with the possible exception of the first dose.

Nurse

The nurse is interested in administering the medication in a safe, timely, and efficient manner. The specific timing of the medication schedule is important to nursing. Nurses also need to document observations made during medication administration and to make this information available to others as they monitor the patient's therapy. Nurses depend on pharmacists to make the medication available when needed.

In sum, physicians, pharmacists, and nurses all need access to medication information; however, they use this information in different ways.

The information flow in the medication process is cyclical, just as the medication process itself. Information from each step feeds the next yet each step requires access to the CPR (see **Figure 13-1**). To support workflows, the correct information needs to be provided to and gathered from each step in the process.

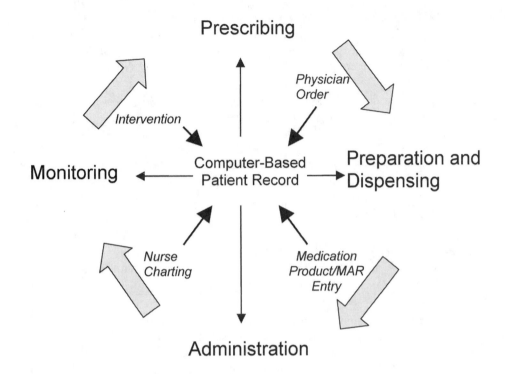

Figure 13-1. Medication Process Information Flow

Integration of communication and clean handoffs between physician, pharmacist, and nurse are essential to the successful implementation of CPOE.

TECHNOLOGY ENABLERS AND BARRIERS FOR CPOE

Many technology tools are available to support CPOE. The speed and reliability of computer hardware and software are now much better than they were in the past. The demands of electronic commerce and banking have supported the development of computer and database systems that eliminate downtimes. Networking and communications technology support faster, more-reliable communications. Devices are getting smaller, and battery lives are becoming longer. Wireless communication is affordable. Concerns surrounding Y2K forced health care organizations to update or replace clinical systems. HL7 standards are used consistently for interfaces.

The biggest barrier to CPOE is the large number of operational, clinical, and technological decisions that need to be made when implementing a CPOE solution. Significant effort is needed to design workflows and to identify how to support them with information technology. These decisions are difficult to make because little evidence is available on which to base them. In an ideal world, there would be ample measures of clinical and operational processes to compare with similar benchmark measures of best practices. Little research has been done to identify the benefits of CPOE. The studies that have been published evaluate "homegrown" systems rather than widely available vendor systems. More research is needed to compare different types of systems.[18,19]

Standardization is also a significant barrier to CPOE implementation. It is very costly for a hospital that has put in place multiple interfaced clinical systems to replace them with a new CPOE system. Interfacing systems is difficult when there are limited standards to support data sharing. HL7 standards support the transmission of data but few standards exist for the coding of much clinical data. Standards are needed for coding medication identification, allergies, dosage units, dosage forms, routes, diagnoses, procedures, and other clinical data. These standards will support medication-process integration between systems and will simplify the implementation of CPOE and clinical decision-support systems.

The result of the lack of best practices and standards is that clinical information technology systems are customized to the organization. Clinical and CPOE systems available from vendors require a significant amount of design, setup, and configuration prior to use. As a result, installing a CPOE system is a costly undertaking. Case-study estimates by First Consulting Group indicate that the cost of implementing a CPOE system in a 500-bed teaching hospital is $7.9 million and that annual operating costs are $1.35 million.[20]

Pharmacy Automation

Replacing repetitive manual tasks with technology can increase the quality of care because of the consistency that technology provides. Robotics for prescription filling, medication unit dose cart filling, and i.v. preparation are examples of such technology. Automated dispensing systems (ADS) are also used to enhance security and tracking of medications as well as to give caregivers quicker access to them.

Automation and information technology are used throughout pharmacy operations. A recent ASHP national survey found that 8 percent of hospitals have a centralized robotic drug-distribution system and that 58 percent use decentralized ADS.[17] Implementation of this technology is normally justified on the basis of labor savings or revenue enhancement. These technologies can also have an impact on medication safety. No studies have been published that compare the safety of a centralized robotic cart fill with that of decentralized ADS.

CENTRALIZED MEDICATION DISTRIBUTION AND PREPARATION

No studies have directly linked the use of centralized unit dose cart-filling technology to reduced medication errors, but studies have shown a reduced error rate in robotic cart filling (0.6 percent) compared to manual filling (2.9 percent).[21]

Though the safety impact of robotic-dispensing equipment may be minimal, this technology serves as an enabler to bar-code medication charting. Until drug manufacturers uniformly put bar codes on unit dose packages, only facilities using robotic cart-fill equipment can easily implement bar-code charting systems.

Automated devices to support compounding of i.v. solutions and parenteral nutrition admixtures were used in 33 percent of the facilities responding to the previously cited ASHP national survey.[17] In addition to automating repetitive tasks, these devices automate the calculations and measuring that occur in i.v. preparation. Proper operating procedures and maintenance are essential to safe use of this equipment. ASHP has published guidelines for safe use of this equipment.[22]

DECENTRALIZED MEDICATION DISTRIBUTION

The cost of unit-based ADS is justified on the basis of labor savings in medication delivery and narcotic tracking. The cost is also justified because it captures charges more accurately and therefore may bring in additional revenue. Most hospitals have interfaced their medication-order profiles to these machines in order to comply with the Joint Commission on Accreditation of Healthcare Organizations (JCAHO) requirement that pharmacists review orders prior to administration. The medication-profile interface not only helps manage overrides from ADS but also may reduce product-selection errors that can be common in unit-based cabinets. Such errors occur when the wrong medication is selected from the list on the system's electronic display. The medication-profile function does not eliminate errors stemming from selecting the wrong product from a drawer containing multiple drugs or from incorrect stocking. Look-alike products need to be monitored carefully for these problems

PRESCRIPTION FILLING AND PRESCRIPTION-WORKFLOW MANAGEMENT

A recent observational study of 50 pharmacies found prescription-filling error rates of 1.7 percent, and of these errors 6.5 percent were judged to be clinically important.[23] Automation includes prescription counting, packaging and labeling automation, workflow automation with scanning, interactive voice-response systems for refill requests, and electronic prescription writers with interfaces to pharmacy computer systems. A high-volume ambulatory pharmacy offers a perfect environment for workflow automation. The process is well defined, and standards have been developed and implemented for data storage and interfacing. Most of the multidose medication packages used in ambulatory pharmacies are bar coded to support automation.

Safety Issues in Pharmacy Automation

ASHP has published guidelines for the safe use of automated medication storage and distribution devices.[24] The document calls for careful planning in advance of the purchase and installation of equipment. Such planning will articulate the goals for the technology, define measures to assess the needs of an automated system, and describe the resources needed for successful implementation. Front-end, back-end, and downtime operations must be analyzed from a patient-safety perspective.[25]

FRONT-END OPERATIONS

Front-end operations are those that deliver the final product or service. With centralized robotics, these would include the i.v.-preparation and cart-filling processes. With decentralized ADS distribution, the front-end operation is the dispensing of the medications. User workflows need to be designed for safe practice. Workflow procedures must be tested to identify shortcuts that can compromise safety. Forced functions to support the workflows can help maintain safe workflows. Where necessary, reports or audits should be developed to monitor workflows. User education and training are important to safe front-end operations. Downtime procedures must be developed and users must be trained on how to perform them. Some facilities schedule downtime drills to ensure that staff members are aware of the procedures.

One front-end issue commonly associated with decentralized ADS is dispensing overrides, i.e., removal of medications without matching orders or patients. The safe use of centralized robotic systems requires that users follow the proper front-end procedures.

BACK-END OPERATIONS

Back-end operations are those procedures that maintain the automation for continued use. Examples of back-end operations are cleaning and maintaining equipment, managing and stocking inventory, removing expired medications, maintaining software, maintaining interfaces, and maintaining internal data files. Good back-end procedures are important for safe front-end operation of the automation. These operations are often understaffed or mismanaged. Errors in the back-end operation can compound into significantly larger errors on the front end. Stringent double checks, audits, and monitoring are needed to maintain safe back-end operations. Examples of safety problems associated with back-end operations are listed in **Table 13-1**.

Table 13-1. Common Safety Problems with Back-End Operations of Automation

- Out-of-stock medications in dispensing equipment
- Expired medications in dispensing equipment
- Repackaging errors and errors with overbagging

- Restocking into the wrong location
- Stocking look-alike medications in close proximity to each other
- Incorrect assignment of stocking and par levels
- Improper cleaning and maintenance
- Improper monitoring of interfaces
- Errors in maintenance of medication data tables
- Management of ADS-dispensing overrides

AREAS FOR IMPROVEMENT

Improvement in pharmacy automation is needed to better support safe workflows. Inventory management, process monitoring, decision-support integration, and best-practice research are necessary to maximize the safe use of automated systems.

Out-of-stock medications, medications that are not stocked, and expired medications in dispensing systems have a negative impact on medication safety. If a medication is not available at a nursing unit at the appropriate time, the nurse may resort to shortcuts in an effort to locate it. At best, the medication will be administered late. Many of today's ADS lack appropriate inventory-management support. These systems need to support accurate stocking and inventory controls through the automated adjustments of par and reorder levels. The systems should also automatically request users to add items to or remove items from the dispensing cabinet on the basis of order activity and use.

Reports are needed that monitor back-end operations and show the link between back-end and front-end operations. An example of such a report in robotic cart filling is one that shows the number of manual cart-fill picks caused by stock outages. A similar report can show out-of-stock and other error conditions for ADS.

Decision-support functionality needs to be integrated into ADS for safer override dispensing. Therapeutic duplication checks and allergy and dose-range checks will create a safer environment for these devices.

Little research has been published on best practices associated with automated systems. Such research is needed. Available technologies must be compared and optimal workflows identified.

Clinical Pharmacy Automation

Medication clinical-order processing tools such as allergy interaction, therapeutic duplication, and dose-range checking are in use at many facilities. There are many additional information tools to assist the pharmacist with safe and efficient clinical practice. These tools support documentation of clinical activities, communication, and identification of medication issues.

ORDER VERIFICATION

The most common clinical tools are the automated checks that occur at the time of order entry. Determining which clinical alerts to present at the time of order entry is difficult. It is important to display important warnings without burdening the user with other warnings. Research is needed to identify best practices in this area.

Expansion of automated checking at many facilities has been limited because the necessary information is not integrated into their systems. Dose calculations require patient height, weight, age, and laboratory results. These data should be available to the pharmacist at the time of order verification.

THERAPY VERIFICATION

The implementation of CPOE has introduced some complexities into the order-verification process. In keeping with JCAHO requirements, most CPOE systems support pharmacist verification of orders prior to medication administration. This verification is accomplished by presenting each order to the pharmacist for review. During verification, the pharmacist is able to view the patient's medication profile. This approach to order review is similar for interfaced and integrated CPOE and pharmacy systems. The problem is that current-order-review methods offer substantially less functionality to the pharmacist than the paper process did. In the paper process, the pharmacist is given an order sheet that contains all orders for the patient. This allows the pharmacist to verify that lab tests and dietary orders are appropriate for the medications ordered. In addition, many hospitals use preprinted order sheets to support specific care plans. Since pharmacists are familiar with these forms, they can easily scan the form and identify changes from the preprinted defaults. This efficiently supports the pharmacist's need to verify the therapy. Rather than receiving just one order at a time, pharmacists need to receive the orders and order sets in a way that supports safe, accurate, and efficient verification of medication therapy. The current application support of CPOE verification makes it difficult for pharmacists to see the forest (therapy) through the trees (orders).

MONITORING OF THERAPY

Many information technology tools are available for medication monitoring.[26] For example, automated reports can make it possible to monitor and detect predefined trigger events. The events monitored can be specific lab results, medication orders, medication-dispensing events, charting events, or error-reporting systems. These reports can be created in batches that include triggers over a defined period of time or they can be displayed immediately. Trigger reports can be used to identify conditions that may require pharmacy intervention or identify a potential adverse drug event (ADE). Examples of trigger events are a laboratory value that exceeds normal ranges or the dispensing of a reversing agent. Error-reporting systems can be audited against trigger reports and chart reviews to identify detection rates and error-reporting effectiveness.

Linking of the laboratory and pharmacy databases can provide many opportunities for enhanced monitoring and ordering. Linkage of medication and laboratory results can support better automated dose verification and monitor the appropriateness of antibiotic therapy and anticoagulation therapy. CPR systems have decision-support engines that can validate new orders against laboratory results and other patient information. Stand-alone systems are available that have databases that receive lab and medication data via standard interfaces. These systems also have rules engines and communications functions to support medication monitoring after an order is entered. Both the CPR and stand-alone systems support the monitoring of lab results against active orders.

Standards for the coding of laboratory results and medications allow vendors to develop databases of standard rules for decision-support systems. Because it is so costly for hospitals to develop their own rule sets, a public database of evidence-based rules would be valuable.[27]

MEDICATION INFORMATION DATABASES

The advent of the Internet and of handheld computing devices has increased the accessibility of medication information. Hospitals are replacing print formularies with online formularies.[28] Most medication references and journals are available online as full text. Many clinical computer applications provide direct links to online reference databases.

Medication references are also available for handheld computers. Such computers can contain the equivalent to many volumes of printed material and provide quick access via search tools. As wireless networks are implemented in more facilities, portable access to online information will become possible.

COMMUNICATION TOOLS

Accurate, reliable, and efficient communication is essential to support medication-process workflows. Careful design of workflows to use electronic communication technology can make them more efficient and safer. Good communication support in clinical systems results in fewer redundancies and better documentation.

Communication is supported in CPR systems via messaging inboxes, outboxes, and work queues. These work in much the same way as e-mail applications do, but the clinical messaging is integrated with the clinical applications. For example, if a pharmacist is reviewing a physician order and needs to intervene for clarification, an intervention message is attached to the order and forwarded to the ordering physician. The physician reviews the message and responds to the pharmacist. The communication occurs quickly and is well documented. These messaging systems also support workgroups and the ability to delegate work and communications. The result is faster response to communications, fewer interruptions, and better documentation.[13,29]

INTERVENTION TRACKING

Intervention-tracking systems provide vital information to support quality improvement in the medication process. The capture of intervention data is difficult unless the process is simple and can be easily incorporated into the clinician's work. To support this need, intervention documentation has been integrated into Internet Web solutions, pharmacy information systems, and handheld computers.[30]

Handheld Wireless Devices and Machine-Readable Coding

Wireless handheld devices have been used in the shipping and delivery industries for many years. These devices support accurate tracking of packages, receipt of goods, and inventory management. Key features of these devices are small screens, small keypads, touch-sensitive screens, integrated bar-code readers, and wireless networking.

These devices provide good support for applications that require minimal textual keyboard entry, need to display only a minimal amount of data, and require mobility. They have been used successfully for electronic-charting applications. Their chief advantage is small size and mobility. The disadvantage for medication administration is that the screens can be hard to read. They also do not support the occasional need to enter textual information when charting medications. It can be difficult for nurses to carry the devices when they are handling several medications at the same time. Many hospitals are using wireless charting devices on small carts to provide more-readable screens, ensure portability, and facilitate keyboard data entry.

Recent mandates by the FDA that machine-readable bar codes be printed on all unit dose medications will enable expanded use of bar-code charting systems.[31] Current bar-code charting implementations are primarily in facilities that repackage medications for robotic dispensing. Lot numbers and expiration dates may one day be added to the bar codes.

In order to close the loop on safety in medication administration, many hospitals print bar codes on patient wristbands. Current devices and software applications support these bar codes in clinical laboratory applications.

New technology using radio frequency identification tags support patient tracking and identification. This technology can also support patient identification for medication charting. These devices can be read without touching or waking the patient and can be read much more reliably than bar codes.

Order Scanning Technologies

Scanning technologies can support faster communication between nursing and pharmacy.

The newer technologies provide better resolution than fax scanning and support new workflows in pharmacy. This technology supports centralization of order-entry processing. It is even possible to consolidate the order processing of several hospitals.[32] Order-scanning systems allow pharmacists to flag problem orders and to assign them to their work queues for follow-up. The system also collects data that are needed to analyze order turn-around times and order activity by time of day.

Integration of Workflows

The health care environment is complex and demanding. It has zero tolerance for errors, demands good communication and coordination between all functional areas, and must provide individual care to each patient. To achieve these goals, work processes need to be well designed and supported by technology. The design of good workflows is difficult because there is little research-based evidence on best processes. As a result, the workflows developed are tightly coupled and in constant flux. Technology support for these workflows is essential not only to ensure efficient and safe operations but to also gather evidence to identify best practices.

Workflow requirements for medications may be categorized into three components: clinical, operational, and financial. Clinical workflows support safe and effective clinical decision making. Operational workflows are the processes needed to implement clinical decisions such as order processing and medication preparation, distribution, and administration. Financial workflows support accurate inventory controls, pricing, charge capture, and patient billing. In many health systems, the technology tools that support each of these workload components reside on a different computer system. Data interfaces provide the technical integration between the systems.

When developing workflows, one must balance the needs of these three components. Designing workflows that meet all three components is difficult, primarily because the software for each system is designed to support its specific component workflows. Integration is easy when the workflows match between systems; the challenges arise when they don't. An example of mismatched workflows is that which occurs between billing and distribution operations in hospitals with centralized cart fills. Additional operations work is needed to credit returned medications. Many times returns cannot be accurately processed because of operational issues. Integration issues are simpler when the systems being integrated are from the same or affiliated vendors because the vendors have designed their systems to support common workflows.

Similar issues exist when integrating workflows between the functional parts of the medication process, i.e., order entry, medication distribution, and medication administration. Workflow design can become extremely difficult when each function resides on a separate system.

The result of mismatched workflows is compromised safety. It is difficult for the information technology to support good communication between physicians and pharmacists when physicians are entering and validating orders on separate computer systems than pharmacists. Additional process and communication issues can develop if nurses use a separate application for medication charting.

Clinical or safety workflow needs are given higher priority than operational or financial concerns if the safety needs are supported by evidence. Most operational and financial needs can be quantified into financial or efficiency savings that are supported by evidence. Because safety needs are not well supported by evidence, they often lose the workflow argument. Therefore, it is important to consider how decisions relating to single versus multiple vendors and interfacing versus integrating can affect the ability to develop workflows to support safe medication use.

The Pharmacy Informatics Specialist

A pharmacy informatics specialist is an individual who is responsible for the bridge between the information systems technology components and the clinical, operational, and business needs in the medication-use process. This requires that the informatics specialist be an excellent communicator. He or she is a patient and medication-process advocate to information services (IS) and a technology advocate to pharmacy. The specialist has an educational role in helping IS personnel understand the safety and operational workflow needs of patient care and, at the same time, helping pharmacy personnel understand how information system tools can best support their needs.

Pharmacy informatics specialists normally have education or experience in a clinical discipline involved in the medication process. Persons with such a background may include pharmacists, pharmacy technicians, and nurses. Most specialists have additional education in informatics, management information systems, or computer science.

Pharmacy informatics specialists can report to IS or to pharmacy departments. In order to be successful, the specialists should attend meetings of the pharmacy management team as well as of the clinical information systems team.

New pharmacy informatics roles will likely develop as CPOE and decision-support systems continue to be implemented. Clinical pharmacists with training in new, rule-based clinical tools will be able to define monitoring criteria for pharmacists as well as physicians.

Conclusion

The use of automation and information technology has had significant impact on enhancing medication safety. The potential for the use of these technologies to support safe medication practice is tremendous. The development of these medication-safety tools is still in its infancy. Significant additional benefits of these tools will occur upon standardization of data, identification of best practice, and refinement of the tools to support best-practice workflows and decision support. The journey has just begun.

References

1. Oren E, Shaffer ER, Guglielmo BJ. Impact of emerging technologies on medication errors and adverse drug events. *Am J Health-Syst Pharm.* 2003;60:1447-58.

2. Bates DW. Using information technology to reduce rates of medication errors in hospitals. *Br Med J.* 2000;320:788-791.

3. Bates DW, Cullen D, Laird N, Peterson LA, Small SD Servi D, et al. Incidence of adverse drug events and potential adverse drug events: implications for prevention. *JAMA.* 1995;274:29-34.

4. Patterson ES, Cook RI, Render ML. Improving patient safety by identifying side effects from introducing bar coding in medication administration. *JAMA.* 2002;9:540-553.

5. Institute for Safe Medication Practices. Medication Error Prevention Toolbox. *ISMP Medication Safety Alert.* June 2, 1999.

6. Murphy N. Safe systems through better user interfaces. 1998. Available at: http://www.embedded.com/98/9808fe.htm. Accessed January 24, 2005.

7. Anderson Consulting Group Inc. System "uptime" study for the Healthcare Industry. Downington, PA: Anderson Consulting Group; December 1, 2001.

8. Kilbridge P. Computer crash—lessons from a system failure. *New Engl J Med.* 2003;348:881-882.

9. Institute of Medicine. *The Computer-Based Patient Record: An Essential Technology for Health Care.* Rev. ed. Washington, DC: National Academy Press; 1997.

10. Kohn LT, Corrigan JM, Donaldson MD, eds. Committee on Quality of Health in America, Institute of Medicine. *To Err Is Human: Building a Safer Health System.* Washington, DC: National Academy Press; 1999.

11. Committee on Quality of Health Care in America, Institute of Medicine. *Crossing the Quality Chasm: A New Health System for the 21st Century.* Washington, DC: National Academy Press; 2001.

12. Handler T. A restatement of Gartner's CPR definition. Stamford, CT: Gartner Group. December 12, 2000.

13. Dadam P, Reichert M, Kuhn K. Clinical Workflows–The Killer Application for Process-oriented Information Systems? Ulmer Informatik-Bericht No. 97-16. Ulm, Germany: University of Ulm; November 1997.

14. Health Level Seven, Inc. What Is HL7? Ann Arbor, MI: Health Level Seven, Inc. Available at: www.lh7.org. Accessed February 12, 2005.

15. Leape LL, Bates DW, Cullen DJ, Cooper J, Demonaco HJ, Gallivan T, et al. Systems analysis of adverse drug events. ADE Prevention Study Group. *JAMA.* 1995;274:35-43.

16. Milstein A, Galvin RS, Delbanco SF, Salver P, Buck Jr CR. Improving the safety of health care: the Leapfrog initiative. *Effect Clin Pract.* 2000;3:313-316.

17. Pederson CA, Schneider PJ, Santell JP. ASHP national survey of pharmacy practice in hospital settings: Prescribing and transcribing— 2001. *Am J Health-Syst Pharm.* 2001;58:2251-2266.

18. Agency for Healthcare Research and Quality. Making Health Care Safer: A Critical Analysis of Patient Safety Practices. Rockville, MD: Department of Health and Human Services; 2001:59-69. AHRQ publication 01-E058.

19. Oren E, Shaffer ER, Guglielmo BJ. Impact of emerging technologies on medication errors and adverse drug events. *Am J Health-Syst Pharm.* 2003;60:1447-1458.

20. First Consulting Group. Computerized Physician Order Entry: Costs, Benefits and Challenges, A Case Study Approach. Long Beach, CA: First Consulting Group; 2003.

21. Perini VJ, Weaver PE. Midyear Poster Presentation, ASHP 1998.

22. American Society of Health-System Pharmacists. ASHP guidelines on the safe use of automated compounding devices for the preparation of parenteral nutrition admixtures. *Am J Health-Syst Pharm.* 2000;57:1343-1348.

23. Flynn EA, Barker KN, Carnahan BJ. National observational study of prescription dispensing accuracy and safety in 50 pharmacies. *J Am Pharm Assoc.* 2003;43:191-203.

24. American Society of Health-System Pharmacists. ASHP guidelines on the safe use of automated medication storage and distribution devices. *Am J Health-Syst Pharm.* 1998;55:1403-1407.

25. Klibanov OM, Eckel SF. Effects of automated dispensing on inventory control, billing, workload, and potential for medication errors. *Am J Health-Syst Pharm.* 2003;60:569-572.

26. Miller, LK, Nelson MS, Spurlock B. A Com-

pendium of Suggested Practices for Preventing and Reducing Medication Errors. Sacramento, CA: California Institute for Health Systems Performance; 2001. Available at: http://www.cihsp.org. Accessed February 18, 2005.

27. Schiff GD, Klass D, Peterson J, Shah G, Bates D. Linking laboratory and pharmacy. *Arch Intern Med.* 2003;163:893-900.

28. McReadie SR, Stumpf JL, Benner TD. Building a better online formulary. *Am J Health-Syst Pharm.* 2002;59:1847-1852.

29. Andrew WF, Bruegel RB. Workflow management and the CPR. *Adv Health Information Exec.* 2003;7(2):49.

30. Clark JS, Klauck JA. Recording pharmacist's interventions with a personal digital assistant. *Am J Health-Syst Pharm* 2003;60:1772-1774.

31. US Food and Drug Administration. FDA rule requires bar codes on drugs and blood to help reduce errors. 2004. Available at: http://www.fda.gov/oc/initiatives/barcode-sadr/default.htm. Accessed January 24, 2005.

32. Cronk J. Digital scanning and consolidated entry of medication orders in a multihospital health system. *Am J Health-Syst Pharm.* 2002;59:731-733.

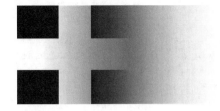

Application of Human Factors Engineering in Process and Equipment Design

Laura Lin Gosbee and
Mary E. Burkhardt

Introduction

The medication-use system is multifaceted, and improving its safety draws on many skills and disciplines. The majority of health care practitioners today have had little or no exposure to the concepts of human factors engineering (HFE), yet there are many areas in which the principles of HFE would be imperative in the medication-use system, in the workplace, and in information system and environmental design. Human factors engineering is the study of human capabilities and limitations and of the application of that knowledge to the design of systems. Technological advances in health care, whether they are new information systems, new medical devices, or new high-alert drugs, introduce new complexities. Complexities often creep in slowly, without drawing much attention. It isn't until disastrous events occur that these complexities are acknowledged, if at all, for the role they play in creating a system that is prone to human error. Complexities in the health care system make HFE relevant to safety practices. Other high-reliability organizations or high-risk industries have built safety cultures around HFE, by recognizing that one must fit the task (or system) to the human, and not vice versa.[1]

HFE is not a discipline that is done "somewhere else." To the contrary, HFE issues are everywhere; they are a part of everyday life.[2,3] HFE comes into play any time a human uses a machine, follows a protocol, reads instructions, interprets guidelines, records information, reads information, sees or hears a warning or alert, makes decisions, or monitors a situation or process. Vulnerabilities exist everywhere. Accordingly, HFE can and should be applied to almost everything.

This chapter reviews general concepts of HFE and illustrates its applicability to the medication-use system. It begins with an introduction that summarizes the general concepts of HFE. Next, it discusses target areas where HFE can be applied and identifies HFE stakeholders, which include both the architects of change that arise from an HFE approach and front-line personnel who are affected by these changes. The third section of the chapter provides an overview of what is involved in an HFE approach and of the activities in the hospital that should incorporate HFE. Finally, the chapter describes how employees in health systems can incorporate HFE into their medication-safety plans.

HFE Considerations

From a human factors perspective, the medication-use process is not just a sequence of activities. It is a complex process that involves the interaction of multiple systems made up of people, equipment (devices, software, paper forms), and organizational culture (policies, procedures, guidelines). Factors that are not always obvious or seen without the aid of a human factors mindset affect the way in which this process unfolds.[4] A systems perspective helps one see the interdependencies and interactions among various systems and system components. A human factors perspective helps one see and analyze the human-system interactions and identify areas that can benefit from human factors interventions.

User-system interaction shapes how work is carried out at both a macro level and a micro level. Carrying out tasks may range from coordinating people, tasks, or equipment to reading a warning label. The design of a system influences whether a user correctly operates a piece of equipment or follows a process (e.g., computerized order entry software, an infusion pump or a syringe, or a patient chart or protocol). The design of any of these system elements, whether intentional or unintentional, provides cues that tell the user how to operate it (e.g., correctly measuring medication or efficiently navigating through computer screens to find information). Cues might include, for example, the shape of a device, the use of color, the content and organization of displayed information, a navigation scheme in a software program, a type of display (e.g., digital or analog), whether information is presented as raw data or at a higher level, the layout of switches or buttons, labeling, or auditory feedback. Collectively, these factors determine how easy or difficult the device is to use and how well it supports the user's task.

Symptoms of poor design can be easily identified (see **Table 14-1**). Symptoms may be due to a combination of factors, but they are usually an indication that human factors issues are at play. HFE can help with identifying the underlying cause of these symptoms.

Table 14-1. Typical Symptoms that Indicate the Need for HFE

- Steps to use a device or to carry out a process seem nonintuitive or overly complex.
- Users find it difficult to learn or to remember how to use a device or to follow a protocol.
- Finding and fixing errors is time-consuming.
- Frequent refresher training is necessary to stay competent in use of a device or software.
- Users frequently mix up items because they look alike or their names sound alike.
- A sequence of activities is tedious, repetitious, or prone to slip-ups.
- Alarms occur for no good reason and are more of a nuisance than a help.
- The user cannot tell what a device or software program is doing.
- Users think the "old" way of doing things is better, even after achieving competence with the new way.
- Many work-arounds are needed (e.g., adding notes, extra warning labels, tape, markings).

Poor design can be considered a latent failure, i.e., a failure that creates a predisposition for errors to occur.[4,5] It lies in wait for a triggering event, usually initiated by an unsuspecting user. **Table 14-2** gives examples of latent failures, or human factors design issues, that may make a system susceptible to user errors. These are the underlying causes that create symptoms such as those listed in Table 14-1.

Table 14-2. Examples of HFE Design Issues that May Cause Symptoms Such as Those Listed in Table 14-1[6]

- Operator has insufficient information on which to make decisions.
- User is confronted with too much information, some of which is irrelevant.
- Critical information is not obvious or is hard to find.
- Information is not in a format that makes it apparent how it influences the operator's decision (e.g., data are not transformed to functionally relevant information, information visualization is not available or is inappropriate to user's goals and tasks).
- Navigation scheme, structure of the tasks, or process flow is not obvious or visible to the user.
- Default settings are not appropriate or are difficult to change.
- Data in the system are difficult to review.

Along with latent failures in design, other factors influence how work is performed in the medication-use process. Examples include

- user characteristics
- work environment
- team characteristics
- nature and complexity of the task
- concurrent tasks or activities

Problems arising from design issues listed in Table 14-2 may be aggravated or accelerated by the factors listed above. For more examples of these factors, see **Table 14-3**.

Table 14-3. Examples of Factors that Influence Human Performance

FACTORS	EXAMPLES
User characteristics	Education and training, which influence expectations and biases; sleep deprivation (influences reaction time, alertness); cultural norms
	Orienting staff after they worked a shift or have other work place fatigue can affect how amenable they are to learning and their subsequent performance.
Work environment	Light levels, layout of work area, interruptions, noise level (e.g., information overload caused by too many irrelevant warnings or irrelevant alarms)
	Ambient noise from printers, phones, doorbells, beepers, radios, work processes, and staff chatter
Team characteristics	Team dynamics, division of responsibility, team communication/coordination (centralized or distributed), team expectations, shared equipment
	Workplace structure, such as team-based versus primary care nursing models, the interface between pharmacy and nursing, cross-departmental teams, centralized versus decentralized pharmacy department structures

cont'd

Nature and complexity	Repetition involved, vigilance demanded (length of vigilance-of the task, related task, amount or nature of stimulation), workload (physical and mental demands of the task, frustration), dependence on short- or long-term memory, expertise required, time pressure, level of automation
	Checking unit dose carts, i.v. chemotherapy orders, in-depth problem solving in drug therapy monitoring, workload distribution during peak times
Concurrent tasks	Interference from other mental demands (e.g., operating other devices simultaneously, communicating with other personnel, following multiple policies)
	Pharmacists simultaneously filling outpatient or discharge prescriptions from the inpatient pharmacy, supervising other workers, and juggling order entry, responding to beepers, and taking charge of and code-cart restocking

Human-system interaction is also influenced by human characteristics. These characteristics include limitations in perception and cognition as well as physical limits such as strength. Collectively, these human limitations define how we interact with systems—for instance, how much we can remember; how well we can differentiate between objects, sounds, and information; how well we can find and integrate information; how long we can remain cognitively alert; and how much interference is experienced when we are interrupted during a task.

While the factors that can adversely affect the human-system interaction may seem unending, there are also human capabilities that can be credited for making things work, despite nonideal conditions and influences.[7] These include abilities for complex reasoning, problem solving, and adapting to new or changing situations.[8] These qualities allow humans to understand complex relationships between various types of data to infer the state of a system (e.g., process control, monitoring vital signs), to detect pertinent information when presented in appropriate formats, to detect trends when data are displayed graphically (e.g., complex process-control tasks), or to draw on experience when handling a crisis. One of the tenets of human factors is to take advantage of these human capabilities when designing a system that supports human work.[1,9]

The understanding of human capabilities as well as limitations as they apply to work forms the basis of HFE design principles (see **Table 14-4**).[10] Efficiency, reliability, and ease of use are best achieved when the design recognizes human limitations and takes advantage of human capabilities. Human factors principles are discussed in detail below in the section entitled "Overview of HFE Approach."

The factors described above and summarized in Tables 14-2 through 14-4 (i.e., latent failures, influencing factors, and human limitations and capabilities) are important in understanding how work is actually, as opposed to should be, carried out. This is central to designing systems that take into consideration human factors as well as understanding why errors might be occurring in a system.[4,10-12]

Table 14-4. Examples of Human Limitations and Capabilities and Their Implications for Design

	NATURE OF LIMITATION	IMPLICATIONS FOR DESIGN
Limitations	**Perceptual** • contrast of lettering to background • differentiation of colors, shapes, and words that look alike or sound alike **Cognitive** • short-/long-term memory • integration of information from spatially separated sources **Physical** • time/accuracy trade-offs of gross motor tasks • reach limitations	HFE principles for design and development of • labels, warnings • software programs • paper forms • process/activity flow • workplace design • training/education • cognitive aids • decision-support systems • policies and protocols
	NATURE OF CAPABILITY	
Capabilities	**Perceptual** • ability to perceive trend information when graphic data are presented • ability to spatially locate auditory or visual signals **Cognitive** • ability to understand complex relationships and make diagnoses • ability to troubleshoot **Physical** • Ability to learn and carry out complex sequences of motor tasks	

Adapted from Gosbee.[6]

Callout Box 1. Breadth and Variety of HFE Applications

Air Traffic Control. Signal detection, communication, and coordination procedures, decision making, situation awareness, information displays, decision-support systems.

Aviation. Cockpit displays, checklists, helmet-mounted displays, 3D auditory displays, training and simulation, communication and coordination, automation, situation awareness.

Computers. Software interface design (e.g., graphical user interfaces such as menu systems, drop-down boxes, icons, links, navigation, data visualization, direct manipulation), speech input and display, manual input devices, software documentation.

Industrial/Occupational. Work schedules, stress, protective equipment, materials handling, job design, organizational design, personnel selection, training, job aids, illumination, noise, climate, vibration, architecture and interior design.

Medical Systems/Rehabilitation. Medical-device design, alarms, information display, situation awareness in patient monitoring, home medical devices, health care informa-

cont'd

tion systems, assistive devices for disabled or elderly individuals, instructions, labeling, and packaging of medication for the elderly.

Process Control (e.g., nuclear power, petrochemical). Information display (e.g., data visualization, navigation), alarms, team coordination and communication, training and simulation, decision making, decision-support systems, procedures (computerized and manual), situation awareness, expertise, and adaptation.

Transportation. Vigilance, head-up displays, road signs and warnings, interference from concurrent tasks (e.g., talking on cell phone while driving), ergonomic design of seating, design and layout of controls.

Callout Box 2. Learning More about HFE

Attend human factors courses offered through universities.

Go to annual meetings of the Human Factors and Ergonomics Society (www.hfes.org), the Association for Computing Machinery (ACM) (e.g., www.acm.org/sigchi/), and the Usability Professionals' Association (www.upassoc.org).

Look for human factors-related periodicals such as *Human Factors, Ergonomics in Design*, ACM journals (e.g., *Transactions on Computer-Human Interaction*), *International Journal on Man-Machine Studies, IEEE Transactions on Systems, Man, and Cybernetics; Human-Computer Interaction*.

Look for HFE guidelines, such as Do It by Design (FDA), Write It Right (FDA), and HFE Guidelines and Preferred Practices for the Design of Medical Devices (AAMI/ANSI).[4]

Look for books that deal with human factors. If you are new to the topic, factors, start with

Norman D. *The Design of Everyday Things*[2]

Cohen M. *Medication Errors*[11]

Casey S. *Set Phasers on Stun—And Other True Tales of Design, Technology, and Human Error*[8]

If you want to know more, then move on to

Wickens CD. *Engineering Psychology and Human Performance*[1]

Nielson J. *Usability Engineering*[10]

Wiklund M. *Medical Device Design and Equipment Design–Usability Engineering and Ergonomics*.[12]

Sanders MS and McCormick EJ. *Human Factors Engineering and Design*.[13]

Meister D. *Human Factors Testing and Evaluation*.[14]

Rubin J. *Handbook of Usability Testing: How to Plan, Design and Conduct Effective Tests*.[15]

Target Areas for Applying HFE

What does HFE have to do with pharmacy practice and medication management? Once a practitioner studies human behavior and the science of human error from a systems approach, it becomes apparent that much of what occurs inadvertently in health care mishaps is related to a design that does not encourage safety (e.g., a lack of engineering controls or fail-safes) and the failure of the work system to communicate impending dangers to the worker (e.g., lack of feedback, poorly designed warning or alarm system).

The next question that comes to mind is, Where can pharmacists and others apply HFE to improve efficiency, reduce errors, and reduce the mental workload of clinicians? The applicability of HFE is more apparent in the dispensing side of pharmacy practice, but it has applicability across the spectrum of pharmaceutical care (for example, see: pharmacy.auburn.edu/cpod/cpod.htm#publications). It is applicable, for example, in equipment, work areas, and work processes.

EQUIPMENT

The most obvious target area to apply human factors is equipment.[12,16] The word *equipment* covers a broad range of items. As used in this chapter, it includes any physical instantiation besides humans that serves a functional purpose in the workplace. This might include devices, whether they are simple or complex, for example: tubing, connectors, magnetic resonance imaging equipment, intravenous (i.v.) pumps, syringes, computer software, and paper forms (e.g., order forms, patient charts, policy manuals, warning or alert signs, checklists).

Equipment can be used to help carry out a physical task or to convey and record information. In all cases, equipment is used to help humans achieve some goal(s). *Equipment design*, in this context, refers to how well the equipment meets the needs of the user. For example, the design of equipment used in the preparation of parenteral products or the administration of i.v. solutions should be mindful of human limitations in perception, cognition, and motor abilities in order for it to be safe and effective, both for the user and for the patient.[4,10,12]

Computer systems are ubiquitous in the medication-use system. HFE deals with the human-computer interface of these systems. This includes information displays, navigation schemes (e.g., moving between screens, links to other areas of the program, the menu system, mechanism used to advance fields or steps in a process), levels of information presented (e.g., overview vs. details), methods of obtaining different views or of sorting information, types of graphical display that best depict information, how best to present the information that is useful to decisions to be made, effectiveness or disruptiveness of alarms,[17] type of user input device (e.g., keyboard, mouse, touch screen), and user feedback.

For instance, many pharmacists can readily identify with order-entry systems that use the "enter" button versus the "tab" button to change fields and know the perils of switching systems back and forth. But HFE is more than that. HFE deals with what and how information is presented to the user. HFE can help guide what information should be provided to aid human decision making, what information is needed to carry out different tasks, what information is needed to help users understand their progress in carrying out a task, and how the information should be displayed and organized so that the users can pick out areas of focus, find information and easily detect when something needs attention, carry out the actions that result from any decisions, and appreciate the implications of their decisions or actions. HFE has been used successfully in industries and high-reliability organizations to design systems that work with humans to maximize safety rather than overtaxing the worker in order to maintain safety.

HFE even applies in the design of paper forms. Well-designed forms, such as standardized order forms, pathways or care maps, and admission and assessment forms, encourage the user to fill them completely because they are easy to use and can be used to rapidly retrieve information. Paper forms can be used as cognitive aids (e.g., checklists or sequence of activities) that help shape the process flow. A cognitive aid can serve as an external mental model that makes explicit any knowledge that is critical to the user's task or decision making. One example of paper forms is the unit dose profile, which, despite its limitations, is extremely useful in helping pharmacists achieve an overview of the patient's care in one glance. Computerization of this functionality brought great business efficiencies. But when it came to researching drug therapy issues (i.e., backtracking to see the progression of orders), pharmacists often had to actively search out more information on such matters as doses returned not administered that was hidden deep within the computerized record and that was formerly readily apparent from glancing at the unit dose profile. Similarly, the 24-hour sign-out sheet for controlled substances gave nurses a broad overview of controlled-substance activity every day in one glance, but such information was often "lost" in the data-storage systems of automated dispensing systems. The information was in the device, but the user had to work harder or actively query in order to access it. Pharmacists' drug therapy monitoring profiles are another example of information that is readily displayable in the paper world but that may not yet be available in an electronic environment.

Overview charts or tables offer a good example of the way in which human factors can play a role in designing information displays. Most pharmacists found these tables easy to use and operationally efficient because drug information was displayed in a logical format that enabled the user to see the differences between and among products in the same category. Other examples of overview displays, including antibiogram charts, renal dosing charts, and compatibility charts, similarly demonstrate how the specific task and goal of the user dictates what information should be displayed and the format in which it should be presented. Human factors analysis is focused on these objectives, i.e., determining the content and format of information so that it best supports the user's decision-making tasks and other goal-oriented activities.

Print and label design (e.g., patient instructions or warning labels) is another target area that can be examined with HFE. The human factors issues are similar to those associated with other forms of information display. The content and format of the information can be analyzed or designed through HFE methods. The text (color, font, size, contrast with background), shape and color of the label, graphics/icons, readability, language, text organization, and content are all aspects of design that can be analyzed through human factors methods. Designing a label to convey risks can benefit from established human factors research in the area of warnings and risk communication.[18-20]

Callout Box 3. A Pharmacy Manager Recalls HFE Failures

When I joined a hospital as director of pharmacy, staff easily let me know which pieces of equipment, such as printers, packagers, and keyboards, that they found most usable. Was it the staff members' love of the task that either wore out the equipment in happy batches of labor or that banished it to the dust-filled corners of the pharmacy?

Retrospectively, I now believe that much of the love-or-hate relationships staff had with equipment were rooted in human factors. The most striking example was a printer that did the line feed so that you didn't waste labels but was designed with a platen (roller) that couldn't be removed but could pinch your fingers. This resulted in countless jams of labels, which required surgical extraction with forceps and a pharmacy spatula, and poor-quality labels. I was happy to toss that printer and its associated problems into the dumpster in favor of the old, standard dot matrix printer that wasted a few labels (that we recycled anyway) but cranked out the work year after year until its parts wore out. I understand that the same love-hate relationships exist between people and their barcode printers and numerous other pieces of pharmacy equipment.

I remember purchasing fancy equipment for packaging unit dose liquids. It was one fabulous machine, with its rotating disk and six-cup filling cycle. The technicians hated it, and setting up the machine was so laborious that they would rather package things by hand. We couldn't keep anyone trained on it, because no one used it enough to remember how to set it up again. A $10,000 investment went down the drain.

Examples of Equipment Design

Unit Dose Packaging

In the early days of unit dose, packaging was a major challenge. Examples of HFE issues can be seen with systems used to package liquids and with various sealing methods. It seems there were two extremes, leaking or impenetrable. Glass containers fell into disuse, having been replaced by plastic cups that were often of poor quality and virtually impossible to open. Packaging for tablets or capsules often required scissors or a pocketknife to open. Countless examples such as this occur in practice and in the over-the-counter world of pharmaceutical packaging.

Epinephrine Auto-Injectors

Imagine thinking you need to click a penlike device to administer epinephrine in the event of anaphylaxis, only to find out that it had been redesigned to require a "stab" motion. From a human factors perspective, the device itself, and the metaphor it conjures, provide misleading cues on how it should work. Countless health care professionals and patients have been handed the device without training. Any device whose operation is not intuitive runs the risk of user error, particularly in an emergency, even though instructions for use are available on the packaging.[21]

Acetaminophen Drops

One company redesigned the packaging for its high-concentration acetaminophen drops so that they could not be poured out of the bottle and accidentally administered in place of lower-concentration acetaminophen liquid. The need to use a dropper to extract the drops was a forcing function to ensure the parent or nurse used the appropriate measuring device. However, design considerations should not stop here. How the dropper is gradated and marked influences whether the user makes the correct measurement. Also, the content and layout of the label and instructions play a role in how the user interprets and understands what measurement to make. For instance, if the instructions specify that "2 droppersful" are to be given, the user may misinterpret this to mean give "2 full droppers." Often one dropperful does not mean a full dropper, but just a portion (i.e., up to a specific notch) of a dropper. This misunderstanding could easily lead to an overdose.

Packaging

Some companies have made efforts to incorporate safety into their packaging. For example, whole product lines of injectable drugs have been redesigned to incorporate color differentiation, in addition to size, shape, and other visual cues to help with identification and differentiation. Some companies have put labels on both sides of the containers. Others have marketed dosage forms that limit the amount in the i.v. bag or that offer drugs only in premade solutions.

Counting Tray

Sometimes, simpler designs are better. Take the standard counting tray in every pharmacy. It is simple yet efficient and outperforms many an electronic counting device for some tablets. There are minimal instructions; the design is so intuitive that someone can use it after observing another person use it only one time.

Syringes

Safety-shielded syringes are designed to protect the health care worker from needle sticks. The sheath moves over the needle after use when the device is discarded. When used in the pharmacy, the sheath can be very clumsy. It tends to move over the needle *before* the user is done using the device to inject drug into an i.v. solution, causing inaccuracy in measurement and leaking of the product all over the user and the i.v. bag or bottle.

WORK SPACES

The application of human factors and ergonomics to work-space design is not new. It has played a role in transforming assembly lines and manufacturing facilities into efficient production systems, using time-motion studies or work-flow analysis pioneered by Taylor[22,23] and Frank and Lillian Gilbreth.[24,25] Many pharmacies have taken little advantage of such approaches to achieve efficiency and reliability in work flow in the pharmacy. Improvement can be made through organizing work areas to match or support the work flow or by organizing products in a way that supports the tasks of locating and retrieving products. Some products should be grouped, while others should be separated to avoid mix-ups. Equipment and storage design should meet the functional needs for tasks. The results of a human factors analysis can inform decisions on spatial organization and positioning so that it supports work flow and movement of people and materials from one area to another. Budgeting and space constraints often impede the director's ability to make improvements in these areas. New construction often will meet building codes and Americans with Disabilities Act requirements, yet fall short of meeting human factors considerations that might improve efficiency, prevent errors, or improve comfort level of workers. For instance, the selection of open rather than closed areas has impact on oversight and supervision, which ultimately has an impact on safety. Open and uncluttered dispensing areas often lend themselves to improved communication among staff and better oversight of ancillary staff. Work areas that are mazelike and chopped up into separate rooms often present challenges to staff in terms of security, efficiency, communication, and workplace morale.

Callout Box 4. Results of Overlooking HFE in Workplace Design

Did you ever think the design of a pharmacy could be a safety hazard? Or that it could make a candidate for employment decide not to join your staff?

I once convinced a terrific candidate to join our hospital staff, but she lost interest the minute she stepped inside the pharmacy. The pharmacy had been designed by the hospital architect, who did not listen to the previous pharmacy director or the staff. In subsequent years, numerous safety hazards were identified, all of which were attributed to poor design. The design-related problems included security issues that resulted in drug theft, supervisory problems, low morale, medication errors, inefficiencies in processing orders, obsolete inventory, drug shortages, staff injuries, and overall unsafe working conditions. After 10 years, the department was renovated, at a cost of more than $500,000. Lack of attention to HFE principles early in the design phase can end up being very costly.

Drug security can also be improved by making work spaces more open. Cluttered and poorly organized areas increase the likelihood of error as well as of theft. Communication and teamwork are easier if employees are in physical proximity and can hear and see coworkers and consult each other.

An emphasis on workplace design is essential to ensure the secure storage of medications, especially controlled substances. Well-lit, well-designed areas are especially important for staff who perform tedious tasks such as counting, packaging, and dispensing controlled substances. Factors such as counter height and depth, seamless work counters, organizational space, counting trays, dispensing records, and storage space for complex and changing inventories also merit attention. An uncluttered, well-lit work space also improves the ability to use video surveillance of the dispensing area, which can be a valuable tool in detecting and preventing drug diversion.

WORK PROCESSES

Many processes in the medication system are geared toward molding or accommodating human behavior. Examples include formularies and protocols and policies on such matters as automatic stop orders (ASOs) and therapeutic substitution. Designing or developing these processes can benefit from HFE concepts. HFE methods can be used to design processes and the equipment or products used to support these processes such that they are more efficient and less prone to error. Understanding the process flow, information flow, material flow, communication and coordination, and supervisory roles involved can help determine the requirements for designing equipment to support the work and materials such as cognitive aids (e.g., cheat sheets, pocket guides, checklists) that serve as external reference sources for the people involved in carrying out tasks or making decisions in a given process. The design of processes is intimately intertwined with the work-space design and equipment design. These system elements are considered "coupled," in that changes in one affect the others. For instance, a change in a process or protocol has an effect on the way in which users might carry out a task in a given work space, or it might change the way in which they use the equipment. This interdependence makes it imperative to examine not just isolated elements in the medication-use system but in the system as a whole, that is, equipment, workspace, and processes.

Standardization and checklists are often used as means to shape the ways in which people work. Sliding-scale insulin protocols that are part of diabetes-management protocols established by health care facilities are an example. HFE is not about standardization and checklists per se, but rather about the analysis that goes into determining what parts of a system would benefit from standardization, what the standard should be, and what work aids (e.g., equipment, tools, checklists, cheat sheets) should be designed and provided to users to support such standardization.

For example, ASOs had an important safety role when patient lengths of stay were longer and drugs changed less frequently. They addressed the danger of therapy being continued too long. Now, orders change more rapidly: Patients move unit to unit more often, and the utility of the ASO policies has come into question. In fact, discontinuation of some newer drugs (HIV drugs, tuberculosis drugs, antithrombotics) may be even more dangerous than accidental continuation of therapy. Pharmacy and therapeutics committees should take a serious look at the utility of the ASO process in total context of the patients they serve.[26] This change in the very nature of drug therapy means that the complexity and basic premise behind ASO are also changing, making it a perfect candidate for examining human factors issues at play. The content of an ASO policy and any supporting software or paperwork (policy manuals, guidelines, checklists, reminders, etc.) should be analyzed and designed using human factors methods. Other interventions that arise from a human factors analysis of work processes include the interjection of forcing functions, use of fail-safes or checklists, and feedback of information. For instance, cardiac-arrest carts often have checklists and are standardized throughout the organization.

Examples of other work processes that have HFE components include order processing subsystems such as new-order processing, reports and communications between and among providers, and a myriad of drug-administration tasks. Drugs administered by the wrong route frequently can be traced back to the failure to "design out" the wrong-route failure mode through the appropriate use of connectors in the medical product industry. Wrong-tube, wrong-hole, and wrong-connector events occur because of the failure to design out errors or to force the user to do it correctly by eliminating alternatives.

Stakeholders

For any target area selected as a candidate for applying human factors analysis, it is necessary to identify (1) who should perform the HFE activity and (2) the users of the end product (i.e., the device or process). Stakeholders may include

- device makers

- pharmaceutical vendors
- software vendors
- group purchasing organizations
- hospitals (e.g., physicians, nurses, pharmacists, respiratory therapists, technicians, biomedical engineers, and staff in procurement, central supply, storeroom)
- patients and their caregivers

Decision makers need to consider how the roles of the various stakeholders are relevant to HFE analysis considerations. For example, with patient-controlled analgesia (PCA) pumps, the manufacturer should perform the HFE activity related to designing the device. But at the facility or health-system level, the end-user population comprises multiple stakeholders. The intermediaries, such as biomedical engineers, perform the initial setup of devices (e.g., set the defaults). Physicians fill in the PCA order sheet. Pharmacists evaluate, enter, and verify the order; they also prepare the products and purchase related drugs and supplies. Nurses assemble the supplies, program the pump, and teach the patient. Patients use the activation button. Each stakeholder group interacts with the device (or related processes) in a different way and has varying goals and tasks. A human factors analysis can be performed with different stakeholders in mind.

Within each stakeholder group may be subgroups. Analysis focusing on different stakeholders and even subgroups will uncover the many layers where human factors issues may reside. For instance, a nurse who works in the recovery room may be programming PCA pumps on an hourly basis, whereas a floor nurse may be programming less frequently. This difference in frequency of use may have implications on the risk for errors and the type of errors that may occur, how frequently refresher training is required, the extent and nature of redesign that is warranted, or the type of cognitive aid that is most effective. Examination of these issues should be performed across a broad spectrum of user groups, since one user group may encounter different difficulties or issues with a device than another does.

Overview of HFE Approach

In describing the human factors process, it is useful first to categorize the activities that are candidates for incorporating a human factors approach. Activities that have an impact on medication safety can be broadly categorized into development and evaluation activities. These two categories include activities that center around (1) developing an in-house product, such as software, paper forms, policies and protocols, guidelines, or training and education; and (2) evaluating products for procurement, risk assessment, and adverse-event investigation.

While these two categories of activities might appear to be vastly different, both types of activities—development and evaluation—employ the same set of human factors tools. The main element that differentiates how the tools are employed is the final product of employing the tools. In development activities, human factors methods can be used to develop design requirements and guide design ideas.[10,12,14,15] In evaluation activities, such as procurement decisions or adverse event investigations, human factors methods can be used to detect and identify user-interaction problems that are born from poor design that might lead to errors.[10,14] Later in this section, we provide a list of activities that are ideal candidates for incorporating human factors methods.

HFE DEVELOPMENT ACTIVITIES

Human factors provides two concepts that can help developers of in-house products ensure that their products are not breeding grounds for errors. The concepts are (1) user-centered design and (2) iterative cycles of design and testing.

User-Centered Design

A design process that incorporates HFE is often referred to as "user centered." In contrast, many products on the market today are "technology centered"—i.e., the design is built around a new technology, with little regard to the prospective user. The latter approach is laden with pitfalls because correct and efficient use of that technology depends on its usability. No matter how groundbreaking a new technology or system is, the human must be able to correctly, efficiently, and safely operate or use it. If this is to happen, human factors must be considered early on in the process- or product-development cycle.

A user-centered approach focuses on the end users. The end user might be an engineer responsible for setting up a device and troubleshooting when problems occur, a care provider who educates the patient on how to use the device, a care provider who assembles the device or attaches it to the patient, or a patient who uses the device without supervision. Each end user has a different set of functional needs; in some cases, these needs overlap. That is, each end user will interact with the device differently, on the basis of his or her goals. These different interactions must be factored into the design. A user-centered approach requires that a product be designed with the end user in mind, including his or her functional needs (what functions does user need to accomplish tasks), characteristics (e.g., education, training, expectations), inherent human limitations and capabilities (as listed in Table 14-4), and characteristics of the user's task and work environment (e.g., task must to performed quickly and concurrently with other tasks, under low lighting and high noise conditions, with little tolerance for error).

Callout Box 5. Real-Life Examples of the Value of User-Centered Design

Cell Phones Many people have more than one cell phone, and the phones' features differ widely. Address books are constructed differently, the "yes" and "no" buttons mean different things, the power buttons have different shapes and icons, etc. Even the steps to dial 911 might be different. Sometimes the user cannot tell whether a call is connected, can't see the buttons in dim light, or see the color screens in bright light. After a short period of experimentation, it is quickly apparent which phones are the easiest to use. In short, despite a number of design variations and embellishments, many of the new phones are no more useful than were models of a decade ago. None seem to have instructions plugged into the menus to assist in its use.

Iterative Design and Testing

User testing that is done in a repeated manner is called *iterative design and testing*. This is the second concept that should guide any efforts to incorporate human factors. An iterative approach specifies that human factors should be considered not only early on in the development cycle of a product or process but also throughout the cycle. (User testing, which is sometimes called "usability testing," is discussed later in this section.) The results from user testing provide input for refinement of the design. An iterative approach ensures that the final design is based on concepts validated in an incremental fashion. This approach has advantages over a single user test at the end, because if major flaws are found at that point, it is difficult to isolate specific design problems and it is more time-consuming to tackle a massive redesign than to make smaller modifications in iterative steps.

HFE FOR EVALUATION ACTIVITIES

This section introduces various methods of analysis (cognitive task analysis, heuristic evaluation, cognitive walk-through) and user testing that are useful for anyone charged with evaluation activities. The same methods can be incorporated into development activities within the user-centered design or iterative design and testing frameworks.

HFE Design Principles

HFE design principles can be applied to practically any type of user interface (e.g., devices, paper forms, software, educational or instructional materials, checklists, cheat sheets, workspace design). The principles describe general characteristics of a user interface that make it more usable and efficient and less error-prone.

This section provides an overview of HFE principles. For more extensive coverage of HFE principles, see Nielson[10] or Sanders and McCormick.[13]

Keep the Dialogue Simple and Natural

The display of information or graphics (or any visual, auditory, or tactile item meant to convey information) must be as simple as possible. More is not always better; providing too much information may lengthen the time that users need to find the information they are looking for or make it overly complex to find at all. The dialogue should be as natural as possible, and the terms (or icons, auditory sounds, color convention, etc.) should be familiar to the user and easily and correctly interpreted. The dialogue should also reinforce how the device or equipment works and be congruent with user expectations.

Minimize Reliance on User Memory

Strategies to minimize user memory load include the following:

1. Make relevant information apparent to the user. For instance, display the acceptable range of values (such as 1–5) or the expected format of the value to be entered (e.g., dd-mm-yy) so that users aren't forced to remember each time.

2. Make it obvious how to navigate to a desired location or page in a software program or paper manual (e.g., menu system, links, table of contents).

3. Automatically fill in information in fields where the user would otherwise have to retype information when filling out several pages or screens, or provide a pull-down list of options from which the user may choose when the values to be filled in belong to a finite list of typical values.

4. Make the expected unit of measurement obvious, or provide functions that help the user translate values into the expected unit (e.g., feet instead of meters or ounces instead of milligrams).

5. Provide cues that help orient users in terms of where they are in the software program or paper manual.

Maintain Consistency

To maintain consistency within a system, a designer must consider both its visual appearance and its functionality, or structure. For instance, the same information should be presented in the same location and formatted to appear the same way, so that users can find it easily. The way in which the elements of a system behave should also be consistent and predictable. This might include how a certain button behaves in different contexts, the method of inputting information (e.g., graphical versus command line), how to navigate between pages or fields (tab, enter, or space bar), or how to execute or cancel a command.

Provide Meaningful Feedback

Feedback is the process by which a user is informed about what a system or device is doing, whether the user's intended commands were executed successfully, whether an error has occurred, or how to recover from errors. This is important when response times are slow, when there are automated functions that the user must monitor or supervise, when the user wants to verify that an action or command has been completed before moving on, or when the user must engage in troubleshooting. Lack of feedback can result in disorientation, duplicated actions or commands, failure to complete tasks that go unrecognized, or frustration when meaningless "error" messages appear.

Offer Clearly Marked Exits

When clearly marked exits are available, users gain a feeling of being in control, that is, being able to cancel a command or action, stop a process, or escape from unintended situations. Allowing users to maintain ability to cancel or undo actions enables them to recover from errors and revert to a previous state without disastrous consequences. It acknowledges that user errors will happen and provides a forgiving buffer zone.

Provide Shortcuts

The design of systems should accommodate the more experienced user by providing short-cuts for frequently used commands or actions. Shortcuts might include function keys or special keystrokes that execute an entire sequence of commands, buttons or links that take the user to a place further along in a process or a frequently accessed screen or page, provide a history or list of frequently accessed functions or links, or provide the option to skip screens or steps that are irrelevant to the task at hand.

HFE Analysis Methods

Analysis methods are pertinent to individuals who must make procurement decisions for medical software or devices, retrospectively examine errors, contribute to in-house development of hospital software, develop or revise hospital policies or procedures, or participate in facility design, development, or reorganization.

The goal of a HFE analysis is to capture information about how a device or system is used or how a process is carried out. The purpose of such analyses is to identify any mismatches between how a device or process was designed and how the user actually uses it. This is sometimes called *human-machine interaction* or *human-computer interaction*. Human factors analysis methods can help determine why errors might be occurring.

There is a wide range of analysis methodologies, varying in focus, depth, and suitability to different systems. One such methodology is a set of analyses collectively called *cognitive task analysis*. Conducting such an analysis may include field studies of users performing the work in the actual setting, simulations or bench tests, heuristic evaluation based on design principles, information-requirements analysis, functional needs assessment, and cognitive walkthrough (see **Table 14-5**).

A HFE analyst may perform some or all of these analyses, depending on the nature of the system being evaluated, the focus of the evaluation, and time and budget constraints. The products of such analyses include mapping of the system structure and an understanding of how a user navigates through the system (e.g., through a work area or through menus of a software program), specific features of a device or process that violate HFE design principles, and identification of factors (e.g., poor lighting, noise, or multiple handoffs) that have an adverse impact on human performance. Further information on these methods can be found in a number of sources.[10,12,14,15] Lin et al.[27,28] provide an example of cognitive task analysis applied to PCA pumps. Horsky et al.[29] employed a cognitive task analysis to characterize the cognitive demands of a computerized physician order entry system.

User Testing

User testing can validate or help guide the development of policies or procedures, assess the usability of prospective software or devices for procurement, or test different theories explaining why errors might be happening in a hospital.

User testing involves putting a product or process to the test with actual end users.[10,15] The focus of user testing may vary.[30] At the micro level, tests evaluate specific characteristics or elements of an interface (e.g., color coding of display elements, readability of text messages); at

Table 14-5. Examples of Human Factors Methods*

HFE Analysis Activity	General Description	Analysis Products
Field Observations	Unobtrusively observe users in the work environment as they carry out typical tasks. Take note of how work is carried out, who carries it out, what they use to carry it out, whom they interact with, and environmental factors (e.g., light levels, noise, crowding from equipment or people).	Characterizes the typical work environment, identifies factors that might affect how clinicians perform (e.g., limitations of equipment, low light levels, high risk or time pressure, frequent distractions), obtains descriptions of how work is actually carried out.
Simulation or Bench Tests	Simulate a process or the operation of a device, using different scenarios (e.g., different tasks time pressure, lighting, errors that one must re-cover from). Simulation involves end users, whereas bench tests can be performed by the analyst.	Involves mapping of the system structure (e.g., Where do all the menus in a software program lead to? Where does the pharmacist or physician have to go to retrieve a certain item? What steps must be performed to use a device?).
Information Requirements and Functional Needs Assessment	Perform information-requirements analysis to identify what information a user needs to carry out specific tasks or activities, from micro to macro (e.g., how can a user tell he must push that button next; how does a user know he must perform that task next; how does he know whom to contact to relay information?). Similarly, a functional needs assessment identifies what tools or informa-tion a user requires to accomplish a task.	Identifies information and functional needs of the user. Identifies task-related activities that depend on short- or long-term memory, identifies where information should be supplied and how it should be supplied, identifies what tools a user needs to accomplish a task.
Heuristic Evaluation	Evaluates equipment or a process against a set of human factors principles. See Gosbee and Lin[4] for a sample list of questions that should be asked when conducting an evaluation. Such questions might include the following: Does the software provide functionality needed by the user? Are buttons grouped in a logical fashion? Is there sufficient feedback to tell the user that he or she has completed a task correctly? Is it obvious what a user must do next?	Identifies areas where human factors principles are violated that may lead to unwanted conse-quences, such as frequent user errors, slips, high mental workload, user frustration, inefficient or inaccurate task completion, misunderstanding of policies, and deviation from prescribed guidelines or procedures.
Cognitive Walk-through	A user is asked to demonstrate or walk through a device or process, thinking out loud or providing commentary on what he or she is doing and thinking at each step.	Characterizes where human decision making is involved in a task and factors that influence decision making, including expertise a user might rely on, where information is retrieved, strategies adopted, and work-arounds developed to circumvent a deficiency.

Adapted from Gosbee.[6]

the macro level, the focus of a test is the integrated system (e.g., ease of learning, operator performance under realistic operating conditions and environmental stressors).

Options for testing platforms are likewise varied and include low-fidelity paper prototypes, rapid prototypes, part-task simulations, and high-fidelity, full-scale simulations that incorporate file-driven delays. Each of these test platforms affords different means for collecting performance data: from direct observation and less obtrusive observation through video recording to electronically logged interaction with the simulations. The following list captures the spectrum of tests and provides a sense of the dimensions of the human-system interaction that can be evaluated:

- user friendliness
- information quality
- display characteristics
- data organization
- data entry
- human performance (e.g., time to perform, error rates, time to respond, mental workload)
- human productivity (quantity produced per unit time)
- ease of learning (time to proficiency)

Planning a human factors test involves the following steps:

1. Identifying the user population. The first step is to identify the population that will be the end users. The importance of involving the people who will be using the product or carrying out the process in the testing cannot be overstated. A user population will have its own unique characteristics, e.g., education, training, knowledge, experience, and expectations. The users might be new to the product or be highly experienced with it. They may work individually or rely on teams. These characteristics influence how the users interact with a new product or process.

2. Defining representative tasks for the test. The next step is to define representative tasks that will be performed by users in the test (e.g., entering, updating, or retrieving information on an ASO). The tasks chosen for testing may be individual tasks or a collection of tasks. They may be completed by an individual or by a team. One may also choose to add a secondary task to the testing to observe a more representative scenario where clinicians are often dividing their time between multiple, sometimes unrelated, tasks.

3. Identifying performance measures. Performance variables need to be identified; for instance, time precision, accuracy, and workload (a measure of physical or mental workload based on an established questionnaire, such as the task-load index developed by the National Aeronautics and Space Administration).

4. Planning data-collection techniques. Data-collection techniques may involve a range of activities, from having an observer take notes and time activities to using computer software to record users' interactions with the software to making a videotape. Often, test runs are needed prior to actual testing with end users in order to perfect the test setup and data collection techniques.

5. Identifying a test site. Conducting the test at a site typical of where the work will be performed adds realism and ability to generalize results of the test to the actual targeted work setting.

Lin et al.[27,28] offer an example of how user testing was used to corroborate findings of HFE analysis that identified vulnerabilities and to evaluate comparative usability of PCA equipment. McLaughlin[31] describes how user testing was used in an iterative fashion to help design and validate the design and organization of medication in a code cart for efficient and reliable retrieval.

Hospital Activities that Should Incorporate HFE

This section provides examples of where practitioners can integrate HFE into the medication-use system in a hospital, clinic, or freestanding pharmacy. Since HFE covers such a wide range, there is an equally wide range of activities that can incorporate HFE (see **Table 14-6**). Depending on the activity, some or all of the HFE methods and tools discussed above can be applied.

Table 14-6. Examples of Hospital Activities that Should Incorporate HFE*

Activity	Applicable HFE Concept	Purpose of Applying HFE Method
Development		
In-house device/software design and development	User-centered design, iterative design and testing, human factors analyses (see Table 14-5), user testing, or simulation	Ensure usability (efficient, functional, easy to learn, easy to use, low mental workload).
Policy, protocol, and guideline design and development		
Training and education; curriculum design and development		
Design and development of paper forms (e.g., labels, order forms, charts, instruction sheets)		
Evaluation Activities		
Procurement (e.g., of devices, software, training programs)	Human factors analyses (see Table 14-5), user testing, or simulation	Identify usability issues with prospective or existing equipment, software, training programs, new or existing policies, or protocols that may lead to errors.
ADE investigation (RCA, FMEA, and reporting systems)		

Adapted from Gosbee.[6]

Hospitals pose a unique challenge regarding usability issues because the users vary widely in terms of core training and experience and because the quality of in-service training offered by hospitals varies widely. Staff are often assumed to be competent in equipment or software use unless they themselves report their lack of knowledge or comfort using the product. Sometimes the equipment and software used in health care facilities is not obviously different from version to version; as a result, the end user does not realize a change or upgrade has occurred until the product fails.

DEVICE PROCUREMENT

HFE can be used to help guide procurement decisions. The various analysis and user-testing methods discussed earlier in this chapter may be performed in order to obtain crucial data on usability of the device and software.[16] This will help the decision maker ascertain prior to the purchase whether a particular device or software meets the functional needs of end users, presents a high risk for user errors, or poses any particular training challenges for novice users, users with extensive experience on another system, users who only occasionally use the device or software, and user groups who may not have the same goals and thus use it differently.

Specific devices where this might be useful in pharmacy departments include infusion devices, bedside or home-monitoring equipment, counting and measuring equipment, automated dispensing cabinets, controlled-substances cabinets, devices used to assist the worker in i.v. admixture compounding, and computer hardware and peripherals.

HFE principles are important not only in the evaluation and procurement phases but also throughout the life cycle of the device. For example, one facility had a number of PCA-related medication events. A team was formed to examine the issues that might be contributing to these events. The team included both the staff who ordered and dispensed the devices from the storeroom and biomedical engineering staff. Once its deliberations started, the team made a startling discovery. The staff nurse reports had varied in terms of what they had reported as "usual" programming patterns for the PCA pumps. The hospital had seen a surge in the use of the devices, and the storeroom had leased a number of pumps to meet the patient need. The biomedical staff then realized that the leased pumps used various versions of software that may not have been the same version as that used by the hospital's own pumps. This pointed out the vulnerability that the leased pumps had not gone through the biomedical department for inspection, and that the processes of leasing equipment needed to be revamped.

In a second example, a health system had purchased several pieces of packaging equipment to provide unit dose packaging for inpatients. During the life cycle of the equipment, the rights to the packaging equipment were sold to another company. In that transition, improvements or upgrades were made that affected functionality and safe use of the equipment. Because the sales forces also changed, there was a lack of continuity between vendor and client. As a result, only some of the facilities using the equipment got the hardware and software upgrades. Some of the equipment at facilities that did not receive the upgrade eventually overheated and failed. The lesson learned is that the vendor should stipulate in the contract language that customers will be notified of all upgrades and that those upgrades should be planned and conducted in cooperation with the facilities in a timely and safe fashion. This should also include any necessary training and implementation tools.

From the HFE standpoint, planning for transitions between old and new equipment can be fertile ground for improvement. Major changes in functionality of equipment and the associated supplies (e.g., parts, batteries, tubing, strips, reagents) could pose significant hidden hazards if not managed appropriately.

IN-HOUSE SOFTWARE DESIGN AND DEVELOPMENT

HFE should be adopted by anyone involved in developing in-house software products. It can provide a framework for the development cycle (user-centered design and iterative design and testing) that can help ensure that user-interaction issues that might otherwise become latent errors are resolved during development. Design concepts and early prototypes should undergo user testing to identify any features that do not adhere to HFE principles. Results of early user testing should be used to guide the refinement of the design. User testing and design refinement should be repeated throughout the design and development.

A designer or developer can also use HFE analysis and user testing to determine functional and information requirements. This will have an impact on physical design, organization, and layout (e.g., of information or controls); the structure and sequence of tasks; the level of detail or higher-level information available to the users depending on their goals, organization, and layout of the menu structure (of software); appropriate graphical presentation of information; and level of online training or help functions necessary. Examples of in-house software products include computerized provider order entry systems, bedside bar-code medication administration systems, pharmacy information systems, clinical decision-support systems, clinical data repositories, and patient-registration and medical record systems.

Decision making in health care is difficult to structure and automate, and the software used to support such decisions is complex. The process of automating the prescribing and production of i.v. fluids is a typical example. Decades after the first pharmacy information systems were developed, hospitals and users still struggle with structuring the decision-making process and effectively communicating orders among the various health care providers involved in this activity. Most tasks in the other parts of health care are discrete orders carried out one at a time, but i.v. solutions undergo a sequence of activities; for example, they are ordered, alternated, held, stopped, slowed, and titrated to response. Each of these steps increases the technical complexity, and therefore the end users' interaction with the software and with and the patient. Seemingly inconsequential and isolated usability issues can turn into major ones when the software is put to use in a clinical setting. Not all design woes can be solved by adding more pop-up boxes. Additionally, although the end users use similar information in decision making in health care, the various disciplines often have markedly different views of that information because the end user needs and functional utility of that information vary.

CURRICULUM DESIGN AND DEVELOPMENT

HFE can be used to help assess or develop training and education programs. The objective in this case would be to identify training needs associated with specific devices or policies that might be challenging because of poor design or complexity. HFE can also be used to help design training materials and to evaluate their effectiveness.

The approach is the same as that used in software development: user-centered design and iterative design and testing. Though the end product differs from other devices and software in that its goal is to teach, rather than to help users carry out a task, curriculum developers can use methods and tools such as user testing and HFE analysis to ascertain functional requirements, information requirements, and similar matters, whether the product is paper based (e.g., a user manual) or electronic (software). Conducting a HFE analysis can help identify training issues or requirements for training. For example, it can help the curriculum developer design training material, determine how often refresher training is needed, and make decisions concerning transfer-of-training issues (e.g., how training with one product or system negatively or positively influences how one gains competency with another system or a system upgrade).

HFE methods can also be used to help identify opportunities where the training available to users is insufficient and should be supplemented with cognitive aids that will either help learning or help guide users in decision making, device operation, following protocols, or similar activities.

Training and education are often woefully overlooked or underrated in health care, even though the safe use of equipment and software is an integral part of patient safety. One unique challenge is timing: If training occurs at the beginning of the year but the product is not on site or used for six months, many of the benefits of training may be lost. Likewise, attempting to train patients or family members while they are seriously ill or preparing for discharge from the facility poses its own set of challenges. Finally, medical information rapidly changes, and programs developed one year may be obsolete the next. These factors converge to put demands on health professionals and health systems for doing the right thing at the right time using the right medium. HFE can assist in putting the necessary information where it needs to be and when it needs to be there in order to safely and efficiently perform a task.

Special attention should be paid to medication use and to ensuring that patients truly understand how to self-administer medications. One look at the modern-day inhalers or the new drug administration devices in use today will emphasize the need for HFE evaluation. While health care practitioners may understand the rationale and mechanism of action of the medication, a good number of them may not be able to administer it to themselves, much less teach a patient or family member to do so. Pharmacies and hospitals are high-traffic environments and patient education challenges abound, yet the patient or family member is the last hope of averting a medication error if a failure occurs upstream in the dispensing or prescribing process.

POLICY, PROTOCOL, AND GUIDELINE DESIGN AND DEVELOPMENT

HFE can be used to help assess or develop policies, protocols, and guidelines. It can also be used to help identify any special training needs with respect to such documents.

Anyone charged with developing a policy or protocol faces a two-part challenge. The first challenge is to develop a policy or protocol that will alleviate some other problem or issue; the second is to develop the material to support this policy or protocol so that carrying it out does not create a new problem or issue. To do this requires an understanding of the nature of two things: (1) the task or area that the policy/protocol is intended to affect, and (2) the actual act of carrying out the policy or protocol and the information, material, and machines that the user must come in contact with to carry it out. The designer or developer of policies or protocols should carry out a human factors analysis of both these areas to develop an appropriate and easy to follow policy/protocol. Evaluation of the policy or protocol is equally important in order to test its readability, ease of learning, prominence of critical steps or information, complexity, and memory load. The approach is the same as that used for software development: user-centered design and iterative design and testing.

HFE can also help identify opportunities where complexity requires that the policy or protocol should be supplemented with cognitive aids (e.g., cheat sheets) either to help learning or to help guide users in decision making, device operation, following protocols, and similar functions. This can be supplemented with various forms of risk communication (e.g., warning signs) whose design and evaluation can be aided by the knowledge base on warnings and risk communication.[18-20]

Organizational culture, which defines the boundaries or accepted practices through policies and procedures, also shapes how the medication-use process functions. The intent is to shape work by setting constraints or providing guidance. Whether policies are followed is influenced not only by the intent of the user but also by a host of HFE issues. These issues might include how a policy or procedure is conveyed (e.g., readability, availability, complexity), how a policy or procedure may interact or interfere with other work processes, how much of an impact it might have on mental or physical workload or on timeliness of other time-critical activities (e.g., added paperwork, tedious or repetitive procedures). By adopting a systems view, one can see how a seemingly simple change in policy might influence or be influenced by other processes, devices, or people.

Examples of HFE utility in policy, protocol, and guideline development in health care abound. Processes in health care are often very complex and tightly coupled (i.e., one step is dependent on the preceding step for completion). These steps are often accomplished by different departments or disciplines, further complicating communication. Much of the medication-use system is technically complex in this exact way. The processes of providing anticoagulation therapy, diabetes care, or cancer chemotherapy are striking examples of this complexity. If one approached a group of seemingly similar practitioners to ask how they provide this care to patients (i.e., exactly what steps they use to go from point A to point B), the variety of answers would be astounding. This has never been so obvious as now, when vendors and hospitals are trying to automate decision support with the use of "smart" i.v. pumps—pumps that have internal software to warn the users of under- or overdoses of medication. Attempts to automate this part function have resulted in the discovery, by vendors and hospitals alike, that what was thought to be standardized is in fact not. Some facilities had more than a half-dozen concentrations of the same drug or several methods to administer a drug, whereas a facility across town had just one concentration and one method. It is no wonder the health care professionals struggle to implement this type of automation near the bedside. Understanding the manual process and how it should be simplified precedes the task of automation.

Medication-use systems in hospitals across the United States are strikingly nonstandardized, which in and of itself creates opportunities for patient injury. The Joint Commission on Accreditation of Healthcare Organizations has made nonstandardized concentrations and infusion methods a focus of its patient-safety goals and new medication-use standards. These standards relate to all policy, protocol, and guideline use, usability, and development.

WORK-SPACE DESIGN

Hospitals and pharmacies are often designed in a rush or on a shoestring, such that little attention is paid to the HFE issues in the work space. Yet once constructed incorrectly, these areas are difficult to fix, and fixes are costly. Because work-space design is such an integral part of efficiency and safety in health care, end users should be involved in every step of the process. Most employees have opinions and suggestions to guide designers to design the workplace around the functional needs of the staff. New design ideas, such as articulating work surfaces, better lighting, and modular workstations, make it easier for today's designs to work well into the future. Many tasks in the medication-use system are tedious and require visual acuity. Work areas designed to minimize fatigue and optimize the worker's ability to check work or detect variations can go a long way toward minimizing risk to patient. Some specific literature exists on pharmacy or health care workplace design, but much of the work may be from other industries. HFE can help hospital staff and design staff choose the right design for the task.

Here are some areas to focus on when applying HFE to the remodeling or construction of new facility, purchase of office furniture and storage equipment, and similar activities:

- HFE can help design the layout of new facility on the basis of process flow of work areas, functional needs of the task and the users, and ergonomic specifications.

- HFE can help assess furniture or storage equipment on the basis of task and user needs.

- User testing can help evaluate the design of the workspace (e.g., distance and accessibility between related work areas, width of pathways to accommodate equipment and personnel, height of shelves so that even people who are shorter than average can read the labels and reach stored products, counter space and shelving in the pharmacy to accommodate typical tasks).

ROOT-CAUSE ANALYSIS, FAILURE MODE AND EFFECTS ANALYSIS, AND REPORTING SYSTEMS

The most striking examples of the need to better incorporate HFE into medication safety occur during the analysis of an actual event or of a close call.[16,32,33]

Pharmacists are uniquely suited to design medication systems and to analyze events related to them. Indeed, medication-related root-cause analyses (RCA) would likely not be considered thorough and credible if a pharmacist were not part of the analysis team. Yet advisers often fail to realize the tremendous benefit that a medication-use expert would bring to a RCA or to prevention of the types of events that RCAs explore. Pharmacists may not always be in the communication loop; as a result, they do not know which events have occurred and which have been scheduled for analysis using RCA techniques. The medication-use system falls under the "medical staff function" authority according to JCAHO standards, and in order to ensure the most efficient communication about vulnerabilities and solutions, all medication-related events should be reviewed by the multidisciplinary group performing the medication-use function oversight. This group is often the pharmacy and therapeutics committee, but other groups can perform this function as well. From a human factors perspective, a drug that presents a look-alike problem to the nurse may pose that same vulnerability to the physician or pharmacist. After all, pharmacists purchase the majority of pharmaceuticals in hospitals and deal with supply and contract issues daily. Events analyzed in silo fashion (i.e., by a single department) have the potential for less-than-thorough analysis and intervention.

RCA teams are in an excellent position to incorporate a human factors conscience into the analysis. Questions such as the following could be extremely important to a thorough and credible analysis of an event:

- What were the working conditions at the time of the event?
- What human factors symptoms or issues are associated with the product or equipment?
- What types of latent errors existed before the active error occurred?
- What aspects of the user's tasks or working environment may have interfered or influenced the event?
- What aspects of the product or equipment are counterintuitive or incongruent with the user's knowledge, training, education, or experience (notice that the equipment design is assumed to be deficient in matching the user and not the other way around)?
- How could the device be redesigned to prevent such an event?

EFFECT OF RAISING CLINICIAN AWARENESS OF HFE

HFE is a complex concept, but experience shows that once caregivers are aware of how useful it can be, they often begin reporting and detecting other events and conditions that have previously gone unreported. Just like an American driving a European rental car (without the same U.S.-mandated safety features), the HFE-aware employee becomes sensitive to the lack of safety-mindedness in his or her work environment. Look-alike products get identified and reported, usability problems with equipment and software get reported, and more cognitive aids and diagrams are requested. Thus, even though not always involved in design decisions, the everyday employee (and the patients) can benefit from HFE awareness.[34,35]

Summary

Medication safety involves layers of complex, interdependent elements that range from humans to work spaces to equipment to processes. It is fertile ground for applying HFE, since all aspects of the medication-use process are entangled with human factors issues. The idea of fitting the tool to the human, rather than the other way around, should be the model when analyzing processes, policies, and work space, as well as equipment. Human factors is both a mindset and a field rich with an in-depth knowledge base, ongoing applied research, practical tools, and a broad range of methodologies. A long-term vision for improving medication safety might include a resident human factors expert at each hospital to help bring this mindset to both proactive risk reduction (e.g., usability laboratories to assess prospective technologies) and reactive risk reduction (e.g., RCA, adverse event analysis). This mindset is essential if we are to advance beyond the "blame-and-train" notions of the past.

References

1. Wickens CD. *Engineering Psychology and Human Performance*. 2nd ed. New York: Harper Collins; 1992.

2. Norman D. *The Design of Everyday Things*. New York: Doubleday; 1988.

3. Casey S. *Set Phasers on Stun—And Other True Tales of Design, Technology, and Human Error. 2nd ed.* Santa Barbara, CA: Eagan Publishing Co; 1993.

4. Gosbee JW, Lin L. The role of human factors engineering in medical device and medical system errors. In: Vincent C, ed. *Clinical Risk Management: Enhancing Patient Safety*. 2nd ed. London: BMJ Press; 2001:301-317.

5. Reason J. *Human Error*. New York: Cambridge University Press; 1990.

6. Gosbee JW. Introduction to the Human Factors Engineering Series. *Jt Comm J Qual Safety*. 2004;30:215-219.

7. Wears RL, Perry SJ. Human factors and ergonomics in the emergency department. *Ann Emerg Med*. 2002;40:206-212.

8. Rasmussen J, Pejtersen AM, Goodstein LP. *Cognitive Systems Engineering*. New York: John Wiley and Sons; 1994.

9. Klein GA, Salas E, eds. *Linking Expertise and Naturalistic Decision Making*. New York: Lawrence Erlbaum Assoc; 2001.

10. Nielson J. *Usability Engineering*. Boston: Academic Press; 1994.

11. Cohen MR. *Medication Errors: Causes, Prevention, and Risk Management*. Sudbury, MA: American Pharmaceutical Association; 2001.

12. Wiklund M. *Medical Device Design and Equipment Design. Usability Engineering and Ergonomics*. Buffalo Grove, IL: Interpharm Press; 1995.

13. Sanders MS, McCormick EJ. *Human Factors Engineering and Design*. 7th ed. New York: McGraw Hill; 1993.

14. Meister D. *Human Factors Testing and Evaluation*. New York: Elsevier; 1986.

15. Rubin J. *Handbook of Usability Testing: How to Plan, Design and Conduct Effective Tests*. New York: Wiley; 1994.

16. Schneider PJ. Applying human factors in improving medication-use safety. *Am J Health-Syst Pharm*. 2002;59:1155-1159.

17. Stanton N. *Human Factors in Alarm Design*. London: Taylor and Francis; 1994.

18. Wogalter MS, DeJoy DM, Laughery KR. *Warnings and Risk Communication*. London: Taylor and Francis; 1999.

19. Isaacson JJ, Klein HA, Muldoon RV. Prescription medication information: improving usability through human factors design. In: Wogalter MS, Young SL, Laughery KR, eds. *Human Factors Perspectives on Warnings*. Vol. 2. Santa Monica, CA: Human Factors and Ergonomics Society; 2001:104-108.

20. Lehto MR. Determining warning label content and format using FMEA. In: Wogalter MS, Young SL, Laughery KR, eds. *Human Factors Perspectives on Warnings*. Vol 2. Santa Monica, CA: Human Factors and Ergonomics Society; 2001:143-146.

21. Gosbee LL. Nuts! I can't figure out how to use my life-saving epinephrine auto-injector. Human factors issues associated with an auto-injector. *Jt Comm J Qual Safety*. 2004;30:220-223.

22. Taylor FW. *The Principles of Scientific Management*. New York: Harper; 1911.

23. Taylor FW. *Principles of Scientific Management*. New York: Harper and Brothers; 1947.

24. Gilbreth FB. *Brick-Laying System*. New York: Clark Publishing Co; 1911.

25. Gilbreth FB. Gilbreth LM. *Applied Motion Study*. New York: Macmillan Co; 1917.

26. Institute for Safe Medication Practices. Let's put a stop to problem-prone automatic stop order policies. *ISMP Safety Alert*. August 9, 2000. Available at: www.ismp.org/msaarticles/stop.html. Accessed December 6, 2004.

27. Lin L, Isla R, Harkness H, Doniz K, Vicente KJ, Doyle DJ. Applying human factors to the design of medical equipment: patient-controlled analgesia. *J Clin Monitor Comput*. 1998;14:253-263.

28. Lin, L, Vicente, KJ, Doyle DJ. Patient safety, potential adverse drug events, and medical device design: a human factors approach. *J Biomed Informat*. 2001;34:274-284.

29. Horsky J, Kaufman DR, Oppenheim MI, Patel VL. A framework for analyzing the cognitive complexity of computer-assisted clinical ordering. *J Biomed Informat*. 2003;36:4-22.

30. Reilley S, Grasha AF, Schafer J. Workload, error detection, and experienced stress in a simulated pharmacy verification task. *Percept Motor Skills*. 2002;95(1):27-46.

31. McLaughlin RC. Redesigning the crash cart: usability testing improves one facility's medication drawers. *Am J Nurs*. 2003;103 (4):64A,64D,64G,64H.

32. Gosbee JW, Anderson T. Human factors en-

gineering design demonstrations can enlighten your RCA team. *Qual Safety Health Care.* 2003;12:119-121.

33. Gosbee JW. Human factors engineering and patient safety. *Qual Safety Health Care.* 2002;11:352-354.

34. Gosbee, JW. A patient safety curriculum for residents and students: the VA Healthcare Systems pilot project. *ACGME Bulletin.* November 2002; 2-6. Available at: www.acgme.org/acWebsite/bulletin/bulletin1102.pdf. Accessed October 27, 2004.

35. Gosbee JW. Importance of human factors engineering in error-and-medicine education. *Acad Med.* 1999;74:748-749.

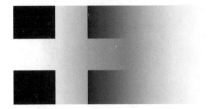

Safe Supply-Chain Management

Marsha K. Millonig and
Bruce R. Siecker

Introduction

The majority of the 3.27 billion prescriptions ordered in this country yearly are handled in a safe and efficacious manner by these three mainstays of the drug distribution system.[1] But increasingly, we are seeing examples of the failure of the marketing system to catch mistakes and deliberate errors within it. Drug counterfeiting, for example, is on the rise. Understanding and combating this phenomenon require an appreciation of how pharmaceutical products are distributed in this country as well as of some of the stratagems now being used by some unscrupulous players in the system.

Elements of the Pharmaceutical Supply Chain

The three primary elements of the pharmaceutical supply chain in the United States are the producer, the distributor, and the dispenser.

PRODUCER

Producers include manufacturers or suppliers of brand-name and generic products and repackagers and labelers that package products under their own or a manufacturer's identity (see **Figure 15-1**). Approximately 100 companies produce the majority of pharmaceuticals,[2] and the top 20 of these companies hold 70.6 percent of the market share.[3] These are followed by several hundred smaller producers. In the United States, the manufacturer or labeler is known by the first field of the three-field drug identification number known as the National Drug Code, or NDC, number.

DISTRIBUTOR

In this country, there are three types of distributors: (1) wholesalers, (2) chain store warehouses, and (3) specialty distributors. Each type of distributor purchases a product from a supplier and sells that product to many customers. Chain store warehouses sell only to stores within their networks. Specialty distributors carry a limited stock (e.g., injectables or antineoplastic agents) or sell only to certain customers (e.g., clinics or freestanding surgery centers). In terms of sales, wholesalers are the largest category of distributors.

DISPENSER

The third element in the supply chain is the dispenser, or pharmacy. The three largest types of dispensers are (1) chain drugstores, (2) independent pharmacies, and (3) food stores or mass merchandisers that have pharmacies on their premises.

More than 90 percent of the sales of drug products are distributed between and among these three elements in an indirect fashion, i.e., the distributor takes physical control of the

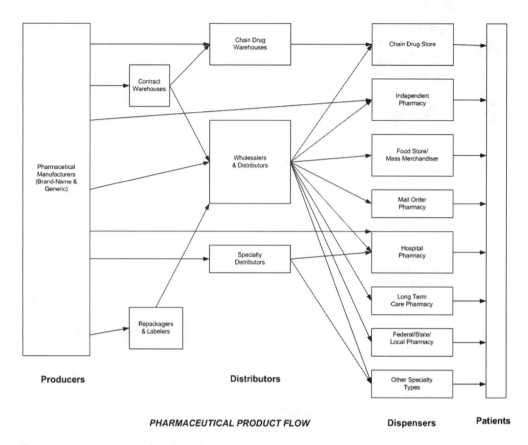

Figure 15-1. Pharmaceutical Product Flow

product from the producer and distributes it to the dispenser.[3] Some sales are still made directly, i.e., from the manufacturer (the producer) to the pharmacy (the dispenser).

Producers, distributors, and dispensers handle the distribution of pharmaceuticals in this country in a safe and efficient way. Each entity is licensed to carry out the duties appropriate to it. Each is a well-known and trusted entity in the distribution system. Each has well-documented procedures and well-defined functions. If errors occur, the solution is generally evident to everyone involved, and error-prevention systems are in place. For example, wholesalers double-check every order before it leaves the distribution center to ensure accuracy. The wholesaler distribution system functions highly efficiently, with more than 12 million items shipped from 233 distribution centers in the United States on an average day. The cost of delivering an individual item is less than $1. Wholesalers' net profit margins are 0.73 percent.[4] Table 15-1 presents additional information on wholesaler volume in the United States in a recent year.

Table 15-1. Wholesaler Order Volume—2002[5]

Number of distribution centers (DCs) in United States operated by HDMA wholesaler members	233
Number of orders* per DC	1,269
Number of invoice† lines per order	12.52
Average number of items per invoice line	3.25
Average number of items shipped per day per DC	51,636

Items shipped per day, all DCs	12,031,097
Items shipped per year, all DCs	3,753 million
Average handling cost per invoice line	$2.84

* A pharmacy sends an electronic order to a DC each day for prescription, over-the-counter, and other items that it needs to replenish.

† An invoice is the total amount of items and their cost for each order. One line of an invoice contains an item, how many of the items were ordered, the price of the individual item, and the total cost for that item = number of items x individual price = total for that item. This is called a *line extension*.

A Secondary Market of Distribution

If the three entities just described were the only components of the pharmaceutical distribution system and the system always worked as described, there would be little room for error. But the system is more complicated than this. Another market exists—one that is dominated by secondary suppliers, discrepancy specialists, and importers that serve to correct anomalies (i.e., if excess inventories accumulate in one part of the system, these distributors buy it and resell it at a discount to "correct" the market). **Figure 15-2** depicts this expanded distribution system. As it indicates, the new supply lines are in competition and are redundant with the major supply lines. Secondary suppliers purchase directly from pharmaceutical manufacturers and wholesalers and distributors. This creates another supply line that competes with the traditional method of distribution. These suppliers are buying the same drug products as everyone else is buying, but at a lower price, and usually in quantity. In addition, importers purchase drugs from foreign sources.

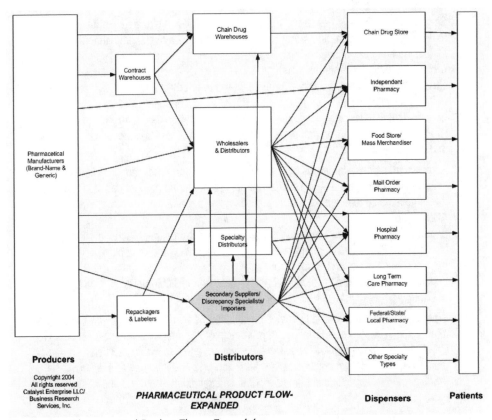

PHARMACEUTICAL PRODUCT FLOW-EXPANDED

Figure 15-2. Pharmaceutical Product Flow—Expanded

These secondary suppliers sell products to chain store warehouses, wholesalers and distributors, specialty distributors, and all types of dispensers—chain drugstores, independent pharmacies, food stores and mass merchandisers, mail-order pharmacies, hospital pharmacies, long-term care pharmacies, nursing homes, federal, state, and local government pharmacies, and others. In some cases, secondary suppliers buy excess inventory from various dispensers, such as hospitals and long-term care pharmacies, in order to get better prices.

This secondary market serves to "share" better prices available in the marketplace and acts as a damper on the whole market by keeping prices more or less the same. It also serves to confuse the market in terms of tracing sales and assigning responsibility.

Secondary Suppliers

Since the late l980s, the drug market has experienced continual price increases. Suppliers often raise prices more than once a year and on a fairly predictable basis. Price increases offer a short-term profit potential to any customer that can afford to buy extra supplies before prices increase, then immediately raise its own prices to reflect the increase. But buying and holding extra inventory comes at a price. Inventory holding costs are significant, and they can quickly offset profit opportunities.

Not surprisingly, market specialists have developed ways to address the need. Secondary suppliers are market specialists that buy large quantities of products in advance at below-normal price (or, when costs are rising, at current prices) and then sell smaller amounts to wholesale distributors, chain warehouses, and pharmacies, in amounts these buyers can use at the time.

DISCREPANCY SPECIALISTS

Since the mid-1990s, it has been increasingly difficult for wholesale distributors to sell to dispensers pharmaceuticals that were slated to expire within six months. An increasing number of hospitals now require that any drugs they purchase under contract have a minimum expiration date of 12 months hence. The World Health Organization now requires that all drugs donated to needy countries and peoples must not expire within a year of receipt. As a result of these changes, wholesale distributors became saddled with significant inventory whose expiration dates are within Food and Drug Administration (FDA) and supplier requirements but that is nonetheless unsellable and not returnable.

At the same time, state boards of pharmacy and third-party prescription drug plans changed long-time dispensing rules and practices regarding product dating. Previously, it was acceptable to dispense a drug if it was not expired at the time it was dispensed. After that practice was changed, pharmacists were not permitted to dispense a drug product if it would expire before the patient had used the entire prescription. This change—and the fact that many state boards of pharmacy and drug plan participation requirements started to require pharmacists to place product-expiration dates on prescription labels—greatly increased the volume of unsellable products held by pharmacies.

Whenever a need arises and becomes significant, the market will find a way to address it, and this issue was no exception. With the help of the Internet and models such as E-Bay®, a new type of market specialist is evolving to address the issue of short-dated, unsellable drugs. These entities, called discrepancy specialists, buy at a discount products due to expire within 6 to 12 months and sell them to buyers who can use them before they expire.

> **IMPORTERS**
> Specialty importers in the pharmaceutical field import either raw material or finished goods inventory for purposes of pharmaceutical compounding. Such importers seek special formulations of the products they sell and serve an important function.

Potential Problems of Distribution

The confusion caused by the multiplicity of supply lines set the stage for the development of a shadow market of pharmaceuticals in this country. That market was fed by profiteers—including criminals, unscrupulous "wholesalers," and rogue Internet sites—that were willing to purchase any drugs available at a special price. The development of a market in illegal trade paved the way for counterfeiters and diverters who fed the industry millions of dollars' worth of fraudulent pharmaceuticals.

The reason this works so well is the presence of multiple channels of distribution, each of which offers a discount or some other incentive to purchase the drug from an alternative source. Often, the incentive is not at all unusual. Consider, for instance, the need to obtain a steady supply of pharmaceuticals that a manufacturer chooses not to sell to a supplier. The supplier thinks there are already enough wholesalers and declines to sell the products. The wholesaler arranges to purchase the pharmaceuticals from an alternative source. The pharmaceuticals may or may not be genuine; in any event, the system has been compromised.

No one is sure whether secondary-source products have been stored and handled correctly. In selling counterfeits, rogue operators are getting quite sophisticated. Often, only one bottle in six contains a substitute product; in other cases, the 80 doses in the bottom of a 100-dose container are fakes; the top 20 doses are real. But most cases involve outright fraud—the entire package is a fake. Many counterfeits are relatively easy to spot by a knowledgeable agent; nonetheless, many counterfeit products are so good that they even fool inspectors of the manufacturing company.

Counterfeit drugs pose significant public health and safety concerns. They may contain only inactive ingredients, incorrect ingredients, improper dosages, or subpotent or superpotent ingredients, or they may be contaminated.[6] The FDA is moving quickly to do something about the problem, but the drug industry—producers, distributors, and dispensers—is still left with the longer-term implications and patient safety.

Recent Errors in the System

Recent examples of counterfeit drugs have been legion, and counterfeits are on the rise. FDA counterfeit drug investigations have increased to 20 per year since 2000, after averaging only per year through the late 1990s.[6]

It is doubtful whether the United States has anywhere near the problems found worldwide, where upwards of 8 percent of all pharmaceuticals are fraudulent.[6] Nonetheless, for the U.S. health care industry, the findings are less than heartening. Epoetin alfa (Procrit®, Epopen®), atorvastatin (Lipitor®), filgrastim (Neupogen®), somatropin (Serostim®), zidovudine (Retrovir®), abacavir/lamivudine/zidovudine (Trizivir®), sildenafil (Viagra®), and olanzapine (Zyprexa®) have been counterfeited by the millions of doses. In one recent case, a wholesaler bought some 2,000 boxes of Epogen® valued at $4,000 each, an $8.5 million transaction. In another case, 110,000 bottles of $22 a bottle Epogen® were repackaged as $445 a bottle Procrit®. The net profit from this single transaction was $46 million.[6] Nearly 90 percent of the product involved in this counterfeit was not recovered.

In response to incidents such as these, the FDA noted that bogus or counterfeit products were produced that are "virtually indistinguishable from the authentic versions," and that they constitute a serious health risk.[6] In July 2003, FDA Commissioner Mark McClellan established a Counterfeit Drug Task Force. The task force was charged with developing recommendations for achieving the following four goals:

1.   to prevent the introduction of counterfeit drugs;

2.   to facilitate the identification of counterfeit drugs;

3.   to minimize the risk and exposure of consumers to counterfeit drugs; and

4.   to avoid the addition of unnecessary costs on the prescription drug distribution system or unnecessary restrictions on lower-cost sources of drugs.

The task force released an interim report in October 2003. The report contains a series of options that might be part of a multipronged approach to combat counterfeit drugs.[6] The options are based on input from other federal agencies, state governments, trade associations, consumer groups, drug manufacturers, wholesale distributors, pharmacies, consumers, academicians, and manufacturers of anti-counterfeiting technologies. They cover five areas: technology, regulatory requirements and secure business practices, rapid-alert and response systems, education and public awareness, and international issues.

Making the Pharmaceutical System Safer

Drug counterfeiting affects all parts of the distribution system, and addressing it will require a collaborative effort. Solutions range from rapid dissemination of information to better means of sorting out the unscrupulous players to all points in between. Some methods rely on electronic technologies such as bar codes and computer-assisted tracking. Some of the best measures of stopping counterfeiting are discussed in the following paragraphs.

Public Education. Using the mass media—newspapers, television and radio news programs, and the Internet—to educate the public about the pharmaceutical supply chain and to inform them of specific incidences of counterfeit medications and attendant problems could be an effective means of limiting problems caused by counterfeits. Notification should include the lot numbers of affected drugs, the distributors (and pharmacies if indicated) involved, how the drug has been copied or replaced, and the health risks involved. This is a reactive, rather than proactive, means of controlling the problem, but one that could be effective.

Pharmacist Notification. Another strategy is to notify pharmacists first. By giving pharmacists current information—rather than just news releases issued to the pharmaceutical press—when shipments of counterfeits have been uncovered, the problem might be stopped at the point of dispensing. Pharmacists should receive information on lot numbers of the affected drugs, the distributors (and pharmacies if indicated) involved, how the drug has been copied or replaced, and the health risks involved. Institutions should name an individual or create an ad hoc team to address these issues.

Enhanced FDA Oversight. More-frequent FDA visits and inspections could help detect the problem at the wholesaler level. This would require expanding the number of FDA inspectors. Improved methods of controlling incoming drug shipments (see below) could be developed and used by wholesalers in grading themselves, or an independent authority could do so.

Strengthening and Standardization of Licensing Requirements. Ethical pharmaceutical distributors support the idea of strengthening licensing requirements and inspections for wholesalers and distributors. They also want standards that are consistent between and among licensing bodies to ensure that disparate laws are not the reason that some entities can cheat the system. Many states have not revisited their distributor regulations for 30 or 40 years.

Best Business-Practice Guidelines. In remarks at the Healthcare Distribution Management Association's annual meeting on November 6, 2003, FDA Commissioner McClellan commended the association and its members for developing and adopting industry "best business practice" guidelines. Institutional practitioners are encouraged to obtain the guidelines (www.healthcaredistribution.org) and discuss them with their prime vendors.

Identification of Unscrupulous Operators. Pharmacists have grown accustomed to trusting their suppliers, especially the distributors. Nonetheless, they must recognize the need for vigilance. Counterfeiters' efforts are becoming increasingly sophisticated. Ensuring that vendors are following industry guidelines and any forthcoming FDA recommendations can help address this issue. Institutional practitioners should ask their prime vendors what error management and safety systems and processes they have in place.

Inspection of Drugs at Time of Receipt. Pharmacists routinely take steps to look at the incoming supply of drugs, but what these steps are is often unknown. A largely forgotten method of inspecting drugs that may have renewed utility today. Called *organoleptic analysis*, this method involves having someone with special training examine the drug for physical properties such as smell, taste, and appearance. Although limited to drug compounds that have distinctive odors, color, or texture, this method could have a role as part of a larger process.

Drug Pedigrees. A *drug pedigree* is a list of all the places that a drug has resided and of all its previous owners. The concept was developed by federal legislators who were trying to identify drugs that have been subjected to unclean and unsanitary conditions. Critics say that drug pedigrees can be faked—and indeed some have been—and can give a false sense of security to the purchaser. Taken in their totality, drug pedigrees can overwhelm a purchaser with paper without offering any guarantee of avoiding counterfeits. They would therefore lose their effectiveness as a mechanism to prevent counterfeits. Moreover, no one is in charge of pedigrees and therefore no one is ultimately responsible for them. Although a recent study showed that 61 percent of responding pharmacists approved of drug pedigrees, there is little if any support at the distributor level or by the HDMA.

Improved Packaging. Better packaging, perhaps involving hidden identifiers and watermarks, is an expensive method of avoiding counterfeits. Hidden identifiers can be materials that are applied to the printing on the package or placed in the folds of wrapping materials, or hidden inks that can be examined. Watermarks are more expensive to produce but harder to duplicate.

An idea that has gained some support is to produce detailed pictures of drug containers, together with the packaging arrangement and labeling material. Packaging pictures would be available on the Internet and from the manufacturer. This is a further attempt to encourage the wholesaler and pharmacy buyer to look more closely at packaging.

Unit-of-Use and Bar Codes. Hospital and community pharmacists, as well as the HDMA, have promoted the use of bar codes and unit-of-use packaging for hospital applications. These technologies could help reduce the number of counterfeit drugs because the counterfeiter would find it difficult to duplicate the bar code and the unit-of-use package. Critics of this method point out that once encased in unit-of-use packages, counterfeit drugs would escape detection efforts because pharmacists and others would assume that packaged products could not possibly be counterfeit.

Bar Coding

In the mid-1900s, as hospitals continued to search for quality improvements, they took a new look at bar codes and began to apply them to reduce errors associated with drug administration. These new uses came to be known as bar code–enabled point-of-care (BPOC) systems. The Institute of Medicine has stated that BPOC is an effective way to reduce medication errors by ensuring that the identity and dosage of a drug are as prescribed, that the drug is given to the right patient, and that all the steps in the dispensing and administration processes are checked for timeliness and accuracy.

Bar coding has many advantages in the delivery of safe health care, especially of safe medication use. Bar coding of patient identification bands, employee badges, and medication forms a closed loop of accountability and safety that is difficult to match. Bar code–enabled systems have helped hospital staff to achieve a 65 percent to 86 percent reduction in medication errors.[7]

The medication-use process offers many points at which unintended and sometimes-undetected human error can produce a serious threat to patient safety. Human mental errors can occur any time, no matter how experienced or well intentioned the practitioner. The only defense is to admit that errors are inevitable and to use methods designed to prevent injury.

Manual redundancies—e.g., having one nurse check another—can reduce up to 95 percent of errors; nonetheless, 5 percent of the errors do get through. To add to the margin of safety, technical solutions have to be used, and the best technical solution is bar coding.

Using machine-readable labeling and scanning safeguards the medication-administration process in the hospital and, in doing so, safeguards the patient. Bar coding enables information to be collected faster and with greater accuracy. Bar-code scanning has an error rate of 1 reading error in 10,000 characters read; keyboards, by contrast, have a 1-in-100 character-error rate.

Computerized Tracking Technologies. One of the most innovative means of tracking inventory is "track-and-trace" technology. Known as electronic product code (EPC) using Radio Frequency Identification (RFID), this technology curtails counterfeiting by applying track-and-trace capabilities from the manufacturer to the patient and would substantially change the way pharmaceuticals are distributed. EPCs are now undergoing development and testing and may prove their merit in the future.

Increased Penalties. The penalties associated with drug counterfeiting are small in relation to the payoff. Penalties for violating controlled-substances requirements are much more severe than those imposed for counterfeiting other drug products. Making penalties for counterfeiting of pharmaceuticals as severe as those for controlled substances might be an effective means of deterring the casual violator.

Price Reductions for Expensive Drugs. Drug counterfeiters make money because there is an economic incentive to cheat the system. An obvious, but less than universally attractive, solution to counterfeiting is to remove the associated economic gain, i.e., to lower the cost of the most expensive drugs so that counterfeiters have fewer incentives. FDA Commissioner McClellan has noted that legislation is needed to address the affordability of and access to prescription medicines. Additionally, he has said, international steps are needed toward sharing the burden of developing medicines.

Conclusion

For the foreseeable future, numerous solutions will be used to thwart counterfeiters, because no one solution works for everyone. Institutional practitioners are encouraged to remember that the logistical management and movement of medications from manufacturer to hospital introduce a number of separate safety issues into the medication process. Hospitals and pharmacists should review issues related to a safe supply chain, including ensuring that their prime vendors are following industry business practice guidelines.

Definitions for Figures 15-1 and 15-2

PRODUCER

Pharmaceutical manufacturer. A company that produces or manufactures drug products; product may be branded or generic.

Contract warehouse. A logistics specialist that distributes a company's product line on the company's behalf. The end user is usually unaware of the logistic firm's role.

DISTRIBUTOR

Chain drug warehouse. An entity that provides a wide range of services to meet the needs of the chain drug industry.

Wholesaler or distributor. A entity that sells every manufacturer's product line to all types of customers.

Specialty distributor. A distributor that sells limited product lines, sells to limited types of customers, or both.

DISPENSER

Chain drugstore. A pharmacy that is under ownership of one company that holds at least four stores.

Independent drugstore. An independently owned and operated community pharmacy.

Food store, mass merchandiser. Food, convenience, grocery, and supermarket stores with pharmacies; any mass-merchandise or discount store with a pharmacy.

Mail-order pharmacy. A facility that fills prescriptions exclusively by mail.

Hospital pharmacy. A pharmacy service for hospitalized patients; includes outpatient pharmacy services serving individuals other than the hospital's own patients.

Long-term care pharmacy. A pharmacy that specializes in treating institutionalized, long-term care patients. A residential care facility not located at a hospital. Includes nursing homes, rest homes and convalescent centers. Includes nursing home providers (usually retail pharmacies whose primary business is selling to nursing homes). Visiting nurses and home healthcare providers are included in this category.

Federal, state, and local government pharmacy. A pharmacy located at a government complex (including family planning, x-ray, dialysis, oncology centers, emergicenters, and alcohol/drug clinics).

Other specialty type. Other clinics and surgery centers.

References

1. Long D. 2004: year in review. Paper presented at: Healthcare Distribution Management Association Marketing Conference; March 21, 2005; Hollywood, FL.

2. Pharmaceutical Research and Manufacturers Association. Membership Web site. Available at: www.phrma.org. Accessed November 11, 2003.

3. Healthcare Distribution Management Association. *HDMA Industry Profile and Healthcare Factbook.* Reston, VA: HDMA; 2003; page 118, chart 186.

4. Healthcare Distribution Management Association. *HDMA Industry Profile and Healthcare Factbook.* Reston, VA: HDMA; 2003; page 8, chart 3.

5. Healthcare Distribution Management Association. *HDMA Industry Profile and Healthcare Factbook.* Reston, VA: HDMA; 2003: page 28, chart 33; page 34, chart 36; page 60, chart 80.

6. Food and Drug Administration. Counterfeit Drug Task Force Interim Report. Rockville, MD: US Department of Health and Human Services; 2003. Available at: www.fda.gov/oc/intiatives/counterfeit/report/interim_report/html. Accessed December 10, 2004.

7. Kohn LT, Corrigan JM, Donaldson MD, eds. Committee on Quality of Health in America, Institute of Medicine. *To Err Is Human: Building a Safer Health System.* Washington, DC: National Academy Press; 1999.

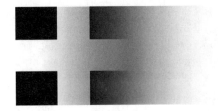

CHAPTER 16

Root-Cause Analysis and Healthcare Failure Mode and Effects Analysis: Two Proactive Harm-Prevention Strategies

John F. Mitchell

Introduction

One result of the 1999 publication of the Institute of Medicine report *To Err Is Human: Building a Safer Health System*[1] was to pique the interest of health care professionals in two industry-proven approaches to error analysis and reduction. The first approach, root-cause analysis (RCA), is a retrospective tool used to delve into the true cause of error. The second, failure mode and effects analysis (FMEA), is a prospective tool that is useful in analyzing potential problems when introducing new systems or equipment or when looking anew at an existing process. Because these strategies are foreign to many in the health care field, they may at first appear overwhelming, but they are more instinctive than they might first appear. A modification of FMEA referred to as Healthcare and Effect Analysis (HFMEA) has been proposed for use in the health care setting and is discussed later in this chapter. In fact, each of us uses RCA and FMEA every day.

Suppose, for example, you turn on a light switch and nothing happens. The room remains dark. The problem is evident: The light does not go on. Your job is to find out why. Many reasons present themselves: The bulb might need to be replaced, the switch might be defective, the wiring might be in need of repair, the wall receptacle may not be working, or the circuit breaker may have tripped. You search until you determine why your light did not go on. In doing so, you perform a root-cause analysis. Once you determine the root cause, you can fix the problem.

FMEA is equally easy to understand. Assume you are about to take a vacation. In planning your time away from home, you probably consider what might go wrong. What is the chance of rain? If you run out of money, how would you access your banking account? If you are visiting a location where Montezuma's revenge may strike, how likely is that to occur, and what should you take with you just in case? These are all examples of anticipating a problem (error) that might occur, determining the relative risk that it may occur, and planning how to prevent it or minimize its impact. In short, you have conducted a FMEA: a failure mode (it might rain) and effects (you would have to stay inside to keep dry if you didn't have the proper rain gear) analysis.

The sections that follow go into more detail about RCAs and FMEAs. Each has a unique role as an approach to improve medication safety. One word of caution. It is easy to become overwhelmed in the minute details that frequently arise during RCAs and, in particular, FMEAs. When that happens, recall the simple examples above and break down the scope of your project into small and achievable tasks.

Root-Cause Analysis in Medication Safety

When should a RCA be applied? The most obvious reason for using a RCA is to determine why an error has occurred. For example, suppose that a patient has been admitted to the intensive-care unit because of the need for intubation after experiencing severe respiratory depression following the administration of a 10-fold overdose of morphine. Though the patient may survive the experience and be discharged without further incident, the seriousness of this error and the possibility that it might recur with less-favorable results may prompt a RCA review. Near misses (i.e., errors that do not reach the patient) usually do not bear the same weight as errors that cause patient harm; nonetheless, their devastating potential may precipitate the need for a RCA.

Consider what might happen in a hospital if many of the automated dispensing machines in the facility were accidentally stocked with 23.4% sodium chloride instead of the normal 0.9% vials. Once the problem is discovered, all the vials may be retrieved, but the potential catastrophic consequences may warrant a RCA. Additionally, repeated errors may raise a red flag that a major event may be imminent. For example, crushing a medication that should not be crushed may not be seen as important enough to initiate an incident report. But how long might it be until a patient experiences an arrhythmia because extended-release propranolol has been crushed and flushed down a nasogastric tube?

On the basis of the scenarios just described, we can identify three types of problems that might initiate a RCA:

1. a serious event that caused, or could have caused, patient harm;
2. a near miss that, had it not been identified, could have caused patient harm; and
3. repeated events that loom waiting to cause a major event.

It can be difficult to determine which errors warrant the consideration of the need for a RCA process and which ones warrant careful observation. Sentinel events almost always prompt a RCA. In the United States, the Joint Commission on Accreditation of Healthcare Organizations (JCAHO) defines a sentinel event as "an unexpected occurrence involving death or serious physical or psychological injury, or the risk thereof. Serious injury specifically includes loss of limb or function. The phrase 'or the risk thereof' includes any process variation for which a recurrence would carry a significant chance of a serious adverse outcome."[2] Table 16-1 suggests sentinel events and other medication errors that might call for an RCA.

Table 16-1. Examples of Events that May Trigger a Root-Cause Analysis

Sentinel Events*
- Unanticipated death or major permanent loss of function, including full-term infants
- Patient suicides

- Infant abduction or discharge to the wrong family
- Rape
- Hemolytic transfusion reaction involving major blood group incompatibilities
- Surgery on the wrong patient or wrong body part

Events or near misses that could cause death or permanent loss of function

- Conscious sedation requiring reversal agents and/or intubation
- Vincristine prepared for, but not given via, an intrathecal route
- Faulty computer software that resulted in mixed patient medication files
- Mass preparation of incorrectly labeled epidural infusions

Events that repeatedly result in medication errors

- Look-alike or sound-alike medications (e.g., MS Contin®, OxyContin®, oxycodone) administered in error from automatic dispensing machine stock
- Wrong patient identification
- Failure to include all special instructions during pharmacy computer order entry
- Incorrect drug selection while using computerized prescriber order entry systems
- Incorrect infusion pump settings

A Sentinel Event Glossary of Terms is available at the Joint Commission on Accreditation of Health Care Organizations' Web site at http://www.jcaho.org/accredited+organizations/hospitals/sentinel+events/ glossary.htm. Accessed December 9, 2004.

RCA Case Study

The case study that follows, based in part, on a real scenario, illustrates the RCA process. While reviewing this section, readers are encouraged to ponder situations that have occurred in their own health care settings and to apply the principles to those situations.

CASE STUDY, PART 1

WD is a 64-year-old female who is brought to the emergency department after her family recognized that she was exhibiting rapidly progressive signs of disorientation. Initial examination and tests suggest a subdural hematoma, prompting her admission to the intensive-care unit. During rounds on the third hospital day, the team notes that she is experiencing increasing hypernatremia. The resident is told to "increase the patient's free water." Unfamiliar with the treatment of hypernatremia, the resident writes an order that reads, "Sterile water IV to be infused at 100 mL/hr." A nurse who is relatively new on the unit calls the pharmacy to ask how to obtain sterile water for infusion. The pharmacy technician who answers the telephone tells the nurse it is obtained from the central stores department. The nurse requisitions the sterile water from central stores and starts the IV as ordered. Eight hours later, a more experienced nurse observes the sterile water at the change of shift, immediately stops the infusion, and notifies the house officer. Laboratory tests later confirm significant hemolysis, most likely caused by infusion of this hypo-osmolar IVsolution.

RCA FACT-FINDING INTERVIEWS

Once an event has occurred and been reported, a RCA may be initiated. To avoid confusion, it is best if a single individual or group is charged with determining the need for a RCA. If the RCA is limited to a single department, such as pharmacy, this responsibility may rest with either the director or the medication-safety coordinator. If the RCA involves multiple departments, someone from risk management, the patient-safety officer, the chief of the medical staff, or an individual with substantial administrative authority should initiate the process. This sets an immediate tone that the incident warrants a high-level review and creates an expectation for both short- and long-term improvement. Although it usually is best to await the findings of the team that will be convened to examine the incident, there are times when circumstances demand immediate corrective actions. For example, if the incident was in part due to the incorrect filling of an automated dispensing machine, a decision may be made to immediately inspect all other units.

The next step is to schedule a fact-finding session for the purpose of identifying all relevant events that led to the error. The individual who leads this session should be a risk manager, a safety officer, or some other individual who has no ties to the participants and can thus be seen as a neutral party. Participants should include any individuals who can provide firsthand knowledge of the events leading to the incident. A representative group might include several physicians and nurses, one or more pharmacists or pharmacy technicians, a unit clerk, and anyone else who can offer factual knowledge directly related to the event. It is best if the participants meet in a single session to review and, most important, agree to the sequence of events as they occurred. At the onset of this meeting, participants should be told that the meeting is nonpunitive, and that all members should feel comfortable presenting their knowledge of the event for the purpose of improving patient safety and avoiding a similar event.

CASE STUDY, CONCLUSION

The patient-safety officer convened a RCA fact-finding session. Participants included the medical resident who wrote the order, both staff nurses who cared for the patient during the time of the event, the pharmacy technician who answered the telephone request from the nurse, the pharmacist who was working in the IV area at the time, a supervisor from central stores, and a risk manager. After roundtable introductions, the patient-safety officer explained that the purpose of the meeting was to gain knowledge of the events leading to the error and to give participants a change to agree on those facts. She stated that this session was nonpunitive and that no one would be accused of wrongdoing. All members were asked to sign a confidentiality form that highlighted the quality-improvement intent of the meeting and emphasized that the knowledge obtained could not be disclosed.

Participants began to outline each step that led up to the incident. Any disagreements as to the factual content were resolved to the satisfaction of all members. A representative from risk management developed a time line depicting each relevant action as it occurred, according to the documentation on the patient's chart or participants' recollections. Because most participants would not be involved in subsequent analyses of the root cause, the chair thanked them and indicated that they would convene upon conclusion of the RCA process to learn of the proposed action plan.

RCA TEAM

Once the facts are known, the next step is to appoint a RCA team. The function of the team is to examine the facts and to develop an action plan that will help ensure that a similar event does not occur.

Team Leader

Selection of an appropriate RCA team leader is extremely important. This individual should be a respected figure within the institution who has the authority to cut through the red tape and serve as a voice of hospital administration. His or her function is to facilitate not only the discussion of the incident but also the development and implementation of the action plan. Typically, the RCA team leader might be the chief or assistant chief of the medical staff, a hospital vice president, or someone who serves in a similar capacity.

Team Members

Team members should include a well-thought-out mix of frontline staff, content experts, and supervisors who represent the areas whose policies or procedures might require change as a result of the event. Because the team members must evaluate the event as objectively as possible, staff members who were directly involved in the event are generally not included. Frequently, the team will also include a risk manager or a quality-improvement individual whose purpose, like that of the team leader, is to keep the team focused on systems improvement. It is best to keep this team to fewer than 10 members.

Team Responsibilities

Rules of conduct should be addressed at the first team meeting. This sets the tone for an open, honest, and nonpunitive discussion. Team rules might include the following: no individual will be identified as a source of blame; each team member is equal and may express his or her opinion without reservation and without fear of reprisal; each member must respect all the others; and no comment is unimportant or insignificant. Other guidelines include the following: criticize only ideas and never individuals; think outside the box and maintain an open mind; and listen constructively.

The RCA team's responsibility is to brainstorm and evaluate the causes leading to the event and to develop an action plan to eliminate or reduce the likelihood of repeat errors. All members should sign a confidentiality statement.

EVENT REVIEW

The first task of the RCA team is to review the event as described during the investigative phase. The team then should discuss each critical step in the event and the processes that might have precipitated the actions of the staff. To assist with this process, it might be helpful to refer to the JCAHO Minimum Scope of Root-Cause Analysis for Specific Types of Sentinel Events,[3] which includes the following areas:

- Patient-identification process
- Staffing levels
- Competency assessment
- Supervision of staff
- Availability of information
- Adequacy of technological support
- Equipment maintenance/management
- Physical environment
- Control of medication (storage and access)
- Labeling of medications

SUMMARIZING RESULTS OF THE TEAM REVIEW

The RCA team determined that a number latent errors contributed to this event. These events and their associated root causes are summarized in **Table 16-2**.

One method that teams often find helpful in analyzing root causes is to create a cause-and-effect, or "fishbone," diagram. Such a diagram is not necessary for a relatively straightforward event, but it is particularly helpful when many issues need to be addressed. It is also an effective way to help prioritize action plans.

To create a cause-and-effect diagram, the team establishes major categories that contributed to the event and diagrams specific problems associated with each category. The end of the diagram identifies the results of the system failures. For an example of how a cause-and effect-diagram might look for the RCA case study discussed here, see **Figure 16-1**.

Table 16-2. Events and Root Causes Identified by the RCA Review Team

Event	Root Cause
A medical resident on rounds misunderstood the discussion of "free water" and assumed this meant administering the product intravenously rather than by mouth.	Residents rotate on a variety of services and may not be familiar with normal procedures on that service.
An inexperienced nurse assumed that sterile water could be given intravenously, despite the fact that she intuitively felt that this was an unusual order.	New employees are frequently intimidated and reluctant to question orders.
The nurse called the pharmacy and assumed she was talking to a pharmacist; the pharmacy technician did not identify herself as such when answering the telephone.	The nurse had no knowledge of how the pharmacy operated and assumed she was talking to a pharmacist. The pharmacy technician did not consider it her responsibility to identify questions that should be forwarded to a pharmacist. The technician did not know the consequences of giving sterile water intravenously.
When asked where the pharmacy obtained sterile water, the technician indicated the product was available from central stores and did not ask the nurse why she was making this inquiry.	The technician did not think about asking why the nurse was asking this question.
Central stores provided the sterile water upon request and had no method to limit the product to pharmacy.	No restrictions were in place to prevent sterile water and similar products from being dispensed by central stores.

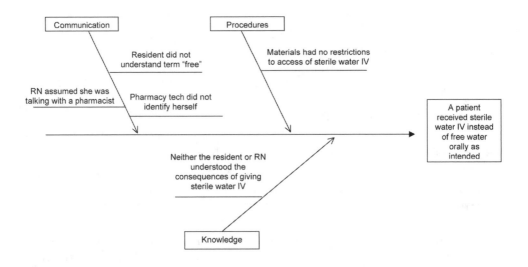

Figure 16-1. Cause and Effect (Fishbone) Diagram

DEVELOPING AN ACTION PLAN

Next, the RCA team develops an action plan to address the issues identified as root causes. Other individuals may be called on to assist at this point. Regardless of group membership, it is important that the team leader have authority to make or, if necessary, to force change. For example, placing a nurse in charge of improving a pharmacy-specific work function is far less effective than is assigning that responsibility to an operations supervisor in the pharmacy. Thus, both the action plan and the leader for that plan must be carefully considered.

One common flaw of RCA teams is the desire to "fix" every issue tangential to the event. Assume, for example, that a hospital has a major error due to a programming problem with patient-controlled analgesia (PCA) pumps. The team's action plan includes a review of every type of pump used in the hospital. While this may be a worthwhile goal, it is likely that the overwhelming task of evaluating all pumps will overshadow a more concentrated effort focused on PCA-pump education. Thus, the RCA team must remain attentive to the problems most directly related to the event. The proximal causes and associated action plans identified by the team exploring this event are summarized in **Table 16-3**.

Table 16-3. Proximal Causes and Associated Action Plans

Proximal Cause	Action Plan
Neither the resident nor the nurse understood the significance of sterile water infusions.	Conduct a hospital-wide educational campaign centering on medical staff, nursing, and pharmacy; encourage additional educational programs within the school of medicine.
Sterile water for infusion was accessible through central stores.	Place a warning flag in central stores' computer that limits access of sterile water to pharmacy; consider moving responsibility for the purchase of sterile water for infusion to pharmacy.
The IV infusion was started before a pharmacist reviewed the order.	With the exception of emergency medications that are required to sustain life, require that a pharmacist review all orders prior to administration.
The technician did not inquire why the nurse was asking the question.	Educate pharmacy technicians as to their role, which includes answering the telephone and knowing when to forward the call to a pharmacist.

For each action, a lead individual should be identified and a measurement tool established to validate the agreed-upon outcome measures.

BRINGING CLOSURE

Once the action plan has been developed, it is important to communicate with the individuals interviewed in the initial phase of the process. This is especially important if the event caused patient harm or was in some way traumatic to the individuals associated with it. This step is best accomplished by bringing together that group of employees and presenting the findings of the RCA team and the action plan to them. If legally appropriate, it would also be helpful to share the event and the action plan throughout the institution as an education process.

RCA SUMMARY

Root-cause analysis is a tool to be used after an event has occurred and is helpful in determining the cause(s) of that event and in developing plans for improvement. To be successful, the analysis should concentrate on system-related issues that precipitated the actions of the employee. This is accomplished by asking a series of "why" questions until the root cause is determined. Once those root causes are identified, action plans focused on elimination of the root cause will help prevent a recurrence of that and similar events.

Healthcare Failure Mode and Effects Analysis

FMEA is a tool that can be used to identify problems that might occur when a new system is being implemented or a current system is being changed or upgraded. FMEA, introduced by the aerospace industry in the early 1960s as a way of identifying potential systems failures, allows designers to anticipate and minimize risks should failures occur. An example of a proactive analysis would be the installation of redundant systems that take over if the primary system fails. FMEA, at its core, isolates

- the failure mode (what could go wrong);
- the effect of a failure (quantification of its severity); and
- an analysis of a failure (detection and ways to minimize the effects of the failure).

Health care adapted a FMEA-like approach in the 1990s, and the JCAHO now requires health care organizations to perform a yearly FMEA on a selected high-risk process. The JCAHO defines a FMEA as a "systematic method of examining a process prospectively for possible ways in which failure can occur."[4] In response to the growing acceptance of the FMEA process in health care, the Veterans Administration National Patient Safety Center (VA NCPS) in Ann Arbor, Michigan, streamlined the FMEA process.[5] This revised process is referred to as health care failure mode and effects analysis, or HFMEA™. For purposes of discussion in this chapter, the HFMEA™ model will be used. Selected definitions of terms used in FMEA and HFMEA™ are listed in **Table 16-4**.[6]

Table 16-4. Definitions of Terms Associated with Failure Mode and Effects Analysis[6]

Criticality	A ranking of a potential failure mode using factors that might include severity, detectability, and probability of the occurrence.
Detectability	Likelihood that a failure will be discovered before it results in patient harm.
Hazard analysis	A process of analyzing collected data to identify risk.
Root cause	The basic reason that initiates a process that results in failure.
Severity	The worst-possible outcome (patient injury) should a failure occur.

The HFMEA™ process includes several distinct steps: selecting the process, assembling an analysis team, developing a flowchart of the process, analyzing each step in the process that could fail, identifying the severity and probability of each potential failure, isolating actions that can be taken to limit the effect of the potential failure, developing outcome measures to test the process, and revamping the process as needed. Each of these steps is described in the following paragraphs.

SELECTING THE HFMEA™ PROCESS

HFMEA™ may be conducted prior to implementation of a new system, program, or piece of equipment. Introduction of a bar-code system to help control and audit automated dispensing machines can serve as an example. A HFMEA™ in this case might include consideration of the risk of electrical or communications failures that would cripple the flow of information. Under these circumstances, orders would still need to be filled, drugs would still need to be accessible to staff, billing would need to continue, and admission, discharge, and transfer would have to be updated, etc. Even a brief failure of the system could have an enormous detrimental impact on the continuity of patient care.

HFMEA™ may also be used to analyze potential failure modes when existing systems, such as a chemotherapy-dispensing laboratory, are revised. Failure modes could be found in each process, from the ordering process to patient administration (e.g., transmission of the order to nursing and pharmacy, preparation and labeling of the drug, the checking process that precedes dispensing, delivery to the nursing station, storage of the drug until used, preparation or acquisition of any special equipment needed, administration of the drug, monitoring of the patient's response, and implementation of drug-wastage procedures as needed).

There is no right or wrong way to select a HFMEA™ process. General topics to consider might include the following:

- a process that is associated with a disproportionally high number of reported errors;
- mandated areas for review by regulating bodies such as JCAHO;
- an error that resulted in a sentinel event;
- systems that may not be associated with high error rates but that could result in a fatality if an error occurred;
- a process that is reported in the literature as error-prone; and
- errors that pose a significant financial burden within the health system.

When selecting the HFMEA™ process, it is important to set reasonable goals. As with a RCA, taking on a process that is too large in scope is a common mistake For example, a HFMEA™ that defines its goal as "reviewing the medication-delivery process" is far too broad. A more reasonable goal would be "reviewing the medication process used in the delivery of PCA." If that goal is still too broad, it could be further narrowed to "reviewing PCA bags or devices stored as floor stock." The point is to select a process that is within the capabilities of the institution, especially if the team does not have extensive experience with the HFMEA™ method.

ASSEMBLING THE HFMEA™ TEAM
Selecting the HFMEA™ team is just as important as is selecting a RCA team, and many of the same principles apply. Membership is ideally limited to 10 to 12 individuals. Larger teams find it difficult to focus. The team should consist of a leader, a facilitator, a recorder, and hands-on experts skilled in the process to be examined. If possible, the team should include a systems engineer who can assist in process analysis and the diagramming of process flow.

- The *leader* must be passionate about improving the process. Ideally, the team leader should also have sufficient authority to acquire resources (e.g., internal and external data, computer support) that the team might need.
- The *facilitator* is charged with keeping the team focused on its objectives and assisting the team leader with the steps used in conducting a HFMEA™. The facilitator need not be familiar with the system being explored. In fact, sometimes it is recommended that at least one team member be "system naive" in order to provide an outsider's view of the process.
- The *recorder* is a detail-oriented individual who will document the recommendations and progress of the team.
- The *experts* are individuals who are intimately familiar the current process and who

will detail every step required to provide the end product. For example, the team experts in the example of a PCA review might include one to two pharmacists, a pharmacy technician who stocks the automated dispensing cabinet, one or two nurses (one from a general floor and one from an intensive-care unit), an anesthesiologist or certified registered nurse anesthetist on the pain team, and supervisors from pharmacy and nursing.

All team members should possess open minds and a willingness to voice their opinions as to where the system is likely to fail. Staff who are threatened by the process may not be effective forces for change. The team leader should make it clear at the first meeting that all opinions will be welcomed, encouraged, and respected.

DEVELOPING A FLOWCHART

The first responsibility of the team is to detail each step in the process. Care should be taken to be as meticulous as possible, as each step is an opportunity for error. Unless the process is well understood or has only a small number of process steps, the process should be diagrammed in a flowchart. A simple flowchart is presented in **Figure 16-2**. It is helpful to number each step; the numbers can later be used as points of reference for its associated risk potential. If the process is very complex, then each major category in the process can be made into a flowchart, resulting in a series of subprocesses.

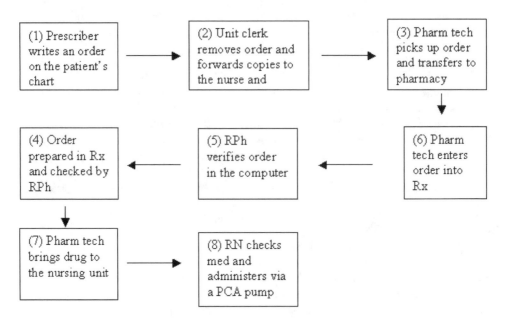

Figure 16-2. Simple Process Flowchart

IDENTIFYING THE PROBABILITY AND SEVERITY OF EACH POTENTIAL FAILURE

The HFMEA™ process uses a matrix that is composed of severity and probability ratings to arrive at a *hazard score*. The hazard score is useful in ranking the importance that is assigned to each potential failure mode in the process. The HFMEA™ hazard score matrix is illustrated in **Table 16-5**.[7]

Table 16-5. HFMEA™ Hazard Score Analysis[7]

		SEVERITY INDEX			
		Catastrophic	*Major*	*Moderate*	*Minor*
	Frequent	16	12	8	4
PROBABILITY INDEX	*Occasional*	12	9	6	3
	Uncommon	8	6	4	2
	Remote	4	3	2	1

Probability Index

Frequent   Likely to occur immediately or within a short period of time (may happen several times yearly).

Occasional   Probably will occur (may occur several times in one or two years).

Uncommon   Possible to occur (may occur sometime in the next two to five years).

Remote   Unlikely to occur (may happen in five to thirty years).

Severity Index

Catastrophic   Death or permanent loss of function; wrong patient or wrong site surgery; infant abduction or discharge to wrong family.

Major   Permanent lessening of body functioning, disfigurement, or surgical intervention required; increased length of stay or increased level of care for three or more patients.

Moderate   Increased length of stay or level of care for one or two patients.

Minor   No injury, increased length of stay, or increased level of care.

As an example of how the hazard score is determined, assume that the pharmacy receives an order for a PCA infusion. One potential failure mode is the selection of the product by the pharmacy technician. Should that step in the process fail and a 10-fold higher concentration of opiate be used to fill the order, the results could be disastrous. After evaluation of this potential failure mode, the HFMEA team agrees to assign it a probability of occurrence of "occasional" and the severity as "catastrophic." The hazard score would thus be assigned a score of 12 using the VA NCPS chart. Each step in the process is similarly evaluated for probability and severity and given a corresponding hazard score.

PERFORMING A DECISION ANALYSIS

The purpose of a decision analysis (see **Figure 16-3**) is to determine which steps in the process are most vulnerable to failure. To do this, the team must answer the following four questions for each process step:

1. Does the process step have a hazard score of significant probability and severity?

2. Does this step in the process represent a single point of weakness?

3. Does an effective control mechanism exist for this point or weakness?

4. Is the hazard so readily apparent (i.e., detectable) that no control mechanism is needed?

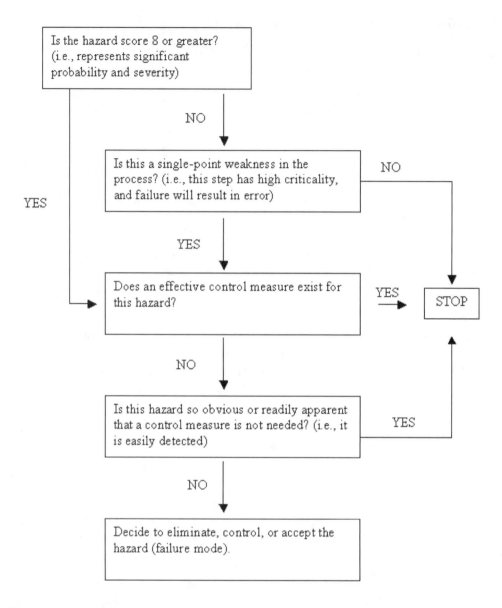

Figure 16-3. Decision-Analysis Tree Used by the VA NCPS

The HFMEA™ team may agree, for example, to conduct an analysis of each process (failure mode) that is ranked with a hazard score of 8 or more. (This number is arbitrary and can be changed if the team members agree.) Teams unfamiliar with the HFMEA™ process may attempt to make the system perfect. While this is an admirable goal, it is advisable to concentrate efforts on only the most critical error points. Using the PCA example, the team assigns a hazard score of 12. Using a decision-support tree, it determines that this failure mode is a single point of weakness. It also determines that an effective control measure exists, because a pharmacist checks the order before it is dispensed and should correct the error. On the other hand, the next step in the process, pharmacist checking, is a single point of weakness that would not have an effective or obvious control measure. Thus, the team must decide whether this failure mode could be avoided or whether the failure mode must be accepted as a potential source of error, given the existing system and available resources.

The failure mode and corresponding information are recorded on the HFMEA™ worksheet (see **Figure 16-4**).[8] Considering the serious patient outcome that could result should this failure mode occur, the team decides that the "action type" should be an attempt to eliminate or minimize the likelihood of occurrence. Only after this decision has been made should the team consider potential causes of the failure mode. Recall that the failure mode identifies only errors that *may* occur and the risk of their occurrence. If the team determines that the failure mode needs an action plan to reduce risk, then, and only then, should the team spend time in determining possible causes. Using the approach will help concentrate the resources of the team.

The possible causes address the reasons why the failure mode could occur. As can be observed in Figure 16-4, each failure mode is given a number and each possible cause is given a letter to tie it to the number. The team can then evaluate each possible cause individually, once again considering the hazard score and decision-tree analysis for that single cause.

DEVELOPING AN ACTION PLAN

Once the HFMEA™ team has decided to try to eliminate or minimize a possible cause associated with a failure mode, its task is to develop an action plan for that possible cause. This often requires the creation of subcommittees that will be asked to suggest alternatives to current procedures. The action plan should be specific and, if possible, should include an outcome measure to demonstrate success or the need for additional improvements. Finally, a lead person should be identified. This individual will be charged with convening the subcommittee and reporting back to the HFMEA™ team.

HFMEA™ SUMMARY

Conducting a HFMEA™ requires a team of professionals who are willing to commit to a process that may take six months to a year. The team will uncover many issues as it examines the process in detail. Team members who are new to the process should be given special instruction so that they can successfully apply the tools and techniques used by the HFMEA™ process. Upper management must demonstrate its support of the process so that adequate resources, both in time and money, contribute to the success of the HFMEA™ team.

Conclusion

RCA and HFMEA™ are powerful tools to be used to reduce the risk of error in our health care environment. Root cause analyses are used to understand why specific errors occurred and how to prevent them from recurring. HFMEA™ is an intensive process that is best used when introducing a totally new system or when considering a wide spread system improvement. Only through the use of these industry-proven methods will our health care system become the safe environment that our patients expect and demand.

HFMEA Step 4 - Hazard Analysis						Decision Tree Analysis				HFMEA Step 5 - Identify Actions and Outcomes				
Failure Mode: First Evaluate failure mode before determining potential causes	Potential Causes	Scoring			Single Point Weakness?	Existing Control Measure ?	Detectability	Proceed?	Action Type (Control, Accept, Eliminate)	Actions or Rationale for Stopping	Outcome Measure	Person Responsible	Management Concurrence
		Severity	Probability	Haz Score									
1 Incorrectly filled PCA syringe not properly checked by RPh		Catastrophic	Uncommon	12	Y	N	N	Y					
	1a Multiple distractions may force the RPh away from the checking process												
	1b Improperly trained techncians may not realize the importance of the RPh final check												
	1c The vial used to prepare the PCA may not be kept with the syringe for the final check												
	1d Crowded work space mading it difficult to determine which ingredients go with each IV												

Figure 16-4. HFMEA™ Worksheet

References

1. Kohn LT, Corrigan JM, Donaldson MD, eds. Committee on Quality of Health in America, Institute of Medicine. *To Err Is Human: Building a Safer Health System*. Washington, DC: National Academy Press; 1999.

2. Joint Commission on Accreditation of Healthcare Organizations. Sentinel Event Policy and Procedures. Rev. July 2002. Available at: www.jcaho.org/accredited+ organizations/hospitals/sentinel+events/. Accessed October 2003.

3. Joint Commission on Accreditation of Healthcare Organizations. Sentinel Events Forms and Tools. Available at: www.jcaho.org/accredited+organizations/ambulatory+care/sentinel+events/forms+and+tools/. Accessed October 2003.

4. Joint Commission on Accreditation of Healthcare Organizations. Sentinel Event Glossary of Terms. Available at: www.jcaho.org/accredited+organizations/hospitals sentinel+events/glossary.htm. Accessed October 2003.

5. Veterans Administration National Center for Patient Safety. Home page. Available at: www.patientsafety.gov/. Accessed October 2003.

6. Spath PL. Using failure mode and effects analysis to improve patient safety. *AORN Journal*. 2003;78(1):16-37.

7. Veterans Administration National Center for Patient Safety. Healthcare Failure Mode and Effect Analysis Course Materials™ (HFMEA™). Available at: www.patientsafety.gov/HFMEA.html. Accessed October 2003.

8. Veterans Administration National Center for Patient Safety. Healthcare Failure Mode and Effects Analysis. Available at: www.patientsafety.gov/worksheets.doc. Accessed October 2003.

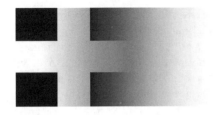

Drug Information Resources and Medication Safety

Gerald K. McEvoy

The single largest proximal cause of medication error is a lack of adequate information about safe drug use during the prescribing, order-transcription, and medication-administration stages. The most common system failure is in disseminating drug knowledge and in making drug and patient information readily accessible at the time it is needed. [1-5]

Introduction

Adverse drug events (ADEs) occur frequently in hospitalized and ambulatory patients, often resulting in serious sequelae.[1,2,6-8] An ADE is defined as any injury resulting from a medical intervention related to a drug, which can be either preventable or unavoidable.[1,2,6-8] One study reported that 6.5 percent of hospitalized patients experienced an ADE during their stay,[1] with incidences in various studies ranging from 1.2 percent to 37.3 percent, depending on the methods used for data collection (e.g., spontaneous reports versus intensive monitoring).[8,9] A study in the ambulatory setting found that 162 of 661 (25%) ambulatory patients at four adult primary care practices experienced a total of 181 ADEs (27 per 100 patients) over a three-month period.[7]

The seriousness of ADEs among these patients varies. In a meta-analysis evaluating data from 39 prospective studies that assessed the incidence of adverse drug reactions (ADRs) in patients who either already were hospitalized or subsequently required hospitalization, the overall incidence for all ADRs of all degrees of severity combined was 15.1 percent.[9] An ADR is defined as an effect that is noxious and unintended but that occurs with an appropriate use at prophylactic, diagnostic, or therapeutic doses, i.e., ADEs *excluding* inappropriate use of a drug such as errors in drug administration, overdose, and abuse.[1,5,8,9] The incidence for serious ADRs was 6.7 percent, and that for fatal ADRs was 0.32 percent.[9] Of the 181 ADEs reported in the study conducted in ambulatory patients, 24 (13%; 3.6 per 100 patients) were considered serious, but none was fatal or life-threatening.[7]

Nearly a decade has passed since the publication of a landmark study in which Leape and colleagues identified the systems failures fundamental to errors that cause ADEs and potential ADEs in the hospital setting.[3] In that study, the investigators found that 39 percent of errors occurred in prescriber ordering and 38 percent in nurse administration.[3] The most common types of errors were dosing errors, which occurred more than three times as frequently as did any other error, and which most commonly included wrong-dose errors and errors in drug choice.[3] More important, Leape and colleagues identified lack of knowledge about the drug as the most common proximal cause of drug errors, accounting for 22 percent of ADEs.[3] In terms of the system failures that produced these errors, the investigators identified the system of disseminating drug knowledge as the one with the highest number of errors.[3] Errors in drug knowledge dissemination reflected a lack of knowledge not only about dosage and routes of administration but also about drug interactions and contraindications in specific patient subsets (e.g., the elderly).[3] The single largest proximal cause of medication error was a lack of adequate information about safe medication use during the prescribing, order-transcription, and medication-administration stages.[3] Other studies have reported similar findings regarding the importance of access to and appropriate application of drug knowledge in preventing ADEs.[1,2,4,5] Therefore, one may conclude that access to reputable, authoritative, current drug information, particularly at the point of prescribing, is critical to safe and effective drug use.

The American Society of Health-System Pharmacists (ASHP) states that, "the provision of medication information is among the fundamental professional responsibilities of pharmacists in health systems."[10] As health-system pharmacists have increased their level of involvement in providing pharmaceutical care, their activities have become less distributive and more information based.[10] Because they are now expected to meet the information needs of the patient care team, either in the hospital or ambulatory care setting, pharmacists today must develop a higher level of competence in this area than may have previously been expected. The pharmacist is key to increasing drug knowledge among health care providers, thereby decreasing the frequency of ADEs through provision of timely, correct, and pertinent drug information.[4]

Pharmacists must not only accumulate and organize drug information literature but also objectively evaluate that information and apply it to a specific patient or clinical situation.[10] An important aspect of this is ensuring that current resources, including representative primary, secondary, and tertiary literature, are available to assist in answering a wide range of medication information requests.[10] This chapter provides an overview of the current state of medication information. It describes the inadequacies of many available information sources as well as the characteristics of dependable, objective, authoritative drug information. Additional discussion focuses on evidence-based medicine and its relevance to sound therapeutic decisions, the current quality of electronic drug information resources, and the challenges associated with off-label drug information and safe medication use. The chapter includes several case reports to illustrate some types of ADEs associated with drug information errors. It concludes with a discussion of the future of drug development and potential medication information risks associated with the more complex and toxic therapies that are likely to become available over the next decade.

Inadequacies of Food and Drug Administration-Approved Labeling

Before a drug can be marketed in the United States, the manufacturer must provide not only data supporting the efficacy of the drug in the treatment of the proposed indication but also labeling consistent with the data and approved by the U.S. Food and Drug Administration (FDA). Under the federal Food, Drug, and Cosmetic (FD&C) Act, a drug approved for marketing may be labeled, promoted, and advertised by the manufacturer only for those uses for which its safety and effectiveness have been established from information submitted by the manufacturer and reviewed and approved by FDA.[11,13] However, FDA acknowledges that the FD&C Act does not restrict the way in which a prescriber may use an approved drug,[12,13] and that a drug may be prescribed for uses or in treatment regimens or patient populations that are not included in approved product labeling (commonly referred to as the package insert) but that are considered appropriate.[11-14] Further, accepted medical practice frequently includes using a drug for purposes not described in its approved labeling.[12,13] As a result, simply relying on drug labeling (e.g., as compiled in the *Physicians' Desk Reference*® [*PDR*®]) does not ensure safe and effective use of a given medication relative to contemporary clinical practice. Alternative, current sources of objective drug information are needed to supplement the information provided in the labeling.[14-17]

A principal deficiency of FDA-approved labeling involves dosage information and reflection of current therapeutic perspectives embodied in guidelines.[16-18,20,21] Although clinicians are taught the importance of individualized dosing, FDA-approved labeling often includes recommendations for only one or two dosages and rarely includes data regarding dosing in relation to mealtimes.[20] Doses typically are set during phase 1 (I) trials (the first step of drug testing in a small group of humans), early in the research process and prior to FDA approval.[19] Dose-ranging studies generally are short in duration and may enroll fewer than 100 patients, thus limiting the investigator's or manufacturer's ability to explore the complete dose and interval ranges that might permit more accurate and complete dosage recommendations.[19] These limitations often lead to knowledge deficiencies that result in unacceptable toxicity or ADE rates, particularly in the context of general medical practice, in which patients for whom these drugs are prescribed do not necessarily meet the inclusion criteria for clinical trials.[18,19] The deficiency of appropriate dosage information in drug labeling is notable given that dosing errors are among the most common reasons for ADEs.

Following FDA approval, new uses for drugs, as well as higher incidences or new types of ADEs, often are revealed.[19,21,22] This often reflects expanded use of the drug in hundreds-of-thousands to millions of patients over several years. In addition, postmarketing research often uncovers the efficacy of doses that differ from the manufacturer's FDA-approved recommendations. Many of these doses are substantially lower than the approved doses and may produce fewer ADEs.[18,19] However, while many of these lower doses are adequately studied, few are added to FDA-approved labeling because manufacturers are not required to update their labeling for such things and may have limited incentive to do so (e.g., anticipated financial return relative to the expense of submitting supplemental data to FDA).[12,13,21] Changes in drug labeling must receive FDA approval, often requiring manufacturers to conduct new studies, a necessity that may hinder efforts to update this information.[12,19,21]

In addition to offering limited dosage information, FDA-approved labeling provides little therapeutic perspective.[11] For example, a drug may no longer be considered first-line, or even alternative, therapy for an FDA-approved indication, but this change is generally not updated in the labeling. Such outdated clinical information can have serious consequences if the labeling, rather than established contemporary practice, were followed, particularly when drugs that are more effective or less toxic or both have displaced the outmoded drug therapy. In addition, drug labeling generally does not include recommendations based on published guidelines. For example, in one study, the initial dosages included in the *PDR* (manufacturer's labeling) for antihypertensive drugs exceeded those recommended by the National Institutes of Health's (NIH) Joint National Committee (JNC) for 58 percent of drugs; 95 percent of the labeling of this latter group of drugs recommended dosages that were at least twice those recommended by JNC.[18] By comparison, certain drug information resources such as *AHFS Drug Information® (AHFS DI®)* that address authoritative guidelines like JNC to reflect contemporary practice do embody such changes in preferred dosing recommendations.[56]

Even if the recommendations of authoritative groups do eventually find their way into labeling, many years can elapse between their establishment as state-of-the-art clinical practice and adoption in labeling. For example, it took three years for labeling to reflect the recommendation of the American Society of Clinical Oncology and the American Society of Hematology that once-weekly dosing of epoetin alfa was an acceptable regimen for the treatment of chemotherapy-associated anemia.[23-26] During this period, the FDA-approved labeling for epoetin alfa (Epogen®, Amgen Inc., Thousand Oaks, CA) continued to state that the drug should be administered three times weekly for this indication; no mention of the once-weekly dosing option was given.[23-25]

These discrepancies between FDA-approved labeling and accepted medical practice provide the basis for the inadequacies of many of the available medication information resources. A primary example is the *PDR*, a drug information resource provided at no charge to physicians, physicians' assistants, nurses, nurse practitioners, medical residents, and students as both an information and marketing medium by pharmaceutical manufacturers and comprising data and recommendations identical to those in the FDA-approved labeling (package inserts).[12,14,20] A negotiated effort of commercial enterprises and government regulators, the *PDR* is the primary drug information resource for unfamiliar drugs for 80 to 90 percent of physicians.[19] Because the information published in the *PDR* replicates FDA-approved labeling, a deficiency in one will also appear in the other.[14]

Wide Array of Drug Information Resources

A wide array of drug information resources is available to both health practitioners and consumers.[10] Information ranges in depth of coverage (e.g., from concise dosing guides such as the *Tarascon Pocket Pharmacopoeia®* to comprehensive drug compendia such as *AHFS DI*); editorial processes (e.g., from drug handbooks and databases that principally glean information from other drug information compilations such as the *PDR* and *AHFS DI* and incorporate unsubstantiated experiential/anecdotal information from practitioners to resources such as the Cochrane Collaboration and *AHFS DI* that employ evidence-based assessments of the medical literature); qualifications, affiliation, and expertise of staff and authors; recognized authoritativeness and incorporation of treatment guidelines from expert groups; independence from the influence of pharmaceutical manufacturers; extent of critical review; currency and updating mechanism; and other key characteristics. Because such a wide array of drug information resources of varying depth, editorial quality, and currency are available, it is critical that practitioners understand the characteristics of the drug information they are accessing and applying to day-to-day patient care decisions and that they use the most dependable, objective, authoritative resources possible.

Although ASHP has identified as key pharmacist responsibilities the evaluation of the medication information needs of health practitioners as well as evaluation of the strengths and weaknesses of available resources,[10] health practitioners often have little guidance about the context and accuracy of the information they are using.[36,38,39,61] (See the discussion under the section on Quality of Currently Available Drug Information Resources, below.) Following is a discussion of some of the key characteristics for evaluating dependable drug information as well as initiatives that are under way to aid in assessing the merits of information, including that accessible via the Web.

Characteristics of Dependable, Objective, Authoritative Drug Information

An ideal source for drug information aimed at fostering safe medication use should provide dependable, objective, authoritative information in the context of sound editorial policies; high-quality, controlled content development; a well-established expert-review process; independence from pharmaceutical manufacturers, health insurers, pharmacy benefits managers, and others who may seek to use the source to promote their own interests; an ongoing updating process; a mechanism for correction notification; and broad-based authoritative guideline incorporation (see **Table 17-1**). A key aspect of such a resource is the evidence-based objectivity that allows the inclusion of uses and dosages that are not included in the FDA-approved labeling (i.e., off-label/unlabeled uses).

Table 17-1. Characteristics of Dependable, Objective, Authoritative Drug Information

Characteristic	Examples/Description
Sound editorial policies	• Evidence-based assessments
High-quality controlled content development	• Preparation by a professional in-house staff • Use of external volunteers limited to expert review, not content development
Expert review	• Participation solicited but voluntary • No honorarium or other benefit provided • Full disclosure of interest by experts
Independence from pharmaceutical manufacturers	• Policies to ensure editorial independence • No financial support • Manufacturer may participate in but does not control review process • Manufacturer information viewed with healthy skepticism
Ongoing updating process	• Published supplements, timely, ongoing electronic updates, or both
Mechanism for correction notification	• Electronic notification via Web site • Other mechanisms (e.g., e-mail, first-class mail) as necessary
Broad-based guideline incorporation	• Centers for Disease Control and Prevention • National Institutes of Health • American Heart Association • American Psychiatric Association • American College of Chest Physicians • American Academy of Pediatrics • Other authoritative groups

Vetting and recognition of the authority of a drug information source by professional, government, legislative, regulatory, and private-sector groups generally speaks to the strength of its editorial process and the dependability of the information it provides. It also is important that the information be free of undue influence of pharmaceutical manufacturers and other third parties who may seek to use the publication to promote their own interests.[11,27,28]

An appropriate process for developing drug information to be included in these types of drug information resources should involve several key steps: information tracking and gathering, evidence-based information analysis, drug information synthesis and development, a review process, and finalization and management of published information (see **Figure 17-1**). As part of maintenance efforts, periodic updating to address the evolving nature of drug information relative to ongoing research and clinical experience, as well as a readily accessible alerting and correction-notification process, are important.

Following is a description of the key elements applied by one well-vetted, recognized source of dependable drug information—*AHFS DI*. Similar elements have been applied in the past by other well-vetted sources of dependable drug information such as *AMA-DE* (no longer published) and *USP DI* (no longer published by USP).

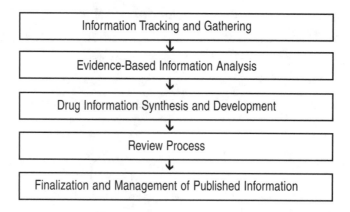

Figure 17-1. Development process for a dependable, objective, authoritative drug information resource.

INFORMATION TRACKING AND GATHERING

It is important in assessing the usefulness and dependability of a drug information resource to understand the sources of information used in developing the content and associated recommendations. Some resources may merely parrot the information compiled by other drug information resources while others may have well-established, evidence-based editorial processes conducted by an experienced full-time professional staff. Parroted resources may have little editorial expertise in evaluating the true merit of the information they publish and may be at considerable disadvantage in maintaining the currency of derived information since it would be difficult for them to contemporaneously monitor revisions and updating of the information upon which their content is derived. For example, dosage recommendations incorporated in the source material from which the parroting originally was derived may change over time to reflect evolving evidence and changes in state-of-the-art practice that may escape the attention of the derived work. Recommended antithrombotic dosages of aspirin have changed over time but depending on when the information was derived from the authoritative drug information source, the derived work may lag behind and not reflect the current state of practice. Likewise, recommended antihypertensive dosages have generally decreased over time but such decreases may not be reflected in derived works that incorporated the information originally years ago and were inattentive to changing recommendations.

For a dependable source of drug information, the information-tracking-and-gathering process should entail monitoring of drug and medical information databases (e.g., MEDLINE/PubMed, TOXNET, www.cancer.gov, www.aidsinfo.nih.gov, www.guidelines.gov, Cochrane Collaboration, MedWatch), as well as monitoring of relevant medical journals, bibliographic and abstracting services, Web sites, and other materials (e.g., government, association, and industry reports and guidelines). Resources such as those available through PubMed and the National Library of Medicine (NLM) provide an expansive array of scientifically based materials for review and analysis. Increasingly, primary and other biomedical literature, such as published clinical studies, may be accessed via the Internet, with hyperlinks from bibliographic and other databases to the full text of the articles themselves.

Information on Unlabeled Uses

A reliable, authoritative drug information resource should include not only information from the FDA-approved labeling but also information on uses, dosages, and routes and methods of administration that may not be included in the FDA-approved labeling for the drug (off-label/unlabeled). As described earlier, reliance on labeled information alone may not reflect contemporary clinical practice. The process of gathering such information should be evidence based and free from the influence of parties with a vested interest in positive or negative commentary.

Many factors can influence the selection of an off-label use for consideration and possible evaluation. The availability of published information, particularly from peer-reviewed journals and expert therapeutic guidelines, is a key factor prompting review for possible commentary on that use in the drug information resource. Evidence from published studies should be given precedence over expert opinion, although the latter may be useful in judging the role of a given drug relative to other therapies. A thorough review of the published medical literature (e.g., via tools such as MEDLINE/PubMed, other NLM databases) should be completed as part of the consideration process. Once evidence from pertinent references is evaluated, a determination can be made regarding the value of further assessment of the use. The advice of expert reviewers may also initiate review and evaluation of an off-label use.

Potential sources of information that may be used in considering off-label uses are shown in **Table 17-2**. Information sources should encompass a wide variety of respected, peer-reviewed sources, as well as authoritative therapeutic guidelines, orphan drug designations, clinical alerts from the NIH and major medical journals and societies, expert advice, and government reports, and may also include presentations from relevant professional meetings (particularly for uses in relatively serious diseases when alternative therapies are unavailable or limited or are toxic).

Table 17-2. Information Sources for Unlabeled Medication Uses

Source	Examples
Major peer-reviewed medical journals	• *New England Journal of Medicine* • *Journal of the American Medical Association* • *Pediatrics* • *Chest*
Bibliographic databases	• MEDLINE (PubMed) • AIDSinfo • PDQ® (www.cancer.gov)
Meta- and Other Pooled Analyses	• Peer-reviewed medical journals • Cochrane Collaboration
Consensus statements and authoritative guidelines	• National Institutes of Health • Centers for Disease Control and Prevention • www.guidelines.gov • American Heart Association • American College of Chest Physicians • American Academy of Pediatrics • American Thoracic Society
Review articles and editorials in peer-reviewed journals	• Long-term experience with the drug not reflected in primary studies
Supplemental new drug application filings	
Orphan use designations	
Approval in other countries with established drug regulatory procedures	• Great Britain
Clinical alerts	• National Institutes of Health • Major medical journals and societies
Other sources	

EVIDENCE-BASED INFORMATION ANALYSIS

In order to reflect contemporary state-of-the-art practice, dependable drug information sources should provide a high-level of evidence-based assessment of evolving drug information (e.g., the primary literature) as well as expert therapeutic guidelines. Less rigorous, ongoing assessments of the published literature may be acceptable if a high-level of attention is paid to contemporary practice reflected in expert therapeutic guidelines and other authoritative sources. Questions to ascertain in evaluating the reliability of a drug information resource should include the procedures employed to evaluate and accurately reflect clinical evidence from the medical literature and expert guidelines.

Analysis of information preferably should be an in-house process performed by a professional staff with strong scientific and therapeutic backgrounds. Such an in-house process potentially provides a high level of quality control and consistency in content development. The process should involve an assessment of the scientific merits of available data, which preferably should be drawn from a large body of references or from alternative sources that have expertly reviewed the evidence. Emphasis should be placed on well-designed, randomized, controlled trials (RCTs). Comparisons with other therapies should be performed where possible; however, because of FDA's emphasis on placebo-controlled studies, most drug research unfortunately does not include comparator drugs in the study design.[11] Alternative sources of expertly reviewed evidence may include published meta-analyses, reviews by the Cochrane Collaboration, and authoritative therapeutic guidelines developed via an evidence-based process (e.g., from the NIH, American Academy of Pediatrics [AAP], U.S. Centers for Disease Control and Prevention [CDC], American Heart Association [AHA], American College of Chest Physicians [ACCP], and similar groups). Consideration also may be given to relevant published cost-effectiveness, cost-benefit, and quality-of-life studies.

Decisions about the merits of various uses, including those that are off-label, should be made on the basis of the evaluation and judgment of a qualified staff, as well as of the advice of clinical and other experts who serve as reviewers or panelists. These decisions should be influenced by the weight of supporting evidence (i.e., the process should be evidence based, with well-designed randomized studies and meta-analyses without heterogeneity weighted more heavily than studies with methodological limitations, case-control studies, uncontrolled studies, or case reports), the importance and severity of the disease, availability of alternative therapies and their relative toxicities, the number of patients affected by the disease, and other factors (e.g., cost considerations). The weight of evidence should be augmented by the strength of efficacy data, availability of independent confirmatory studies, support in other peer-reviewed literature (e.g., editorials, disease and drug therapy reviews), recommendations of authoritative groups (e.g., CDC, NIH, AAP, ACCP), and evidence of an improved risk/benefit ratio (including patient compliance), a new mechanism or site of action, or improved pharmacokinetics or pharmacodynamics relative to existing therapeutic alternatives. Positive commentary should depend on the level of such evidence and on the clinical importance of the drug as part of good medical practice and care. A drug information resource that is narrative in nature or that has a well-defined structure for evidence-level presentation allows a description of the strengths and limitations of available evidence as well as provision of information on any lack of a consensus about the specific role of the drug for a given use.

DRUG INFORMATION SYNTHESIS AND DEVELOPMENT

Dependable drug information resources should guide clinicians in making informed decisions, presenting recommended courses of action wherever possible (e.g., is it a drug of choice, an alternative, a use for which evidence is limited).

Pertinent information, including data from the literature, recommendations of authoritative expert groups, data from FDA-approved labeling, solicited opinions of experts, and other data, should be synthesized and incorporated. The information analysis and presentation should be aimed at guiding clinicians in making informed decisions from a highly dependable and objective source. Data on response indicators and rates, anticipated outcomes, and therapeutic perspectives (e.g., the specific role of the drug) may add valuable insight to clinicians in weighing decisions derived from the drug information resource. Information should be thoroughly documented and referenced, preferably directly in the drug database, or at least be readily available from the publisher. If the drug information is descriptive, information interpretation does not need to be black or white, and limitations can be clearly stated. Any controversy can be addressed and stated at this stage.

Incorporation of the therapeutic perspectives of extramural experts can add to the dependability and relevance of the drug information provided. (See the discussion under the section on the Review Process below.)

REVIEW PROCESS

In assessing the dependability of a drug information resource, information on the rigor of both the internal and external review of draft information prior to publication should be considered.

This process preferably comprises a multistep internal evaluation and review by qualified staff and, as appropriate, a solicited external review involving multiple experts for a given use or drug. The external evaluation and review preferably should include leading medical scientists, clinicians (e.g., physicians), pharmacists, pharmacologists, and other qualified individuals. Depending on the drug and areas of therapy addressed, experts from various professional and governmental settings, including the NIH, CDC, and other areas, may be solicited to participate. The solicited opinions of external experts may be particularly important in gauging the clinical role of the drug in medical practice and as an indicator of the level of consensus on specific therapeutic issues. Participation preferably should be voluntary, and no honorarium or other benefit preferably should be provided. Full disclosure of interest, including any affiliation with or financial involvement in the manufacturer of the drug(s) under consideration and directly competitive products, should be made.

FINALIZATION AND MAINTENANCE OF PUBLISHED INFORMATION

In determining the dependability of drug information resources, the mechanisms for finalizing draft material and maintaining published information should be considered.

A master database of published information preferably should be maintained and updated on a continuous basis, allowing periodic electronic updates (ideally issued at least monthly). Because of the evolving nature of drug information secondary to ongoing research and clinical experience, a high-level monitoring and updating process should be in place. Documentation, including appropriate archival records, should be maintained by and available from the publisher to respond to inquiries about source information. Such documentation should include a high level of reference to published, reputable sources and should rely only minimally on local, anecdotal, and personal experience.

INFORMATION FROM PHARMACEUTICAL MANUFACTURERS

Because drug information sources shape treatment decisions made by clinicians and influence public and private health care policies and decisions, drug information sources should maintain editorial independence from pharmaceutical manufacturers who may seek to use the publication to promote their own vested interest.[11,27,28] Editorial decisions should be evidence based and be made independently of manufacturers and other third parties. Interactions between reputable drug information sources and pharmaceutical manufacturers should be limited to the legitimate exchange of scientific and medical information and should be directed at the scientific and medical areas within the companies, avoiding undue promotional interests.

Because clinicians are overwhelmed at keeping up with drug-related advances, they continue to rely on pharmaceutical marketing, including company-sponsored continuing education, as important drug information sources.[11,28] Therefore, it is critical that reputable drug information resources subscribe to an evidence-based, objective editorial process that refutes unfound claims and that can serve a key role in assisting clinicians at making informed, objective decisions.

Unfortunately, some widely used drug information resources may be less rigorous at maintaining editorial independence, and may actually seek out formal relationships with the pharmaceutical industry (e.g., providing seats on editorial boards) and not exercise sufficient disclosure from external authors to avoid use of those with direct financial ties (e.g., consulting and speakers' fees) to the drug companies.[11,27] Other drug information resources may rely heavily on the contribution of outside authors and local hospital formularies and perform little evidence-based evaluation in a controlled, internal editorial environment. As a result, it is important that the editorial policies and standards of drug information resources be evaluated and considered in the selection of dependable sources. Likewise, some educational programs aimed at prescribers and others involved in the medication-use process continue to promote uses for which limited sound evidence of efficacy and safety has accumulated, despite guidelines aimed at curtailing such practices.[11,28] Unsubstantiated uses, including those derived anecdotally or evaluated in only a few patients, when promoted through such positive commentary,[11,27] potentially expose patients unnecessarily to ADEs.[29] Therefore, a balance should be struck between the level of efficacy and safety evidence and clinical practice.

When a drug is initially approved for marketing in the United States, the manufacturer may be the only source of certain information (e.g., chemistry, stability, pharmaceutical data) about it. For this reason, it is appropriate for a drug information publication to request the current labeling, journal reprints, bibliographies, and other information from the scientific or medical information section of the manufacturer. The manufacturer may be provided a copy of draft material on its drug for comment and may be specifically requested to provide clarification and additional details about both published and unpublished information originating under its auspices. Balancing the manufacturer's comments with those of nonmanufacturer experts as part of the review process and/or with other sources of expert knowledge and advice (e.g., accepted therapeutic guidelines) is particularly important when off-label information is being considered. Any comments from the manufacturer should be clearly attributable to it during the review and evaluation.

Dependable sources of drug information should view all data from pharmaceutical manufacturers with healthy skepticism, with an overriding assumption that each study is sponsored by the manufacturer unless determined otherwise. In certain situations, it may be necessary to ask the manufacturer to identify which studies they sponsored. Such sponsorship should be considered in the interpretation of the study conclusions, especially in cases where these conclusions differ from those of other available information. Interpretation of results from these studies also may be affected if the results, particularly details about study design or data, appear to be incomplete or misrepresented. A disclosure of interest should be requested from all authors of published studies, as well as all others who serve as reviewers, to establish any potential conflict. These disclosures should be weighed accordingly in any evaluation of author or reviewer comments.

Recognition of a bias favoring publication of positive clinical findings should strengthen the healthy skepticism employed in evidence-based assessment of data published on drugs. Suppression of negative findings also can directly or indirectly affect issues surrounding drug safety, as reportedly was the case with pediatric use of selective serotonin-reuptake inhibitors.[30]

Evidence-Based Medicine

Evidence-based medication use draws on the results of controlled clinical trials and consensus advice on best practices. Unfortunately, a high proportion of prescription medication use is not evidence based, which compromises the quality and raises the cost of health care. Many national quality initiatives have developed evidence-based guidelines (see National Guideline Clearinghouse at www.guidelines.gov) on the use of medications (e.g., ACCP guidelines on antithrombotic therapy,[31] the Centers for Medicare & Medicaid Services [CMS] National AMI [Acute Myocardial Infarction] Project,[32] Cochrane Collaboration[33]), and many more are forthcoming. However, there is an immense gap between the publication of these guidelines and their application by practitioners.

Well-defined medical practice standards that specifically identify experimental therapies and established standards of care will likely always be somewhat lacking, mainly because of the continually increasing pace of advancement in medical science and the dynamic nature of medical practice.[34] Practice standards for certain drug therapies, specifically biotechnology-produced drugs, cancer chemotherapy, and treatments for diseases with rapidly evolving dynamics, such as human immunodeficiency virus (HIV) infection, are constantly changing. The nature of these drug therapies challenges professional societies and other authoritative groups to review scientific data expeditiously and to develop standards that continue to be up to date.

Clinical pharmacy specialists and scientists play an important and a growing role in the generation of new knowledge related to the appropriate use of medications. Their expertise is invaluable in developing, adapting, implementing, and monitoring compliance with clinical guidelines and in the development of clinical decision-support systems, including those incorporating computerized prescriber order entry applications. Pharmacists can expand evidence-based medication use by improving their knowledge of scientific breakthroughs, ensuring the use of reputable drug information resources that employ sound editorial standards, and appropriately applying new scientific knowledge in practice. The ultimate primary beneficiary of pharmacists' involvement in these processes is the patient.

Quality of Currently Available Drug Information Resources

Despite a highly advanced medical research establishment and a thorough peer-review process for publishing research results, mechanisms to translate published findings into general medical practice remain rudimentary.[28,35-38] Clinicians are expected to stay abreast of current medical journal articles, government guidelines and reports, therapeutic guidelines from authoritative groups such as AAP and ACCP, clinical alerts from pharmaceutical manufacturers and others (e.g., medical journals and societies), scientific conference proceedings, and reports from the popular press regarding unpublished results. The volume of information is staggering.[37-39] For example, in 2003, the FDA issued 449 safety-related drug labeling changes and 66 safety notifications for clinicians.[40] The NLM indexed 526,000 articles for all its databases in 2003; MEDLINE alone now includes more than 12 million references from more than 4,700 journals.[37,41,42] In terms of ongoing research, in 2004, NLM's clinical trials database (www.clinicaltrials.gov) included information on more than 6,000 trials for a wide range of diseases and medical conditions conducted at 70,000 locations, and the National Cancer Institute's (NCI's) PDQ database included information on an additional 1,800 active and 120,000 closed clinical cancer trials.[37] Adding to the complexity are the 20,000–50,000 health and medical Web sites with varying reliability accessible through the Internet. Eighty percent of physicians use the Internet for health information and about 66 percent use it routinely in their practices, with 86 percent of this latter group searching for drug information.[38]

The advances in drug research, the rate at which FDA is approving ever more potent and potentially toxic therapies, and the exponential growth in published medical information make it nearly impossible for physicians and other health care providers to grasp this enormous volume and array of resources to glean the information relevant to safe and effective drug therapy in their clinical practices.[36,38] Although certain information may suggest that immediate changes are necessary in clinical practice, a clinician may learn of the information only by chance (e.g., if he or she subscribes to the journal in which the data are reported and actually reads it, hears about it from a colleague, or listens to a news report discussing the information). More important, clinicians often have insufficient advice regarding the perspective and accuracy of the information. This is particularly true for information originating on the Internet, where determining the quality and relevance of medical information is a monumental and, in many cases, nearly impossible task.[38,39,43] For these reasons, important, substantiated medical advances are often overlooked by clinicians, making the disparity between knowledge and practice massive.

A wide range of drug information resources is available to pharmacists and clinicians. ASHP states that "up-to-date drug information shall be available, including current periodicals and recent editions of textbooks in appropriate pharmaceutical and biomedical subject areas. Electronic information is desirable."[44] Of the information sources, the most respected are primary references from peer-reviewed journals. However, because of the sheer volume of peer-reviewed journals published,[42] pharmacists often must rely on secondary or tertiary sources (e.g., textbooks, drug information compendia such as *AHFS Drug Information* [*AHFS DI*]) that provide dependable, objective, and authoritative drug information. In addition, the federal government recognizes through legislation and regulation three currently available compendia for information on medically accepted uses of drugs:

- *AHFS DI*, published by ASHP;[45-52]

- *Drugdex® System*, published by Thomson MICROMEDEX™;[45] and

- *USP Dispensing Information®* (*USP DI®*)[45-52] published by Thomson MICROMEDEX originally under license from USP but no longer subject to USP's editorial standards or contributions.[53, 54]

The editorial standards of two of these compendia (i.e., *AHFS Drug Information* and *USP DI* [when it was published by USP]) have been widely vetted by the U.S. Congress, the Center for Medicare & Medicaid Services [CMS], national health insurance groups (e.g., Health Insurance Association of America [HIAA, now America's Health Insurance Plans] Health Care Technology Committee, Medicaid's national medical directors, the National Blue Cross and Blue Shield Association), and many others and have been subject to public comment on several occasions via the *Federal Register*. Similar vetting occurred with *AMA-DE*, but the compendium no longer is published. *Drugdex* has not undergone such a broad-based vetting nor an opportunity for public comment via *Federal Register* notification.[11,27,46,77] Several other differences also should be considered when evaluating the strengths and weaknesses of each.

For example, while *AHFS DI* relies (and *USP DI* previously relied) on an in-house staff of drug information analysts and editors to develop monographs and routinely has requested disclosure of interest from all independent expert reviewers for decades, *Drugdex* reportedly has relied on an internal staff as well as external authors, some of whom may have had business relationships with the pharmaceutical industry.[27] This difference can result in significant variations in the quantity and quality of information included in each monograph. For example, gabapentin (Neurontin®, Pfizer Inc., New York, NY) is an anticonvulsant approved by the FDA for epileptic seizures and postherpetic neuralgia.[55] In addition to the approved indications for this drug, *Drugdex* listed 48 off-label uses for the product in 2003 (e.g., hiccups, nicotine withdrawal, bipolar disorder, migraines), far greater than the number included in *AHFS DI* and *USP DI*.[27,55-57]

Thus, conducting a sound, evidence-based drug information development process, addressing authoritative therapeutic guidelines, and soliciting the expertise and experience of independent expert reviewers become even more critical to ensuring that the information included in these compendia represents the standard of care in medical practice.

INTERNET-BASED INFORMATION RESOURCES

Many of today's drug information resources bear little resemblance to those on the shelves of drug information centers in the 1960s and 1970s. Technologic advances during the past four decades have completely revamped the medication-use process, including delivery of drug information.[37,38,58] Electronic media have become standard sources of drug information, with the Internet emerging as a significant resource for pharmacists, physicians, and patients. These electronic tools, particularly the Internet, allow clinicians to find answers to therapeutic questions in real time,[38,58] an advantage that historically has been considered desirable but difficult to attain.

The Institute of Medicine has stated that access to comprehensive health care information is critical to the delivery of high-quality care.[59] Very few clinicians, however, have ready access to the data needed to make good decisions for their patients. Everyone involved in health care is impatient for technologies that streamline bureaucracy, enhance communications, and improve the effectiveness of medical care.[35] These public benefits, however, have been slow to develop. A principal reason is that medical care is one of the most complex of human undertakings, making computerization of medical tasks and information provision a massive challenge.

Recent advances in computer technology and information management have started to demonstrate the value of this technology as well as areas for progress. However, major impediments to optimal use of information technology, particularly of the Web, remain, because of difficulty in identifying sites that are subject-specific and relevant as well as in determining whether retrieved information is reliable.[38]

Efforts are under way to address many of the concerns described above. Companies such as WebMD (www.webmd.com), Medscape from WebMD (www.medscape.com), Physician Online (now a part of WebMD), MDConsult (www.mdconsult.com), SKOLAR MD (www.skolar.com), and Skyscape (www.skyscape.com) are attempting to assimilate information from the vast array of resources (e.g., medical journals, government reports, FDA alerts, scientific conferences) and provide data to clinicians that are tailored to their specific medical practices.[36]

Drawbacks to Internet-based medical information services may include an inability to supply patient-specific information in a timely way and the lack of disclosure regarding how the data are compiled, reviewed, digested, and reported to the end user (e.g., the clinician). Without such information, an accurate assessment of the quality of such Web sites and the information provided cannot be made.

Many sites provide information on drug- or medication-related topics. The sheer number of Internet results obtained as a result of using the Google™ search engine when searching for both "medication" and "information" (3.02 million) or for both "drug" and "information" (8.1 million) is staggering (Google search November 1, 2004). In addition, a disturbing amount of inaccurate and even potentially life-threatening medical information is readily accessible to anyone with an Internet connection and Web browser.[39,43,60] Overall, information technology aimed at improving patient care has been lacking in scientific evaluation and critique. In addition, there remains a dearth of evidence on how Internet usage can influence health-related decisions and outcomes.[60] Early studies evaluating the quality of health information available on the Internet found that very little of the information was consistent with current standards of practice and that some information would actually be harmful to patients if followed.[38,43,60-63] Information posted on Web sites from traditional medical sources (e.g., major academic institutions) was no more likely to adhere to clinical practice standards than was information on nontraditional sites.[63]

Although much has changed in the years since these studies were published, concerns remain regarding the quality, validity, and reliability of Internet-based medical information sources.[38,39,43,64,65] Adding to these concerns is the absence of a recognized authority for Internet oversight and the absence of a consensus on standards for drug, health, and medical information Web sites.[38,39,43,61] Approximately 70 million Americans were using the Internet for health-related reasons in 2002, a number that undoubtedly continues to increase, and the potential for harm from inaccurate, inferior quality, and inappropriate information is significant. The attendant risks associated with the wide variability in medical information quality are of particular concern in the context of direct patient and consumer access, since these individuals likely will not have the knowledge and judgment to readily determine the trustworthiness of the information.

Internet use is proliferating so rapidly that establishing some means for readily determining the quality and relevance of medical information is critically important.[38,39,43,61] In the absence of uniform guidelines for information publication on the Internet, many clinicians, scientists, and editors have proposed standard evaluation schemes that employ core criteria used to evaluate print literature (**Table 17-3**).[65-67] The appeal of these evaluative tools is that they provide a framework that pharmacists and others may use to assess the content, objectivity, and reliability of each Web site. The reality, however, is that few pharmacists have the time to evaluate each aspect of every Web site they access and still provide timely responses to information queries. In the short-term, it may be advisable for pharmacists to limit Internet information retrieval to a few specific Web sites that they use in their daily practices and have thoroughly evaluated. Additional sites could be added to the Internet "repertoire" as necessary, following evaluation and content validation. However, this practice seems unwieldy in the long-term, with a vastly increasing number of Web sites to evaluate and increasing time constraints.

Table 17-3. Examples of Criteria for Evaluating Medical Information on the Internet[65-67]

Criterion	Description
Authority	• Authors and credentials are clearly identified • Those responsible for developing and maintaining the Web site are listed
Content	• The site considers the depth of material presented versus lists of links or repetitious information • Standards include depth of evidence, strength of recommendations, accuracy, clinical usefulness, quality of references (e.g., published or unpublished data) • Scientific standards are applicable (e.g., peer-review, adherence to clinical practice guidelines and standards)
Objectivity	• Material is free of commercial influence, or advertising is presented separately from informational content
Attribution	• References and ownership/copyright data are clearly identified
Currency	• Material is dated and updated regularly

Accessibility/Ease of Use

- Information is able to be accessed quickly (e.g., time required to download information, ease of navigation)
- Site search capabilities are straightforward and clearly understandable
- The site can be accessed without charge
- Registration requirements are limited and clearly defined

Although there currently is no consensus among information specialists regarding a definitive set of criteria for evaluating Web site quality, many initiatives are under way to promulgate quality standards.[38,39,64] As one of the U.S. Department of Health and Human Services' (HHS) objectives for the Healthy People 2010 goal of using communication strategically to improve health, HHS established the need to increase the proportion of health-related Web sites that disclose information that can be used to assess the quality of the site.[64] HHS recommended that health-related Web sites disclose publicly the following information about their sites:

- the identity of the developers and sponsors of the site (and how to contact them) and information about any potential conflicts of interest or biases;
- the explicit purpose of the site, including any commercial purposes and advertising;
- the original sources of content on the site;
- how the privacy and confidentiality of any personal information collected on the site is protected;
- how the site is evaluated; and
- how the content is updated.[64]

An expert panel convened by HHS describes high-quality health information as accurate, current, valid, appropriate, intelligible, and free of bias.[64] Professional associations (e.g., American Medical Association, American Telemedicine Association, Health Internet Ethics, Health on the Net Foundation, Internet Healthcare Coalition's Health Code of Ethics initiative, MedCIRCLE Collaboration funded by the European Union) are issuing guidelines and recommendations, the Federal Trade Commission is sanctioning false and misleading sites, and developers and purchasers of online health resources are being urged to adopt standards for quality assurance.[38,39,64]

The great expansion of clinical and medical research information and the immense migration of such information to the Web, with its inherent deficiencies, pose a major challenge to health care providers in their attempt to keep up with advances.[38] When this information is used to support medical decisions, public health and safety issues arise.[38] As a result, the NLM has proposed a mechanism by which it would objectively review drug and medical information sites and develop a drug information catalog of Web sites (DRUGINFOFOCI database).[38] Under this proposal, Web sites would need to meet a standard set of quality indicators prior to being cataloged; the quality indicators would be used to identify credible sites and would be consistent with criteria widely used to assess Web site authority and data reliability.[38] NLM's Specialized Information Services Division would evaluate drug information databases that emphasize clinical use according to five selection criteria: authority, content (e.g., currency, reliability, scope, documentation, alerting mechanism), design (display aesthetics, ease of use, navigability), purpose, and support (presence of quality information links, contact information, disclaimer and privacy policy).[38] In part, NLM hopes that this initiative will address the many challenges posed by the Internet—a highly unstructured and unsupervised medium with a vast but disordered method of posting information that may vary widely in quality.[38]

Relationship between Quality of Drug Information and Quality of Patient Care

Gaps exist in current biomedical knowledge of most drugs, thus diminishing the end results of drug therapy.[68] For example, the potential for thalidomide to cause phocomelia, a severe birth defect, when administered to pregnant women was unknown when the drug was initially introduced in 1958,[69] and the link between aspirin use in children and adolescents and Reye's syndrome was not uncovered until many decades after the drug had been available.[70] Understanding the relationships between administration of these drugs and subsequent appearance of these ADEs was a key aspect of expanding the knowledge base about these two drugs, and filling these knowledge gaps contributed substantially to the elimination of new cases of both phocomelia and Reye's syndrome. In addition to gaps in understanding the potentially dangerous or toxic effects of drugs, gaps exist in our understanding of the beneficial effects of medications. An example of this type of gap is the lack of knowledge about the benefits of thalidomide in treating aphthous ulcers in patients infected with HIV,[71] a use for the drug that was not known when the drug was first introduced.

Occasionally, gaps can be identified prospectively, allowing clinicians to address them proactively rather than waiting for a problem to occur.[68] For example, HIV is known to become resistant to antiretroviral agents, but clinicians have not yet developed a satisfactory combination of agents to completely prevent or overcome this known resistance problem. Identifying knowledge gaps such as this provides specific opportunities for gathering information in an effort to improve medication use.

QUALITY OF INTERPRETATION AND CASE REPORTS

Among the many challenges of increasing the quality of drug information is improving the way in which that information is interpreted, particularly given the fact that pharmacists are not always the ones doing the interpreting.

An example of this is a case in which a newborn infant died after having inadvertently received a 10-fold overdose of penicillin G benzathine via the intravenous (i.v.) route as treatment for possible congenital syphilis.[72] An investigation into this case revealed a wide range of system errors, including many relating to misinterpretation of published drug information by a neonatal nurse practitioner (NNP) as well as by the dispensing pharmacist. Part of the error stemmed from the fact that this drug was not on the formulary and therefore not commonly dispensed. Other contributors were incomplete information in several referenced drug information sources (e.g., not specifying the salt [the benzathine] and not specifically precautioning against i.v. use of this salt). Even after consulting two drug information sources, the pharmacist misread the dose as 500,000 units/kg, instead of 50,000 units/kg. This led to the pharmacist misreading the actual drug order as 1,500,000 units instead of 150,000 units; the 10-fold overdose would have required 5 separate injections, which should have prompted the pharmacist to suspect a possible error, but did not. Misinterpretations of drug information also occurred several times when a NNP tried to verify the appropriate treatment for syphilis as penicillin G benzathine.[72] In particular, one drug information source consulted by the NNP (*1994 AAP Red Book®*) did not specifically warn that penicillin G benzathine should be administered *only* intramuscular (i.m.); another publication (*Neofax® 95*) neither specifically mentioned the benzathine salt in the penicillin G monograph nor warned about the importance of route of administration for the various forms of the drug. (Since these errors, the publishers of these resources have made numerous corrections to the text.[72]) To avoid the pain of multiple i.m. injections in a neonate, the NNP changed the administration route to i.v., ultimately resulting in the infant's death. This case confirms the importance of appropriate drug knowledge dissemination as a means of avoiding ADEs.

Another concern with regard to drug information interpretation is the way in which drugs are ordered or prescribed. In an effort to improve patient safety and quality of drug information, the Joint Commission on Accreditation of Healthcare Organizations (JCAHO) has developed a "minimum list" of dangerous abbreviations, acronyms, and symbols that should not be used for handwritten, patient-specific communications (see **Table 17-4**).[73] Although medical publishers and printed or electronic information are not subject to these JCAHO standards and the likelihood of misinterpreting the typeset versions of these abbreviations is small, at least one resource (*AHFS DI*) has voluntarily elected to eliminate the offending abbreviations from its publication in order to reinforce the standards for good handwritten clinical documentation, with the ultimate goal of decreasing medication errors.[56]

Table 17-4. JCAHO List of Dangerous Abbreviations, Acronyms, and Symbols[73]

Abbreviation	Potential Problem	Preferred Term
U (for unit)	Mistaken for zero, four or cc.	Write "unit."
IU (for international unit)	Mistaken as i.v. (intravenous) or 10 (ten).	Write "international unit."
Q.D., Q.O.D. (Latin abbreviations for once daily and every other day)	Mistaken for each other. The period after the Q can be mistaken for an "I" and the "O" can be mistaken for "I."	Write "daily" and "every other day."
Trailing zero (X.0 mg), lack of leading zero (.X mg)	Decimal point is missed.	Never write a zero by itself after a decimal point (X mg), and always use a zero before a decimal point (0.X mg).
MS, MSO$_4$, MgSO$_4$	Confused for one another; can mean morphine sulfate or magnesium sulfate.	Write "morphine sulfate" or "magnesium sulfate."
μg (for microgram)	Mistaken for mg (milligrams), resulting in 1,000-fold overdose.	Write "mcg."
H.S. (for half-strength or Latin abbreviation for bedtime)	Mistaken for either half-strength or hour of sleep (at bedtime). Q.H.S. mistaken for every hour. All can result in a dosing error.	Write out "half-strength" or "at bedtime."
T.I.W. (for three times a week)	Mistaken for three times a day or twice weekly, resulting in an overdose.	Write "3 times weekly" or "three times weekly."
S.C. or S.Q. (for subcutaneous)	Mistaken as SL for sublingual or "5 every."	Write "Sub-Q," "subQ," or "subcutaneously."
D/C (for discharge)	Interpreted as discontinue whatever medications follow (typically discharge meds).	Write "discharge."
c.c. (for cubic centimeter)	Mistaken for U (units) when poorly written.	Write "mL" for milliliters.
A.S., A.D., A.U. (Latin	Mistaken for OS, OD, and OU, etc.	Write "left ear," "right ear,"

abbreviations for left, right,   or "both ears."
or both ears)

Using outdated information can also contribute to ADEs, since drug information is constantly evolving. One such example was the i.v. administration of large volumes of hypotonic albumin human solutions on the basis of dilution information contained in out-of-print editions of a drug information resource (*Handbook on Injectable Drugs®*). In the edition that was current at the time of the ADEs, specific warnings about the risk of hypotonicity (e.g., hemolysis) had been added to the albumin monograph in the *Handbook*.[74,75] Also contributing to these ADEs was a lack of appropriate drug knowledge dissemination to the pharmacists involved about the risks of administering large volumes of highly hypotonic solutions i.v. under any condition.[75] The basis of the information on diluting albumin human originated with even older drug information published by FDA in the *Federal Register* as part of the final rule on albumin.[74,75] Because the FDA had never retracted this original information,[74,75] the agency took a number of steps to warn practitioners about the risks of hypotonic albumin human solutions subsequent to the case reports of ADEs.[74]

As noted earlier, information in FDA-approved labeling may not be current. While the focus of this discussion has been dosing information and the therapeutic perspective, the failure of FDA to ensure timely revision of all associated drug labeling for cautionary information can also contribute to the risk of ADEs. For example, in a July 2003 analysis of information provided for patients and for professionals on nitroglycerin, a contraindication about combined sildenafil (Viagra®) and nitroglycerin use was not included in most of the patient information provided by nitroglycerin manufacturers five years after FDA approval of the Viagra® contraindication. An examination of the professional labeling for 10 nitroglycerin products revealed that only two included the contraindication while three included a warning rather than the stronger contraindication. In other words, half of the FDA-approved professional labeling for nitroglycerin included no mention of risk with sildenafil.[76]

Earlier discussion in this chapter described concerns about the widely variable quality and reliability of drug and medical information accessible via the Internet, with the possibility that some such information may be dangerous. In one case report in which the parents of a dehydrated child with diarrhea followed the advice of a pediatric Web site, the child's course was complicated by misinformation provided on this site. The advice did not reflect evidence-based clinical practice guidelines, resulting in a prolonged course of recovery for the child.[60] In this case, it clearly was not misinterpretation of the information obtained by the parents but the provision of information that did not conform to established standards of care.[60]

Future of Drug Development

In the future, drugs and drug regimens are likely to become more complex and more toxic, particularly when certain drugs are used in combination. For example, even in the current environment, the management of HIV infection is extremely complex.[66] Patients who receive highly active antiretroviral therapy generally take three or more such agents. Given that there currently are five different drug classes of antiretroviral agents, with more likely to follow, the combination possibilities are seemingly endless. Moreover, agents in some of these drug classes (e.g., protease inhibitors, nonnucleoside reverse transcriptase inhibitors) may interact with each other, as well as with other drugs, herbal agents, and recreational drugs. Adding to this complexity is the frequency of drug administration that may be necessary to maintain or enhance virologic suppression. Staying current with the possible HIV drug interactions is difficult, in part because data are often presented at scientific meetings in abstract or poster form, with a significant lag time until peer-review publication. Despite this drawback, these data are of immediate clinical relevance to pharmacists and physicians treating these patients, and the information needs to be accessible in a timely manner. The Internet currently serves as a key medium for disseminating HIV drug interaction data,[66] and its use is likely to increase. Therefore, it is imperative that pharmacists be able to judge the validity, objectivity, and authority of the content and content provider for these sites.

Another change that is occurring is a shift in responsibility for certain risks associated with specific drugs from the prescriber or pharmacist to the patient. For example, with the increasing use of thalidomide for aphthous ulcers in patients with HIV infection, women who are infected with HIV and experience aphthous ulcers face a dilemma. If they take thalidomide and become pregnant, their fetus has a greatly increased risk of phocomelia. Assuming the clinician prescribing the medication provided appropriate information about this risk, it may then become the woman's responsibility to take appropriate contraceptive precautions to avoid becoming pregnant in order to avoid this risk.

Another way to limit ADEs that result from errors in interpreting medical or drug information is the increasing practice of restricting distribution of certain drug to those prescribers who have been credentialed or authorized to prescribe them. A form of credentialing could be specific training (e.g., limited to certain board-certified specialists) or continuing medical education with appropriate knowledge assessment that must be completed on a regular basis.

Summary

A landmark study conducted by Leape and colleagues identified lack of drug knowledge as the most common proximal cause of ADEs.[3] Since that publication, and as pharmacists have increased their involvement in pharmaceutical care, provision of correct (and correctly interpreted) drug information has taken a more prominent role in advancing the safety of medication use, not only in the hospital setting but in all settings where pharmacists are integral to patient care.

A wide array of drug information resources is available, both in print and electronically, some applying the traditional quality control mechanisms typically associated with highly regarded and trusted peer-reviewed medical literature with others applying little if any such controls. The safe use of medication information requires that pharmacists and other health care providers critically evaluate drug information sources not only in terms of content but also in terms of their editorial processes and potential influence from pharmaceutical manufacturers and others. Unfortunately, determining the standards and editorial policies applied is not always obvious or easy.

In the current environment of overwhelming information and limited time for evaluation, the Internet has become a real-time source for drug information, albeit without many (or any) of the editorial processes that are the foundation for reliable information sources to which health care providers have historically turned. Without these processes, pharmacists should view information from Internet resources, and any other resource lacking these characteristics, with healthy skepticism. Regardless of the tools available, it remains the pharmacist's responsibility to provide reliable, up-to-date, authoritative, objective information to other health care providers and to patients.

References

1. Bates DW, Cullen DJ, Laird N, et al. Incidence of adverse drug events and potential adverse drug events. Implications for prevention. ADE Prevention Study Group. *JAMA.* 1995;274:29-34.

2. Bates DW, Leape LL, Cullen DJ, et al. Effect of computerized physician order entry and a team intervention on prevention of serious medication errors. *JAMA.* 1998; 280:1311-1316.

3. Leape LL, Bates DW, Cullen DJ, et al. Systems analysis of adverse drug events. *JAMA.* 1995:274:35-43.

4. Lesar TS, Briceland L, Stein DS. Factors related to errors in medication prescribing. *JAMA.* 1997;277:312-317.

5. Phillips J, Beam S, Brinker A, et al. Retrospective analysis of mortalities associated with medication errors. *Am J Health-Syst Pharm.* 2001;58:1824-1829.

6. Brennan TA, Leape LL, Laird NM, et al. Incidence of adverse events and negligence in hospitalized patients: results of the Harvard Medical Practice Study I. *N Engl J Med.* 1991;324:370-376.

7. Gandhi TK, Weingart SN, Borus J, et al. Adverse drug events in ambulatory care. *N Engl J Med.* 2003;348:1556-1564.

8. van den Bemt PM, Egberts TC, de Jong-van den Berg LT, et al. Drug-related problems in hospitalized patients. *Drug Saf.* 2000;22:321-333.

9. Lazarou J, Pomeranz BH, Corey PN. Incidence of adverse drug reactions in hospitalized patients: A meta-analysis of prospective studies. *JAMA.* 1998;279:1200-1205.

10. American Society of Health-System Pharmacists. ASHP guidelines on the provision of medication information by pharmacists. *Am J Health-Syst Pharm.* 1996;53:1843-1845.

11. Angell M. *The Truth about Drug Companies: How They Deceive Us and What to do about It.* New York: Random House; 2004.

12. Blum RS. Legal considerations of off-label medication prescribing (letter). *Arch Intern Med.* 2002;162:1777-1779.

13. Food and Drug Administration. Use of approved drugs for unlabeled indications. *FDA Drug Bull.* 1982;12:4-5.

14. Oddis JA. The PDR is Food and Drug Administration-approved labeling (letter). *Arch Intern Med.* 1997;157:576-577.

15. Cohen JS, Insel PA. The PDR is Food and Drug Administration-approved labeling (reply to letter). *Arch Intern Med.* 1997;157:577.

16. Cohen JS. Pharmaceutical manufacturer sponsorship and drug information (reply to letter). *Arch Intern Med.* 2001;161:2626.

17. Hooper PL. The American Hospital Formulary Service information books beat the PDR (letter). *Arch Intern Med.* 1997;57:575-576.

18. Cohen JS. Adverse drugs effects, compliance, and initial doses of antihypertensive drugs recommended by the Joint National Committee vs. the Physicians' Desk Reference. *Arch Intern Med.* 2001;161:880-885.

19. Cohen JS. Dose discrepancies between the Physicians' Desk Reference and the medical literature, and their possible role in the high incidence of dose-related adverse drug events. *Arch Intern Med.* 2001;161:957-964.

20. Cohen JS, Insel PA. The Physicians' Desk Reference: problems and possible improvements. *Arch Intern Med.* 1996;156:1375-1380.

21. Rajpal A, Reidenberg MM. Drug labeling should be kept current. *Clin Pharmacol Ther.* 2003;73:4-6.

22. Topol EJ. Failing the public health—rofecoxib, Merck, and the FDA (editorial). *N Engl J Med.* 2004;351:1707-1709.

23. Amgen Inc. Epogen® (epoetin alfa) for injection prescribing information. Thousand Oaks, Calif. May 7, 2003.

24. Amgen Inc. Epogen® (epoetin alfa) for injection prescribing information. Thousand Oaks, Calif. June 30, 2004.

25. Keegan P. Approval supplement letter to Amgen Incorporated for epoetin alfa (STN: BL 103234/5053). Rockville, MD: US Food and Drug Administration; June 30, 2004.

26. Rizzo JD, Lichtin AE, Woolf SH, et al. Use of epoetin in patients with cancer: evidence-based clinical practice guidelines of the American Society of Clinical Oncology and the American Society of Hematology. *J Clin Oncol.* 2002;20:4083-4107.

27. Armstrong D. How drug directory helps raise tab for Medicaid and insurers. *Wall Street Journal.* October 23, 2001:A1.

28. Avorn J. *Powerful Medicines: The Benefits, Risks, and Costs of Prescription Drugs.* New York: Knopf; 2004.

29. Food and Drug Administration. Citizen petition regarding the Food and Drug Administration's policy on promotion of unapproved uses of approved drugs and de-

vices; request for comment. Notice; request for comments. [Docket No. 92N-0434] *Fed Regist.* 1994; 59:59820-598226.

30. Wesseley S, Kerwin R. Suicide risk and the SSRIs. *JAMA.* 2004;292:379-381.

31. Hirsh J, Dalen JE, Guyatt G, for the American College of Chest Physicians (ACCP). The sixth (2000) ACCP guidelines for antithrombotic therapy for prevention and treatment of thrombosis. *Chest.* 2001;119 (Suppl 1):1-370S.

32. Burwen DR, Galusha DH, Lewis JM, et al, for the US Centers for Medicare & Medicaid Services. National and state trends in quality of care for acute myocardial infarction between 1994-1995 and 1998-1999: The Medicare Health Care Quality Improvement Program. 2003;163:1430-1439.

33. Cochrane Collaboration. Available at http://www.cochrane.org. Accessed November 1, 2004. Oxford, United Kingdom.

34. American Society of Hospital Pharmacists. ASHP statement on the use of medications for unlabeled uses. *Am J Hosp Pharm.* 1992;49:2006-2008.

35. Gawande AA, Bates DW. The use of information technology in improving medical performance—part I. Information systems for medical transactions. *Med Gen Med.* 2000;2:E14.

36. Gawande AA, Bates DW. The use of information technology in improving medical performance—part II. Physician-support tools. *Med Gen Med.* 2000;2:E13.

37. Knoben JE, Phillips SJ, Szczur MR. The National Library of Medicine and drug information. Part 1: Present resources. *Drug Inf J.* 2004;38:69-81.

38. Knoben JE, Phillips SJ, Szczur MR. The National Library of Medicine and drug information. Part 2: An evolving future. *Drug Inf J.* 2004;38:171-180.

39. Risk A, Dzenowagis J. Review of Internet health information quality initiatives. *J Med Internet Res.* 2001;3(4):e28. Available at http://www.jmir.org/2001/4/e28/. Accessed November 1, 2004.

40. Food and Drug Administration. Index of safety-related drug labeling change summaries approved by FDA; January–December 2003. MedWatch. Available at www.fda.gov/medwatch/SAFETY/2003/jan2003_quickview.htm. Accessed June 23, 2004.

41. National Library of Medicine. MEDLINE®

42. Fact Sheet. Bethesda, MD: National Institutes of Health; September 18, 2002. Available at www.nlm.nih.gov/pubs/factsheets/medline.html. Accessed June 23, 2004.

42. National Library of Medicine. Fact Sheet. Bethesda, MD: National Institutes of Health; March 2, 2004. Available at www.nlm.nih.gov/pubs/factsheets/nlm.html. Accessed June 23, 2004.

43. Risk A, Petersen C. Health information on the Internet: Quality issues and international initiatives (editorial). *JAMA.* 2002;287:2713-2715.

44. American Society of Health-System Pharmacists. ASHP guidelines: minimum standard for pharmacies in hospitals. *Am J Health-Syst Pharm.* 1995;52:2711-2717.

45. Balanced Budget Act of 1997. PL 105-33.

46. Health Care Financing Administration. Medicare program; catastrophic outpatient drug benefit. 21 CFR Part 410. Proposed rule. [BPD-613-P; RIN 0938-AD91] *Fed Regist.* 1989;54:37190-37208.

47. Health Care Financing Administration. Medicaid program; drug use review program and electronic claims management system for outpatient drug claims. 42 CFR Part 456. Interim final rule with comment period. [MB-050-IFC; RIN 0938-AF67] *Fed Regist.* 1992;57:49397-49412

48. Health Care Financing Administration. Medicaid program; drug use review program and electronic claims management system for outpatient drug claims. 42 CFR Part 456. Final Rule. [MB-050-IFC; RIN 0938-AF67] *Fed Regist.* 1994;59:48811-48925.

49. Food and Drug Administration. Dissemination of information on unapproved/new uses for marketed drugs, biologics, and devices. 21 CRF Parts 16 and 99. Proposed rule. [Docket No. 98N-0222] *Fed Regist.* 1998; 63:31143-31161.

50. HCFA Section 9401 of the State Medicaid Manual.

51. Omnibus Budget Reconciliation Act of 1990. PL 101-508.

52. Omnibus Budget Reconciliation Act of 1993. PL 103-66.

53. United States Pharmacopeial Convention, Inc. Drug Information. Frequently asked questions: *USP DI* and Thompson Healthcare, Inc. Available at /www.usp.org/druginformation. Accessed November 1, 2004.

54. Williams RL. Memo from the USP chair and

executive vice president and CEO to the USP Council of Experts and Expert Committee members regarding drug information at USP. Rockville, MD: USP; May 24, 2004.

55. Pfizer Inc. Neurontin® (gabapentin) prescribing information. New York, NY; May 2004.

56. McEvoy GK, ed. *AHFS Drug Information 2003*. Bethesda, MD: American Society of Health-System Pharmacists; 2003.

57. *USP DI. Volume I: Drug information for the health care professional*. Greenwood Village, CA: Thomson MICROMEDEX; 2003.

58. Murray MD. Information technology: the infrastructure for improvements to the medication-use process. *Am J Health-Syst Pharm*. 2000;57:565-571.

59. Kohn LT, Corrigan JM, Donaldson MS, eds. *To Err Is Human: Building a Safer Health System*. Washington, D.C.: National Academy Press; 1999.

60. Crocco AG, Villasis-Keever M, Jadad AR. Two wrongs don't make a right: harm aggravated by inaccurate information on the Internet. *Pediatrics*. 2002;109:522-523.

61. Eysenbach G, Powell J, Kuss O, et al. Empirical studies assessing the quality of health information for consumers on the World Wide Web: A systematic review. *JAMA*. 2002;287:2691-2700.

62. Impicciatore P, Pandolfini C, Casella N, et al. Reliability of health information for the public on the world wide web: systematic survey of advice on managing fever in children at home. *Br Med J*. 1997;314:1875-1879.

63. McClung HJ, Murray RD, Heitlinger LA. The Internet as a source for current patient information. *Pediatrics*. 1998;101(6). Available at: www.pediatrics.org/cgi/content/full/101/6/e2. Accessed June 23, 2003.

64. U.S. Department of Health and Human Services. *Healthy People 2010*. 2nd ed. With understanding and improving health objectives for improving health. Volume I. Washington, DC: U.S. Government Printing Office, November 2000.

65. Purcell GP, Wilson P, Delamothe T. The quality of health information on the internet (editorial). *Br Med J*. 2002;324:557-558.

66. Sheehan NL, Kelly DV, Tseng AL, et al. Evaluation of HIV drug interaction web sites. *Ann Pharmacother*. 2003;37:1577-1586.

67. Wainright BD. Clinically relevant dermatology resources and the Internet: An introductory guide for practicing physicians. 1999;5(2):8. Available at http://www.dermatology.cdlib.org/DOJvol5num2/special/wainright.html. Accessed June 17, 2004.

68. Hennessy S. Potentially remediable features of the medication-use environment in the United States. *Am J Health-Syst Pharm*. 2000;57:543-548.

69. Dally A. Thalidomide: was the tragedy preventable? *Lancet*. 1998;351:1197-1198.

70. Hurwitz ES. Reye's syndrome. *Epidemiol Rev*. 1989;11:249-253.

71. Jacobson JM, Spritzler J, Fox L, et al. Thalidomide for the treatment of esophageal aphthous ulcers in patients with human immunodeficiency virus infection. *J Infect Dis*. 1999;180:61-67.

72. Smetzer JL, Cohen MR. Lesson from the Denver medication error/criminal negligence case: look beyond blaming individuals. *Hosp Pharm*. 1998;33:640-657.

73. Joint Commission on Accreditation of Healthcare Organizations. 2004 National Patient Safety Goals—FAQs. Available at: www.jcaho.org/accredited+organizations/patient+safety/04+npsg/04_faqs.htm. Accessed June 24, 2004.

74. Pierce LR, Gaines A, Varricchio F, et al. Hemolysis and renal failure associated with use of sterile water for injection to dilute 25% human albumin solution (letter). *Am J Health-Syst Pharm*. 1998;55:1057,1062,1070.

75. Trissel LA. Hemolysis and renal failure associated with use of sterile water for injection to dilute 25% human albumin solution (letter). *Am J Health-Syst Pharm*. 1998;55:1070.

76. American Society of Health-System Pharmacists. Comments at FDA's public meeting on the current status of prescription drug information for consumers. Washington, D.C. July 31, 2003.

77. Legislative history for compendial designation for Drugdex: 104th Congress Balanced Budget Act of 1995 (vetoed by President); 105th Congress H.R. 3507 Personal Responsibility and Work Opportunity Act of 1996 (not passed).

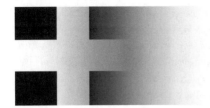

Patient Safety in Clinical Trials

William R. Hendee

Introduction

Clinical trials are conducted to evaluate the safety and effectiveness of new drugs, medical devices, and procedures in human volunteers, including patients. These trials are essential in determining the usefulness of new technologies in health care. But such trials must be carefully designed and deployed so that they yield viable results, do not expose volunteers to unnecessary risk, and satisfy the principles of respect for persons, beneficence, and justice.

In the United States today, approval and oversight of clinical trials is the responsibility of institutional review boards (IRBs), which function autonomously without influence from researchers or administrative officials. This chapter providers a brief history of experimentation with research volunteers, reviews the ethnical principles of research with humans, and describes the role of IRBs in ensuring the safety of participants in clinical trials.

Patient Safety before the Nuremberg Code

For many centuries, medicine in the Western world was largely the product of observational evidence, practitioner experience, and common beliefs and traditions. According to Hippocrates (460–377 BCE), whose teachings guided medicine during this era, health was the product of a balance among the body's four humors (blood, phlegm, yellow bile, and black bile). Disease occurred when these humors became unbalanced. Medical treatments, such as bloodletting, dieting, bathing, and medicating with herbal remedies, were intended to bring the humors back into balance. In these efforts, the welfare of the patient was paramount. The Hippocratic principles of medicine stressed the importance of patient benefit and the avoidance of patient risk, which is encapsulated in the phrase, "First, do no harm."

In the sixteenth century, Western medicine began its evolution from traditional practice toward a scientific process that included experimentation with animals and humans. Examples of the better-known anecdotes of scientific experimentation with humans include the following:

- the discovery that inoculation of fluid from a cowpox pustule provided immunity from the smallpox virus—an experiment performed in 1796 by the English physician Edward Jenner on an 8-year-old boy;

- Louis Pasteur's injection of a suspension of minced spinal cord taken from a rabid rabbit to treat a boy who had been bitten by a rabid dog;

- recruitment of human volunteers by U.S. Army physician Walter Reed for purposeful exposure to mosquitoes to demonstrate that the insects were responsible for yellow fever; and

- introduction of the leprosy bacillus into the eye of a 33-year-old uninfected and unknowing woman by Amauer Hansen, who discovered the bacillus.

From the perspective of today's standards of ethical experimentation with humans, each of these anecdotes raises concern. The events just described, however, pale by comparison with experiments on humans conducted in Germany and German-occupied countries by the National Socialists (Nazis) during World War II. The Nazi experiments were organized by government officials and conducted on Jews, homosexuals, criminals, gypsies, political dissidents, and captured soldiers, among others. Many of the experiments were poorly designed and executed, and often the results were shoddily recorded, if recorded at all. Examples of Nazi experiments are

- hypothermia experiments where naked subjects were immersed in ice water for hours, or penned outside and sprayed with cold water in subfreezing weather;

- decompression experiments in which individuals were subjected to low pressure and lack of oxygen duplicating conditions at altitudes up to 65,000 feet above sea level;

- wound-healing experiments in which subjects were shot, stabbed, burned, or experienced amputations, after which the wounds were infected and then treated with various remedies;

- experiments in which individuals were exposed to chemical- and biological-warfare agents in order to identify effective remedies;

- exposures to high levels of electricity, ionizing radiation, and other stresses in order to test human endurance;

- studies on twins (e.g., exchanging blood between identical twins, forcing fraternal twins to copulate in order to produce children, creating conjoined twins by sewing them together); and

- studies that entailed isolating children from their families in order to distinguish the roles of nature and nurture in human development.[1]

The irony of the Nazi experiments is that Prussia, one of the states in Nazi Germany, had been a leader in ethical experimentation with humans. At the end of the nineteenth century, Prussia passed national statutes to protect the rights of citizens in experimental medical treatments. Of course, the victims of Nazi experiments were seldom Prussian citizens; those killed were, in fact, regarded as inferior life-forms according to Nazi theories of eugenics.

At the end of World War II, an international military tribunal was held in Nuremberg, Germany. After trying Nazi officers, the tribunal conducted the "Nazi doctors" trial in which 15 of 23 defendants were found guilty of human experimentation that constituted atrocities against humanity. The trial produced a set of standards against which the defendants were judged and their guilt determined. These standards, now known as the Nuremberg Code,[2] state that

- Participation in medical experimentation must be entirely voluntary, and informed consent of volunteers must be obtained without coercion in any form.

- Volunteers must be free to withdraw from a study at any time without penalty.

- Experiments with humans should be preceded by experiments on animals.

- Expected results should justify experiments on humans and should be unobtainable by other means.

- Human experimentation should be conducted only by qualified scientists.

- Physical and mental injury and suffering should be avoided whenever possible.

- Death or disabling injury should not be anticipated.

- A study must be terminated immediately if its continuation is likely to cause injury, disability, or death.

The Nuremberg Code represents the beginning of the modern era of protection of human participants in biomedical research.

PATIENT SAFETY SINCE THE NUREMBERG CODE

The Nuremberg Code established an ethical foundation for medical research with human participants. Nevertheless, many examples of abuses of the code have occurred in the past half-century. Examples include the following:

- the Tuskegee, Alabama, syphilis study (1932–1972) in which African-American men with syphilis were followed without treatment with penicillin in an effort to characterize the etiology of the late stages of the syphilis[3];

- the Willowbrook, New York, hepatitis experiments (1956–1980) in which mentally retarded children were infected with viral hepatitis to follow the natural progression of hepatitis and the effectiveness of gamma globulin in preventing and treating it[4];

- the Jewish chronic disease study, conducted in Brooklyn, New York, in 1964, in which live cancer cells were injected into unsuspecting patients in order to study the immune response to cancer[5];

- human radiation experiments between 1944 and 1974 in which U.S. government funds were used to study the effects of exposure to ionizing radiation in thousands of individuals[6]; and

- studies of perinatal transmission of the human immunodeficiency virus in developing countries in the 1990s, in which some subjects were given no medication to inhibit transmission and others were given a dosages of zidovudine that were known to be ineffective.[7]

In 1953, the World Medical Association initiated a debate on the ethical principles of human experimentation. The product of this debate was the Declaration of Helsinki,[8] first issued in 1964. The declaration, which has been revised and reissued many times since its initial publication, expanded the Nuremberg Code to permit enrollment of patients in therapeutic research protocols without their consent under certain specific circumstances. It also allowed legal guardians (i.e., legally appointed representatives) to grant consent for research participation in place of consent by individuals themselves.

In 1974, the U.S. Congress passed the National Research Act, which created the National Commission for the Protection of Human Subjects in Biomedical and Behavioral Research. In 1979, the commission released a report entitled Ethical Principles and Guidelines for the Protection of Human Subjects of Research.[9] This report, commonly referred to as the Belmont report, serves today as the foundation for protection of human research participants in the United States. The Belmont report emphasizes three fundamental principles that serve as the cornerstone of experimentation with human subjects (see Table 18-1).

Table 18-1. Ethical Principles of the Belmont Report[9]

Principle	Application of Principle
Respect for Persons	Reflected in the informed consent process, which includes conditions for ensuring privacy of personal information as well as informed and voluntary participation in research.
Beneficence	Reflected in the assessment of benefits and risks of a study, according to rules of human experimentation, to (1) do no harm, (2) maximize benefits, and (3) minimize risks to participants.
Justice	Reflected in the selection of research participants so that benefits and risks are fairly distributed across a population, and that certain individuals or groups are not denied participation without scientific or legal justification.

Ethical Principles of Human Experimentation

The three principles of the Belmont report provide several guidelines for human experimentation. These guidelines have been compiled from several sources by Shamoo and Resnik[1] and are repeated here as guidance for institutions and individuals conducting or overseeing research with human participants.

- Informed consent. When individuals are capable of making decisions about participation in research protocols that involve a degree of complexity or risk, researchers should obtain informed consent. When individuals lack the capacity to make such decisions, researchers should obtain informed consent from the study participant's legally authorized representative. Subjects should be able to withdraw without penalty from a study at any time and for any reason.

- Respect for persons. Researchers should respect the privacy, dignity, and rights of research volunteers, and they should take steps to protect the confidentiality of personal information.

- Beneficence. Researchers should make every attempt to minimize the harms and risks of research participation, maximize benefits to participants, and strive for a justifiable risk:benefit ratio. Researchers should not conduct experiments that have a high probability of causing death or significant harm, nor should they harm participants in order to benefit society. Researchers should be prepared to end experiments in order to protect participants from harm.

- Social value. Researchers should conduct experiments that have scientific, medical, or social worth; they should not use human beings in frivolous research.

- Justice. Researchers should promote a fair and equitable distribution of benefits and harms in research. Participants should not be excluded from participation in research without a sound moral, legal, or scientific justification.

- Protection for vulnerable subjects. Researchers should take extra precautions when dealing with vulnerable participants (see below) in order to avoid harm or exploitation.

- Scientific validity. Research protocols should be scientifically well designed; experiments should yield results that are replicable and statistically significant. Researchers should strive to eliminate biases and disclose or avoid conflicts of interest. Research personnel should have the appropriate scientific and medical qualifications.

- Resources. Research institutions should have the appropriate resources, procedures, and safeguards to protect volunteers participating in research protocols.

- Data monitoring. Researchers should monitor data to promote the welfare of participants and ensure scientific validity, and should immediately report harms and unanticipated problems in implementing the research protocol.

Over the past few years, several cases of human experimentation have been reported in which one or more of these guidelines have been compromised. These cases include

- a suicide by a participant in a research study of schizophrenia in California in 1994 that raised questions about the adequacy of the informed consent process;

- the 1994 death of a healthy 19-year-old student at the University of Rochester while undergoing bronchoscopy as part of a study in which more samples were taken, and more anesthesia was used, than called for in the approved protocol;

- the 1999 death of 19-year-old Jesse Gelsinger during a gene-transfer trial at the University of Pennsylvania, in which the possibility of serious adverse events was inadequately explained both to the patient and to the Food and Drug Administration

(FDA) and in which the principal investigator had a financial interest in the company sponsoring the research;

- facelift experiments in the early 1990s at a New York City hospital in which surgeons performed two different procedures, one on each side of the patient's face, in order to compare results; and

- eye-surgery experiments on 60 patients at the University of South Florida in which IRB approval and patient consent were not sought and in which both the university and the investigator had a financial stake in the device used in the experiments.

These cases and several others have received substantial press coverage over the past decade. This coverage has stimulated enhanced surveillance by institutions and government agencies over research involving human participants. Without question, this enhanced surveillance is important and justifiable; however, it has greatly increased the workload and cost of overseeing clinical research in institutions and organizations. This added burden has been absorbed as institutions and organizations struggle to apply the ethical guidelines described above in order to help ensure that further ethical breaches do not occur in research with human participants.

Operational Challenges of Ethical Principles in Human Experimentation

The guidelines for human experimentation just described raise several challenges and conflicts in their deployment within institutions and organizations conducting and sponsoring research involving human participants. Four of the most important challenges are discussed in the paragraphs that follow.

THE WELFARE OF THE INDIVIDUAL VERSUS THE GOOD OF SOCIETY

This classic conflict often arises in human experimentation. The intrinsic value of each and every person is fundamental to the principle of respect for autonomy and privacy in research with human participants. It is also important, however, to promote the welfare of society at large (i.e., the public good).

At times, these two goals are in conflict. For example, suppose that a promising drug for Alzheimer's disease is being studied in a clinical trial by randomly separating participants into two groups. Participants in one group receive the drug and the traditional treatment for the disease, and those in the other group receive a placebo plus the traditional treatment. Partway through the trial, the patients receiving the drug are faring noticeably better than those in the placebo group. This phenomenon raises the question of whether the trial should be stopped and all patients should be given the drug and, if so, when this action should be taken. Stopping the trial prematurely will compromise the statistical quality of the trial results and possibly affect the drug's chances for approval; however, continuing the trial will deprive some participants of the drug's benefits.

In some situations, the mere act of informing patients of their participation could compromise study results. This conflict frequently arises in behavioral studies in which knowledge of the study might cause participants to alter their conduct. In this case, the investigator would probably wish to conduct the study without the participants' knowledge, provided that the study did not expose them to substantial risk.

There are different viewpoints on the relative weights that should be assigned to the welfare of the individual and to the good of society.[11] Some persons argue that the individual's dignity and welfare should never be compromised, because to do so puts society on a slippery slope—a situation in which individual rights can be increasingly compromised. Others argue that although human rights are very important, they must sometimes give way in order to advance research conducted in the interests of society as a whole.

ASSESSMENT OF RISKS AND BENEFITS

For an individual, the overall risk of participation in a research study is a product of two factors: the magnitude of the risk and the severity of the risk. A study may have a relatively high probability of an adverse consequence, but that consequence may be relatively minor (e.g., temporary short-term memory loss, dizziness, or feeling flushed). A study that produced consequences such as these might be considered to be minimum or low risk. Minimum risk is defined in the Common Rule, a guideline to which many federal agencies subscribe. The rule defines minimum risk as "the probability and magnitude of harm or discomfort anticipated in the research are not greater in and of themselves than those ordinarily encountered in daily life or during the performance of routine physical or psychological examinations or tests."[12]

Minimum-risk studies sometimes are exempt from institutional review or can be reviewed in an expedited fashion.

Severity of risk is the second part of the equation. A study may have a relatively low probability of an adverse consequence, but the consequence, when it does occur, may be severe (e.g., death or permanent disability). The risk may be considered moderate or high even though the probability of occurrence is low. In such a case, the potential benefit of the study must be substantial in order to outweigh the moderate or high risk. Further, the study protocol must be thoroughly reviewed and approved, and an ongoing monitoring process must be established to ensure that the benefit-and-risk estimates of the study do not change as data are accumulated during the study itself. If these estimates shift, the protocol should be reviewed again to determine whether the study should continue.

VULNERABLE POPULATIONS

A *vulnerable* research subject is one that cannot give adequate informed consent or defend his or her own interests and welfare. Vulnerable populations include children, prisoners, students, employees, seriously or terminally ill patients, people who are mentally ill or disabled, and poor and illiterate people. Pregnant women are also a vulnerable population, in the sense that the fetus is unable to give informed consent. These populations of individuals must be protected from recruitment practices that violate their rights and freedoms. In many cases, a legally authorized representative (e.g., a court-appointed guardian) must consent before an individual belonging to a vulnerable population may participate in a research study.

THE GRAY AREA BETWEEN CLINICAL RESEARCH AND MEDICAL PRACTICE

Clinical research is a component of medical and health research that produces knowledge essential for understanding human disease, preventing and treating illness, and promoting health. In this definition, the goal of research is the production and dissemination of new knowledge, not the treatment of an individual patient. Medical practice, on the other hand, is the application of preventive, diagnostic, and therapeutic measures to benefit an individual patient. Distinctions between these two definitions are frequently not clear to patients and, occasionally, to health care providers. For example, patients often wish to participate in research because they believe it is the pathway to a possible cure, or at least to improved medical care. This belief, referred to as a "therapeutic misconception," must be guarded against in the recruitment of patients into a study. Just because a physician introduces an innovative, perhaps unusual, interventional procedure in caring for a patient does not necessarily mean that the physician is conducting research. The physician may simply be exercising his or her best judgment in caring for the particular patient. Unless the procedure is being evaluated scientifically and results are being collected for dissemination to a wide audience, the practice does not constitute research. Whether or not the procedure is research, it should be explained to the patient, and the patient should consent to it before entering the study.

Federal Regulations Governing Research with Human Participants

Ethical codes such as the Nuremberg Code, the Declaration of Helsinki, and the Belmont report have a high level of moral authority and are very influential in guiding the conduct of research with human participants in the United States and many other nations. Codes, however, have no enforcement mechanism other than societal expectations and peer pressure. Enforcement comes only when ethical principles are codified into laws and regulations. In the United States, this codification mechanism has occurred in a stepwise fashion over many years.[1]

The first step toward regulation of human experimentation in the United States occurred with the opening of the Clinical Center at the National Institutes of Health (NIH) in 1953. The center was responsible for overseeing experiments with human participants anywhere on the NIH campus. In 1965, this oversight responsibility was expanded to include review and approval of all human-experimentation protocols before their initiation. One year later, the U.S. Surgeon General extended the review and oversight responsibility to all NIH-supported research, whether conducted on the NIH campus (intramural research) or at other institutions (extramural research). In 1971, the FDA issued its own regulations for human experimentation involving new drugs and medical devices.

In 1974, the U.S Congress enacted the National Research Act, which mandated that the Department of Health, Education and Welfare (DHEW, now the Department of Health and Human Services [DHHS]) combine all its human experimentation policies into a single document (45 Code of Federal Regulations [CFR] 64). This document requires that each institution or organization conducting DHEW-funded research on humans establish or use an IRB to review and pass judgment on the research according to DHEW requirements. These requirements specified the composition of the IRB and also outlined its duties, which were to (1) review proposed protocols, (2) document the findings, and (3) oversee the conduct of the research by periodic review of progress reports from the investigator.

In 1976, the NIH established the Office for Protection from Research Risks (OPRR) to oversee human subjects research. In 1991, the government issued the Common Rule policy (see earlier), which is applicable to all NIH institutes and centers conducting or funding research involving human participants. The rule applies not only to research on the NIH campus but also to DHHS-funded research taking place in academic institutions and other organizations. Most of these institutions and organizations have extended the applicability of the Common Rule to all research involving human participants.

In 2000, the name of the OPRR was changed to the Office for Human Research Protections (OHRP). The newly named office was also moved from the NIH to the DHHS to give it more authority and autonomy. The OHRP has authority to conduct oversight investigations of institutions where it suspects that compliance with federal regulations governing human experimentation is inadequate. Table 18-2 lists the institutions investigated by OHRP between 1996 and 1999, the reasons for those investigations, and the outcomes. As the table illustrates, each institution was instructed to take certain actions and make certain improvements in its process for protecting participants in research protocols before the restrictions would be removed.[10]

Table 18-2. Summary of Results of Office for Protection from Research Risks Compliance Oversight Investigations, 1996–1999

1996

- Cook County Hospital Hektoen Institute for Medical Research: Revision of IRB review procedures required.

- Cornell University Medical Center: Modification of IRB review and record-keeping procedures; a plan for increased staffing; a plan for education of IRB members and investigators; and a mechanism for investigation of noncompliance required.

- University of Rochester: Review and development of written operating procedures and an investigator handbook; a finalized organization structure of institutional human participant protections; and development of an education program for IRB members and investigators required.

- Wayne State University: Increased staffing and resources for the IRB, development of a mechanism for prompt review of adverse-event reports; development of an educational program for IRB members and investigators; and review and revision of IRB policies and procedures required.

1997

- City University of New York: Development of an educational program for IRB members and investigators; review and revision of IRB policies and procedures; revision of sample informed consent documents to comply with DHHS regulations; and revision of IRB record-keeping procedures required.

1998

- University of Maryland–Baltimore: Review and revision of informed consent documents for psychiatric research to ensure compliance with DHHS regulations; development of an educational program for IRB members and investigators; and revision of IRB review procedures, including procedures for research involving vulnerable participant populations, required.

- University of California–Irvine: Modification of initial review process to ensure compliance with regulations; revision of continuing review and oversight procedures; increased documentation of IRB actions in accordance with regulations; enhanced education for investigators, IRB members, and staff; and increased support for social and behavioral sciences IRB required.

- Western Carolina Center: SPAs required for DHHS-supported human participant research; deactivation of the MPA.

- Rush Presbyterian St. Luke's Medical Center: Suspension of the MPA for five days pending development of adequate corrective action plans. (The MPA was subsequently reinstated with restrictions requiring correction of 17 identified deficiencies.)

- Scripps Clinic and Research Foundation–The Scripps Research Institute: Correction of 20 identified deficiencies in systemic human participant protections; re-review of all DHHS-supported human participant protocols to include review of complete grant application; development of an educational program for IRB members, IRB staff, and research investigators, and quarterly progress reports required.

- Duke University: Restriction of MPA and several corrective actions required.

- Duke University Medical Center: Restriction of MPA and several corrective actions required.

1999

- Friends Research Institute: Removal of coverage under existing MPA of all performance sites outside the Maryland area; removal of recognition of one IRB under the MPA; and withdrawal of approval of all interinstitutional and cooperative amendments to the MPA.

- Mt. Sinai School of Medicine: Satisfactory implementation of a series of corrective actions required.

- Veterans Affairs, Greater Los Angeles Health Care System (formerly Veterans Affairs Medical Center, West Los Angeles): MPA deactivated; suspension of enrollment of new participants in all federally supported research programs; and continued involvement of previously enrolled participants allowed only when in the best interests of participants.

- Fordham University: SPAs required for all DHHS-supported human participant research, and MPA deactivated.

- Duke University Medical Center: MPA suspended for five days, then reinstated with several restrictions, including re-review of all DHHS-supported research by the IRB; implementation of a second IRB; and implementation of education programs for IRB members, IRB staff, and all investigators.

- University of Illinois-Chicago: Corrective actions required in response to 29 identified deficiencies. New enrollments in all federally supported research protocols suspended pending re-review of all protocols.

- St. Jude Children's Research Hospital: Submission of a progress report describing implementation of several corrective actions three months after a site visit.

- Virginia Commonwealth University: New participant enrollment suspended pending development of an educational program for IRB members, IRB staff, and research investigators, and submission of a list of all federally supported research protocols.

Extracted with permission from Ethical and Policy Issues in Research Involving Human Participants. *Vol 1. Bethesda, MD: National Bioethics Advisory Commission; 2001:54-56.*

The FDA has additional regulations of its own that are consistent with the principles of the Belmont report that apply to the ways in which drugs, biological products, and medical devices may be used in clinical research. The FDA regulations are codified in 21CFR Parts 312, 314, 600, 812, and 814. Disregard of the FDA's regulations may lead to various sanctions, including the following:

- longer, more-detailed review cycles of FDA applications;

- warning letters that document concerns and require an institutional response;

- temporary or permanent disqualification or debarment of individuals from research involving human participants;

- temporary or permanent disqualification or debarment of institutions from research involving human participants; and

- other actions, including property seizures, injunctions, criminal charges, and monetary penalties.

Institutional Review Boards

An IRB has full authority within an institution or organization to

- function as an autonomous agency without influence from investigators or institutional administration;

- review and approve or disapprove research protocols for research involving human subjects;

- require modifications in human-research protocols;

- monitor the informed consent process to ensure compliance with approved protocols;

- gather and review information on serious adverse events and unanticipated adverse events;

- stop clinical research protocols or accrual of patients into protocols;
- examine institutional or investigator conflicts of interest;
- require compliance with federal and institutional regulations; and
- serve as a privacy board to ensure patient privacy and the confidentiality and security of protected health information of research participants, as called for in regulations developed as a result of the Health Insurance Portability and Accountability Act of 1996.[13]

To protect institutional interests, an institution can disapprove a study that has been approved by an IRB. However, the reverse is not true; an institution cannot override the decision of an IRB to disapprove a study or to require modifications in a research protocol.

IRBs typically consist of 12 to 20 members who are employees of the research institution, together with one or two nonemployees who represent the public interest in research with human subjects. The composition of the IRB should be characterized by a reasonable mixture of men and women from diverse medical specialties, including physicians, nurses, and research or clinical specialists. To handle the workload and represent the interests of affiliated institutions, many organizations have more than one IRB. At the author's institution (the Medical College of Wisconsin), there are 10 IRBs for the college and its principal clinical affiliates. The review process of a prototypical IRB is outlined in **Figure 18-1**.

In its review of proposed clinical research protocols involving human participants, an IRB considers many questions,[1,14] including the following:

- Is the proposed protocol truly research, or is it an innovative therapeutic intervention that does not contribute to generalizable knowledge?
- Does the research involve living human participants, deceased human subjects, or tissues from human subjects, living or dead? Research with living human participants requires IRB approval. IRB approval of research with deceased human subjects or with human tissues is principally an institutional decision. Research with human tissues that can be traced to their origins raises troubling ethical issues concerning confidentiality and privacy of personal and family information. Because of these issues, IRBs increasingly require review of research protocols involving tissues of human origin, whether from live or deceased individuals.
- Does the research require IRB review? If so, can the review be expedited or is full review required?[7] Investigations for which IRB review is not required include some types of educational research, research using publicly available data that cannot be linked to individual patients (so-called de-identified data), research on public-benefit programs, and food-quality research. Research that exposes participants to minimum or low risk often can be reviewed by an expedited process that bypasses full committee review.
- Have physical, privacy, psychosocial, financial, and legal risks to participants been minimized?
- Do the benefits of the study to participants or society at large justify the risks to the participants?
- Is the selection of research participants equitable? Are certain potential participants excluded from the study, and, if so, are the reasons for exclusion justifiable?
- Are representatives of vulnerable populations included? If so, are measures adequate to ensure freedom of choice for participation without coercion?
- Do participant-recruitment practices protect against coercion, exploitation, or deception?

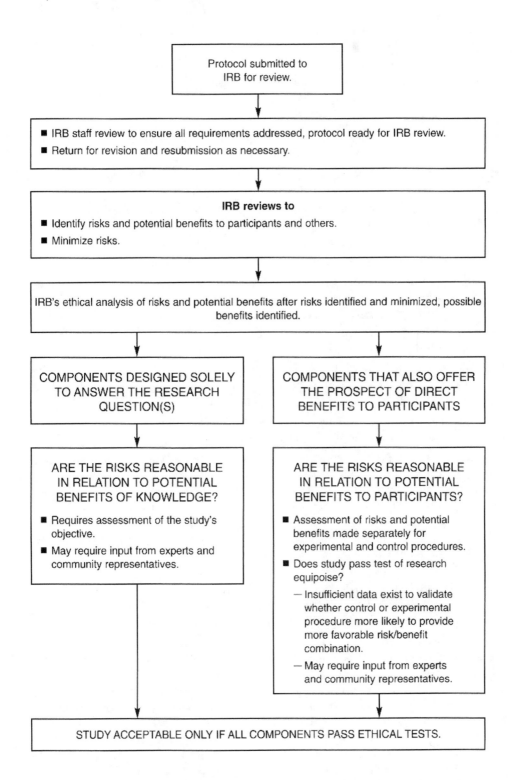

Figure 18-1. Process of IRB Review, Including Analysis of Risks and Potential Benefits

Extracted with permission from Ethical and Policy Issues in Research Involving Human
Participants. *Vol 1. Bethesda, MD: National Bioethics Advisory Commission; 2001:79.*

- Is the privacy of patients respected, and are confidentiality and security of personal health information ensured?

- Does the informed consent practice meet the IRB's standards? In cases where a legally appointed representative provides informed consent, is the practice by which such consent is obtained adequate?

- Does the process of documenting informed consent meet the IRB's standards?

- Are the forms and practice for obtaining informed consent sufficient to ensure that consent is truly informed and voluntary?

- Is the proposed research protocol scientifically valid, and are sample selection and size sufficient to ensure meaningful results?

- Is the knowledge to be gained by the study potentially important to the participants or to patients in general?

- Is there a data safety–monitoring plan to ensure that the safety of participants is not compromised during the study?

- For studies of moderate or high risk to participants, is there an oversight group (e.g., a data safety–monitoring board) in place to ensure that participants are not exposed to greater-than-anticipated risks?

- Is there a monitoring process in place to periodically review study data and to notify the IRB if the risk:benefit analysis of the study needs to be reexamined?

- Are there any institutional or investigator conflicts of interest associated with the study (e.g., does the institution or investigator stand to benefit financially in any way if the study results turn out to favor a product or procedure)?

- Are other institutions or organizations involved in the study, and does that involvement compromise the quality or safety of the study in any manner?

In addition to its initial review, the IRB must review progress reports submitted at least annually by the study's principal investigator. Further, the IRB must be notified of allegations of research misconduct by anyone associated with the study. In response to such notification, the IRB has the option of suspending, closing, or terminating a study. If the allegations result in a full investigation of alleged misconduct, the IRB may be required to notify other organizations, including the NIH Office of Research Integrity, the OHRP, the FDA, the data safety monitoring board (if one exists for the study), and the editors of all journals in which reports of the study have been published or to which results have been submitted.

Often allegations of misconduct are filed by a whistle-blower. An institution must not retaliate against a whistle-blower who has filed an allegation of misconduct in good faith. Such retaliation could in itself be interpreted as an act of research misconduct.

Before a federal grant or contract can be awarded to an institution or organization for research involving human subjects, it must file an Assurance of Compliance with the OHRP. This assurance may be for a single project (a single-project assurance, or SPA) or for multiple research projects (a multiple-projects assurance, or MPA). The assurance states that the institution and its researchers agree to comply with federal regulations, to monitor research involving human participants, and to report instances of serious or repeated noncompliance of regulations. If the OHRP determines that an institution has violated the conditions of an SPA or MPA, it may restrict, suspend, or terminate the assurance. Until the assurance is reinstated, no federally funded research involving human subjects may be conducted at the institution.

The OHRP may also impose sanctions on individual researchers for noncompliance with federal regulations. Possible sanctions include the following:

- recommending to the DHHS that the researcher be barred from receiving funding in support of research;

- requiring OHRP approval for every study conducted by the researcher;
- forcing the researcher to obtain remedial training or education; and
- restricting the investigator's ability to conduct research (e.g., by requiring supervision of the researcher).

Safety in Research with Human Participants: Restoring the Public Trust

Over the past several years, research with human participants has come under heightened public and governmental surveillance, as projects with inadequate protection of participant safety and insufficient attention to ethical norms have been reported to federal agencies and publicized in the media. Research volunteers have been injured and, in a few cases, have died in experiments of questionable ethical merit. Respected institutions have had their clinical research programs suspended by federal agencies.

Organizations conducting research with human participants have ratcheted up their review and surveillance programs in efforts to ensure compliance with federal regulations and ethical standards. As stated in a report of the National Patient Safety Foundation's 2002 meeting, "In the end, the research community must come to grips with the reality of these difficulties. We must find ways to communicate truthfully and effectively to the public and to dialogue with the public as a partner in these issues. We cannot be afraid of public scrutiny or public involvement. The public is our most important partner in creating systems of protection and furthering biomedical progress."[15]

As described in the National Patient Safety Foundation report, these are the steps to restoring public trust:

- Acknowledge problems.
- Involve the public in all phases of research.
- Lead in the promotion of ethical conduct.
- Create protection programs that enforce the principle of respect for individuals.
- Provide adequate resources to IRBs so that they can do their job of protecting research subjects.
- Remove negative disincentives and create positive incentives for institutions and investigators to do the right thing.
- Involve and engage investigators and investigative teams in the bioethics process.
- Fully disclose all potential conflicts of interest.
- Invest IRBs with the power to prevent research where conflicts exist.
- Promote transparency in all phases of research.
- Develop high ethical standards for process and conduct that exceed basic compliance.
- Enforce high ethical standards through leadership.
- Evaluate programs and processes and strive for continuous improvement.
- Tell the truth.
- Acknowledge and correct mistakes when they occur.
- Avoid "spin" and "hype."
- Learn and practice more-effective communication with potential participants.

- Fully disclose all potential risks.
- Provide leadership in research with human volunteers.[15]

Conclusion

Everyone involved in research with human participants has an obligation to ensure that the research plan is viable, the safety of participants is protected, and the research is conducted according to fundamental ethical principles. Past lapses in meeting these requirements serve as reminders of the importance of this obligation. The safety of patients is always important, but nowhere is it more so than in experiments where the subjects may not experience a direct benefit of participation and the technologies being evaluated may present unknown risks to the volunteers. Persons conducting such experiments must keep the design, safety, and ethics of human experimentation foremost in mind.

References

1. Shamoo AE, Resnik DB. *Responsible Conduct of Research*. New York: Oxford University Press Inc; 2003:86,196-199.

2. Annas G, Grodin M, eds. *The Nazi Doctors and the Nuremberg Code: Human Rights in Human Experimentation*. New York: Oxford University Press; 1992.

3. Beecher H. Ethics and clinical research. *N Engl J Med*. 1966;274:1354-1360.

4. Munson R. *Intervention and Reflection*. 4th ed. Belmont, CA: Wadsworth; 1992.

5. Levine RJ. *Ethics and Regulation of Clinical Research*. 2nd ed. New Haven, CT: Yale University Press; 1988.

6. Advisory Committee on Human Radiation Experiments. Final Report. Stock No. 061-000-00-848-9. Washington, DC: Superintendent of Documents, US Government Printing Office; 1995.

7. Lurie P, Wolfe S. Unethical trials of interventions to reduce perinatal transmission of the human immunodeficiency virus in developing countries. *N Engl J Med*. 1997;337:853-856.

8. Eckstein S, ed. *Manual for Research Ethics Committees*. 6th ed. New York: Cambridge University Press; 2003.

9. National Commission for the Protection of Human Subjects of Biomedical and Behavioral Research. The Belmont Report. Washington, DC: US Department of Health, Education and Welfare; 1979.

10. National Bioethics Advisory Commission. *Ethical and Policy Issues in Research Involving Human Participants*. Vol 1. Bethesda, MD: National Bioethics Advisory Commission; 2001:79.

11. Bronzio J, Smith V, Wade, M. *Medical Technology and Society: An Interdisciplinary Perspective*. Cambridge, MA: MIT Press; 1990.

12. Emanual EJ, Crouch RA, Arras JD, Morena JD, Grady C, eds. *Ethical and Regulatory Aspects of Clinical Research: Readings and Commentary*. Baltimore, MD: Johns Hopkins University Press; 2003:39-55.

13. Amdur R, Bankert E. *Institutional Review Board: Management and Function*. Sudbury, MA: Jones and Bartlett Publishers Inc; 2002.

14. Dunn C, Chadwick G. *Protecting Study Volunteers in Research: A Manual for Investigative Sites*. Boston, MA: CenterWatch Inc; 1999.

15. National Patient Safety Foundation. Accountability in Clinical Research: Balancing Risk & Benefit: Forum Report. Chicago, IL: National Patient Safety Foundation; 2002.

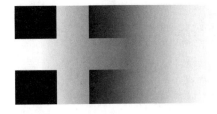

Poison Centers: A Key Component of the Patient-Safety System

Daniel J. Cobaugh

Introduction

The goal of patient-safety initiatives is to optimize the medication-use process and, through the use of technology and system changes, to provide an errorfree environment for patient care. As with traditional injury-prevention models, these preventive efforts focus on those factors that predispose to injury and the system breakdowns that can occur at the actual time of injury.

In an effort to provide guidance for the development of injury-prevention strategies and models, the Haddon matrix delineates the preexposure, exposure, and postexposure phases surrounding an injury event.[1] Medication-safety efforts can be integrated into this framework. For example, root-cause analysis[2] can be categorized as a postexposure activity using the Haddon matrix.

Breakdowns related to the medication-use process result in development of some type of toxicity in the patient. The American Association of Poison Control Centers (AAPCC) noted in 2000 that 75 percent of digoxin-related fatalities reported to U.S. poison centers in 1999 resulted from a therapeutic error.[3] Screening for and diagnosis of toxicity following a patient-safety event and a well-coordinated approach to management of the toxic sequelae are critically important components of the Haddon postexposure response.

This chapter reviews clinical toxicology resources available through the U.S. poison centers and describes the activities performed by staff of these centers in the care of patients who have developed toxicity as a result of a medication error. Although this chapter focuses on the poison center's role in supporting health professionals caring for patients who are the victims of medication errors, it is important to recognize that the poison center's role in medication safety begins in the home. The centers often receive calls from the public regarding medication errors and adverse events. Another role for these centers is the provision of preventive and clinical services targeted at unintentional medication exposure.

History of Poison Centers

The first poison center in the United States was established in Chicago, Illinois, in 1953 by Gdalman and Press. The decision to create such a center followed recognition by the Accident Prevention Committee of the American Academy of Pediatrics (AAP) that 49 percent of accidents treated by AAP members were the result of poisoning.[4] By 1957, there were 17 poison control centers in the United States, and by 1978, the number had risen to 661. Many of these centers delegated poison center responsibilities to staff in hospital emergency departments (EDs) and pharmacies that were responsible for other patient-care activities. This resulted in inconsistencies in the scope of the centers' activities and in the quality of information they provided to callers.

Beginning in the early 1980s, a number of factors converged to dramatically change the landscape for provision of poison control services in the United States. First, the AAPCC developed criteria for the certification of regional poison control centers that focused on levels of service, staff requirements, documentation, data collection, prevention programs, health professionals education, and quality improvement.[5] At the same time, state governments and the poison centers' host organizations, primarily hospitals, began to grapple with the escalating costs of providing poison control services. This resulted in a consolidation of centers in an effort to maximize on economies of scale. In 2000, the Poison Center Enhancement and Awareness Act was signed into law. This act authorized federal grant support to poison centers as well as funds to establish a nationwide toll-free poison center number, enhance poisoning data collection, and establish a nationwide prevention program.

In 2004, there were 61 poison centers in the United States. It is likely that there will be further compression in the number of centers over the next decade. The majority of these centers are located in academic medical centers and have missions that focus on patient care, education, and research. Some poison centers provide services to multiple states. This is an economical alternative in states with smaller populations. To generate additional income, some centers have developed contractual arrangements with pharmaceutical and chemical manufacturers. Among the services provided under these contracts are tailored responses to exposures involving the manufacturers' products and postmarketing surveillance.[6]

In 2004, the Institute of Medicine completed a comprehensive review of poison center services in the United States.[7] Foremost among the IOM's numerous recommendations was that the U.S. Congress amend the Poison Center Enhancement and Awareness Act to provide adequate funding to support a national network of regional poison control centers.

Scope of Poison Center Services

Misconceptions about the scope of services provided by poison control centers are common. Given the centers' historic roots, many members of the public, as well as health professionals, assume that services are limited to responding to accidental exposures in children and pediatric poison prevention programs. It is important to recognize that poison centers provide information regarding toxicologic emergencies across the age spectrum (see Table 19-1). Between 1998 and 2002, the AAPCC's Toxic Exposure Surveillance System (TESS) received more than 3.7 million calls involving patients 20 years of age or greater.[3,8-10]

Table 19-1. Calls to Poison Centers by Patient Age, 1998–2002[3,6-8]

Year	≤ 5 years	6–2 years	12–19 years	≥ 20 years
1998	1,181,006	158,351	158,518	732,421
1999	1,154,799	154,606	157,993	722,243
2000	1,142,796	151,221	160,505	696,171
2001	1,169,478	156,612	165,657	759,401
2002	1,227,381	159,487	171,731	803,520
Total	5,875,460	780,277	814,404	3,713,756

Poison control centers receive calls from health professionals as well as from members of the public. Health professionals who call poison centers are most commonly physicians or nurses in EDs or intensive-care units. Of the 2.38 million calls to poison centers in 2002, 76.6 percent were received from the general public, and 14.3 percent were received from health care facilities.[8-10] The latter included clinicians seeking guidance on the care of patients who had developed toxic sequelae as a result of a medication error.

Requests for poison center consultations can generally involve either an accidental or an intentional exposure. Pediatric poisonings, therapeutic errors, adverse reactions to drugs and foods, occupational poisoning (e.g., lead poisoning), and environmental poisonings (e.g., carbon monoxide poisoning) are representative of types of accidental exposures managed by poison centers. TESS defines a therapeutic error as an "unintentional deviation from a proper therapeutic regimen that results in the wrong dose, incorrect route of administration, administration to the wrong person, or administration of the wrong substance." It defines an adverse reaction as an "event occurred with normal, prescribed, labeled or recommended use of the product." Between 1998 and 2002, more than 811,000 therapeutic errors and more than 172,000 adverse drug reactions were reported to TESS.[3,8-10] In 2000, TESS began to collect more-detailed information on therapeutic errors reported to poison centers. In 2002, the top three reasons for a therapeutic error were administration of an additional dose, a dosing error involving more than one additional dose, and administration of the wrong medication.[10] Attempted suicide is the most common reason for intentional exposures that result in a poison center consultation.

Education of members of the public and of health professionals is another service provided by poison control centers. The centers use a variety of techniques to enhance public awareness of poison prevention and access to the center. Training of health professional students—pharmacy students, medical students, pharmacy residents, emergency medicine residents, pediatric residents, and others—has been a core activity of poison centers for decades.[11] The value of these experiences has been confirmed by pre- and post-test assessments.[12] Poison centers also provide continuing education for a wide variety of health professionals who practice in the facilities in their geographic regions. These educational experiences provide an opportunity to heighten health professionals' awareness of the contributions that poison centers and clinical toxicologists can make when patients develop toxicity as a result of a medication error. This commitment to health professional education provides the centers with an opportunity to expose health system–based patient-safety officers to the clinical toxicology consultation programs available under their auspices. This could enhance the safety officers' knowledge of toxicities associated with the medications most frequently involved in patient-safety events and could provide opportunities for them to establish a relationship with the poison center and to integrate clinical toxicology expertise into their organizations' patient-safety plans.

Figure 19-1. Logo of the American Association of Poison Control Centers

Poison Center Operations

Poison centers are available to provide toxicology consultation 24 hours per day, 7 days per week. Use of a widely advertised nationwide poison center number (see **Figure 19-1**) connects the caller to the poison center that serves his or her geographic area. This enables the centers to be constantly accessible to health professionals. Poison centers are positioned to provide service to all hospitals throughout their regions; services are not limited to the host institution. The centers regularly survey health care facilities in their regions to collect information on each organization's capabilities. This includes each facility's ability to care for critically ill patients, the types and quantity of antidotes stocked, and its ability to provide extracorporeal-elimination procedures such as hemodialysis.

Several types of health professionals staff the centers. The frontline responders are specialists in poison information (SPIs), who are pharmacists or nurses with specialized toxicology training.[13] The AAPCC offers a certification examination for SPIs who have worked for at least 2,000 hours in a poison center and have managed at least 2,000 human-exposure cases. Some poison centers also use poison information providers (PIPs) to support the SPIs. The PIP, who is supervised at all times by a SPI, is not necessarily a licensed health professional. Often, pharmacy students and paramedics are trained for the PIP role.

Clinical and medical toxicologists provide 24-hour on-call support to the frontline center staff. Clinical toxicologists are most often pharmacists who have completed fellowship training in clinical toxicology and are certified by the American Board of Applied Toxicology.[14] Each poison center has at least one physician on staff who serves as the medical director and who is responsible for all clinical supervision within the center. Following completion of residency training in a primary medical specialty (e.g., emergency medicine, pediatrics, or internal medicine) these physicians complete a two-year medical toxicology fellowship and then gain certification from the American Board of Medical Specialties subspecialty board in medical toxicology.[15]

Case Management

Upon receipt of a call, the poison center initiates a comprehensive case-management process. Initially, the SPI conducts a thorough assessment of the history of the exposure and determines the potential for development of toxicity. If there is a risk for toxicity, the SPI makes a decision regarding the most appropriate location for care of the patient. In 2002, more than 74 percent of the cases were managed at the site of exposure, most often the home.[10] Approximately 520,000 (22.2 percent) of all cases reported to poison centers in 2002 were managed in health care facilities.[10]

After the most appropriate treatment site has been determined, the center makes additional recommendations for patient management. In many cases, the poison center recommends use of a decontamination procedure in the home. For example, in more than 1.1 million cases in 2002, poison centers recommended some type of oral dilution of an ingested substance or irrigation, either ocular or dermal, following an exposure by one of these routes. Historically, ipecac syrup was often recommended for gastric decontamination. However, the use of ipecac syrup to induce emesis has decreased dramatically over the last two decades, and some poison centers no longer recommend it.

In some cases, observation is the only intervention required. If observation and decontamination procedures are recommended, the poison center will follow up to verify that the patient's status has improved. If the expected response to home treatment does not occur or if a patient begins to display signs or symptoms of toxicity, the center will recommend transport to an ED. Most poison centers are equipped to interface with the community 911 emergency call system to arrange patient transport and to provide recommendations for out-of-hospital care to paramedics and emergency medical technicians. When transport to the ED is required, the poison center routinely apprises the staff of the patient's status and provides initial recommendations for care.

The poison center may have advised transport to a health care facility upon receipt of the call, or it may have received a request for consultation from the facility, as occurs in cases of iatrogenic toxicity. In these cases, a clinical or medical toxicology consultation, either at the bedside or via telephone, is often provided.[20] These consultations address multiple aspects of the patient's care, including the physical examination and ongoing patient assessment, laboratory monitoring, gastrointestinal decontamination, antidote administration, the use of extracorporeal-elimination measures, and employment of other treatment strategies that are specific to the toxicity that has occurred.

The clinical or medical toxicologist is a critical member of the care team. If the patient is hospitalized within the poison center's host institution, this consultation is often available at the bedside. If the hospitalization involves another health care facility in the poison center's region, this consultation and the follow-up occur by telephone.

The decision to use a specific antidote (e.g., digoxin immune Fab) or an extracorporeal-elimination procedure (e.g., hemodialysis) can be complex. The clinical or medical toxicologist can also contribute to decisions about whether the patient needs to be monitored in a critical-care setting or in a medical or surgical unit. While timely use of interventions can be key to good patient outcomes, decisions about their use must be based on a thorough understanding of the toxicologic characteristics of the implicated substance. The clinical/medical toxicologist is well positioned to provide guidance on the appropriate use of toxicologic interventions. The following three vignettes provide examples of interventions by the clinical/medical toxicologist.

- In a patient who becomes severely ill because of a drug-drug interaction involving digoxin and who has received digoxin immune Fab as an antidote, the total serum digoxin concentration may increase because of a shift of digoxin from tissue to the central compartment, with subsequent binding to the digoxin immune Fab.[21] The elevation in digoxin concentrations is an artifact and does not require treatment. In this case, the toxicologist could provide the team with toxicokinetic information that would prevent the unnecessary administration of additional doses of an expensive antidote.

- In the case of a patient with lithium toxicity who has undergone hemodialysis, resolution of signs and symptoms of toxicity does not necessarily correlate with decreasing lithium serum concentrations.[22] Additional hemodialysis treatments may be required to enhance clearance of the lithium. The clinician who is unfamiliar with the distribution kinetics of lithium might react only to the initial postdialysis serum concentration and not institute additional hemodialysis.

- Concomitant administration of agents that affect serotonin (e.g., monoamine oxidase inhibitors and meperidine) can result in a drug-drug interaction that precipitates the serotonin syndrome and a profound hyperthermia.[23] In these patients, aggressive cooling measures, including ice baths, and benzodiazepines to minimize motor activity are often required.[24] Given the relative rarity of the serotonin syndrome, the physician may not be aware of all of the interventions that might be required to care for these patients.

All poison centers interventions are documented and stored in an electronic medical record to document and maintain patient information.

The AAPCC Toxic Exposure Surveillance System (TESS)

All U.S. poison centers participate in TESS, which was developed by the AAPCC in 1983. The data are collected at the time of the initial poison center call, during follow-up calls, and when bedside consultation occurs. The data-collection software is integrated with the centers' electronic medical records. The database contains extensive epidemiologic information about all poisoning-exposure cases reported to centers. Collected data include demographic information, substance(s) implicated in the exposure, signs and symptoms of toxicity exhibited by the patient, treatments provided, and a determination of the patient's medical outcome.

Each year, the AAPCC publishes a report that provides a comprehensive summary of the data collected through TESS. **Table 19-2** lists selected TESS data elements from these annual reports, which can be accessed at http://www.aapcc.org/annual.htm. Annual reports dating back to the creation of the system in 1983 can be accessed at this site.

Table 19-2. Selected TESS Annual Report Tables

Age and Gender Distribution of Cases

Age and Gender Distribution of Fatalities

Chemicals Substances Implicated in Human Exposure (Organized in Category and Sub-Category Format)

Detailed Fatality Table

Exposure Site

Management Site

Medical Outcome by Age

Narrative Abstracts of Selected Fatalities

Pharmaceutical Substances Implicated in Human Exposure (Organized in Category and Subcategory Format)

Reason for Exposure

Route of Exposure

Substance Categories with the Greatest Number of Deaths

Substances Most Frequently Implicated in Human Exposures

Substances Most Frequently Implicated in Pediatric Exposures

Therapies Provided

TESS data have been used for a variety of purposes, including real-time toxicosurveillance, postmarketing surveillance, regulatory review, toxicology research, and development of poison prevention campaigns.[18] Drug manufacturers often include TESS data in their submissions to the U.S. Food and Drug Administration (FDA), when proposing that a product be moved from prescription to over-the-counter status, and when conducting regulatory reviews.

TESS data have many practical safety applications. For example, they were used in efforts to persuade the FDA to mandate packaging of over-the-counter iron supplements in unit dose containers. Analysis of TESS data over an eight-year period indicated that iron supplements were the single most frequent cause of pediatric unintentional ingestion fatalities and that they accounted for 30.2 percent of reported pediatric fatalities involving ingestion of a medication.[19] A recent study used TESS morbidity and mortality data to calculate hazard factors for substances involved in geriatric poisoning.[23] Data for more than 180,000 cases reported from a 10-year period were reviewed. The analysis of cases in which therapeutic error was the reason for exposure revealed that (in order of occurrence) heparin colchicine, aminophylline/theophylline, lithium, and aspirin had the greatest number of cases in which the medical outcome was coded as major or death. When adverse reactions were reviewed, the authors found that biguanide hypoglycemics, cardiac glycosides, warfarin, antineoplastics, and heparin were associated with significant morbidity and mortality.

In the post–September 11 environment, the AAPCC has worked closely with the Centers for Disease Control and Prevention to develop systems for real-time toxicosurveillance. Data are uploaded from poison center sites to a central repository every 15 minutes. Toxicosurveillance systems have been developed to identify syndromic and product-specific trends in specific geographic locations. This real-time toxicosurveillance technology could also be used for early recognition of emerging safety-related threats related to medications.

Summary

Ideally, the health care system and all its stakeholders must advance to a point where all appropriate systems are in place to prevent medication errors. Patients will be best served if health professionals focus on prevention, or Haddon's preexposure phase. However, we also need to acknowledge that medication errors will occur and that patients will be the victims of these breakdowns. Given the likelihood of toxic sequelae following a medication error, it is essential that the treatment team have access to toxicology expertise. The U.S. poison centers are equipped to provide toxicology consultations that will support providers and will enhance the care of patients who are the victims of medication errors.

References

1. Haddon W Jr. The changing approach to the epidemiology, prevention, and amelioration of trauma: the transition to approaches etiologically rather than descriptively based. *Inj Prev.* 1999;5:231-235.

2. Rex JH, Turnbull JE, Allen SJ, Vande Voorde K, Luther K. Systematic root-cause analysis of adverse drug events in a tertiary referral hospital. *Jt Comm J Qual Improv.* 2000;26:563-575.

3. Litovitz TL, Klein-Schwartz W, White S, Cobaugh DJ, Youniss J, Drab A, Benson BE. 1999 annual report of the American Association of Poison Control Centers Toxic Exposure Surveillance System. *Am J Emerg Med.* 2000;18:517-574.

4. Botticelli JT, Pierpaoli PG. Louis Gdalman, pioneer in hospital pharmacy poison information services. *Am J Hosp Pharm.* 1992;49:1445-1450.

5. Lovejoy FH Jr, Robertson WO, Woolf AD. Poison centers, poison prevention, and the pediatrician. *Pediatrics.* 1994;94:220-224.

6. Krenzelok EP, Dean BS. A program of poison center services to business and industry. *Vet Hum Toxicol.* 1987;29:172-173.

7. Institute of Medicine. Forging a poison prevention and control system. IOM Report. 2004.

8. Litovitz TL, Klein-Schwartz W, Caravati EM, Youniss J, Crouch B, Lee S. 1998 Annual Report of the American Association of Poison Control Centers Toxic Exposure Surveillance System. *Am J Emerg Med.* 1999;17:435-487.

9. Litovitz TL, Klein-Schwartz W, Rodgers GC Jr, Cobaugh DJ, Youniss J, Omslaer JC, et al. 2001 Annual Report of the American Association of Poison Control Centers Toxic Exposure Surveillance System. *Am J Emerg Med.* 2002;20:391-452.

10. Watson WA, Litovitz TL, Rodgers GC Jr, Klein-Schwartz W, Youniss J, Rose SR, Borys D, et al. 2002 Annual Report of the American Association of Poison Control Centers Toxic Exposure Surveillance System. *Am J Emerg Med.* 2003;21:353-421.

11. Jordan JK, Dean BS, Krenzelok EP. Poison center rotation for health science students. *Vet Hum Toxicol.* 1987;29:174-175.

12. Cobaugh DJ, Goetz CM, Lopez GP, Dean BS, Krenzelok EP. Assessment of learning by emergency medicine residents and pharmacy students participating in a poison center clerkship. *Vet Hum Toxicol.* 1997;39:173-175.

13. Mrvos R, Dean BS, Krenzelok EP, Herrington L. A demographic profile of the specialist in poison information. *Vet Hum Toxicol.* 1994;36:330-331.

14. American Board of Applied Toxicology. http://www.clintox.org/Abat/Index.html. Accessed July 2003.

15. Wax PM, Donovan JW. Fellowship training in medical toxicology: characteristics, perceptions, and career impact. *J Toxicol Clin Toxicol.* 2000;38:637-642.

16. Lemke T, Wang R. Emergency department observation for toxicologic exposures. *Emerg Med Clin North Am.* 2001;19:155-167.

17. Litovitz T. The TESS database. Use in product safety assessment. *Drug Saf.* 1998;18:9-19.

18. Litovitz T, Manoguerra A. Comparison of pediatric poisoning hazards: an analysis of 3.8 million exposure incidents. A report from the American Association of Poison Control Centers. *Pediatrics.* 1992;89:999-1006.

19. Gibb I, Adams PC, Parnham AJ, Jennings K. Plasma digoxin: assay anomalies in Fab-treated patients. *Br J Clin Pharmacol.* 1983;16:445-447.

20. Jaeger A, Sauder P, Kopferschmitt J, Jaegle ML. Toxicokinetics of lithium intoxication treated by hemodialysis. *J Toxicol Clin Toxicol.* 1985-86;23:501-517.

21. Browne B, Linter S. Monoamine oxidase inhibitors and narcotic analgesics. A critical review of the implications for treatment. *Br J Psychiatry.* 1987;151:210-212.

22. Carbone JR. The neuroleptic malignant and serotonin syndromes. *Emerg Med Clin North Am.* 2000;18:317-325.

23. Cobaugh DJ, Krenzelok EP. Geriatric poisoning severity: An analysis of poison center cases. *J Toxicol Clin Toxicol.* 2004;42:131.

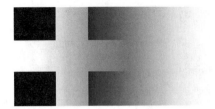

Medication-Safety Self-Assessments

Bruce M. Gordon

In order to get to a destination, you need to know the location of your destination and where you are relative to it. An organizational self-assessment provides the means to establish both a destination (what your organization needs to be) and a current position relative to that destination. It also tells you what things you need to accomplish to get there.

Why Self-Assessment?

When we care for patients, we make a diagnosis and then develop a treatment plan. The diagnosis is determined by taking a history and performing a physical examination, then comparing the results to those that would be typical of healthy individuals or of individuals with disease. When initial examination findings are inconclusive, we do further studies.

Similarly, when the goal is to make an organization safer, we must do the necessary assessments before we can reach a diagnosis and develop a treatment plan. We need to know what treatments have proved successful for organizations with similar diagnoses. We also need to know the costs of these treatments.

In performing a self-assessment, we must first consider the driving force behind it or, to continue our patient care analogy, "Where is your pain?" If meeting regulatory or accreditation standards is the primary driving force, then we will need to focus on specific areas and develop corresponding strategies within a fixed time frame (often 6 to 18 months). For guidance in this work, we may often turn to the Web site of the regulatory or accreditation body in question. FAQ (frequently asked questions) sections of these groups are a great source of information. Listservs on the organization's Web site or on the sites of similar health care organizations (e.g., the American Society of Health-System Pharmacists [ASHP], group purchasing organization, specialty practice groups) likewise provide valuable information.

In another case, the driving force behind a self-assessment may be an organizational response to an adverse event. The self-assessment might be limited to a specific part of the medication-use system and the time frame may be as short as 30 days. An example of this situation would be an organizational response to the Joint Commission on Accreditation of Healthcare Organizations (JCAHO) following a sentinel event.

Either of the situations just described may make an organization's leaders desire to perform a detailed review of the entire medication-use system. If a broad organizational assessment is desired, a larger project team and a longer time frame may be expected. Participants should be prepared to develop an action plan and a time line. This chapter primarily addresses this type of broad organizational self-assessment as applied to the medication-safety system.

Types of Self-Assessments

A self-assessment may be internal or external. The advantages and disadvantages of each type of assessment are described below and summarized in **Table 20-1**.

Table 20-1. Advantages and Disadvantages of Internal and External Self-Assessments

	Internal Assessment	External Assessment
Advantages	Opportunity to gather new skills, knowledge and experience	Efficient, shorter time to impact
		Less impact on staff
	Opportunity for cross-functional team and alliance development	Experienced, knowledgeable consultants
		Knowledge and skills transfer
	Less expense	Provides prioritization schema
		Provides solutions and strategies
Disadvantages	Extensive staff commitment	Higher cost
		Possibility of lack of objectivity

INTERNAL SELF-ASSESSMENTS

An internal assessment entails using published literature, references, surveys, case reports, and internal data to establish a self-assessment methodology and to define its direction and scope. The value of this method is limited by the relatively small number of experienced medication-use system analysts available in-house and by the extensive resources required to plan, prepare, and perform the assessment and implement any resulting recommendations. One key advantage of internal assessments is that they create subject-matter and process-improvement experts within the organization during the course of the project. Members of multidisciplinary project teams often learn a great deal about the medication-use system. The development of knowledge, skills, and cross-functional alliances will prove extremely valuable during the development and implementation of the action plan.

The Institute for Safe Medication Practices (ISMP) has produced the most comprehensive and best-known medication self-assessment tool available today. Called the ISMP Medication Safety Self-Assessment® for Hospitals, it has recently been updated and is available on the ISMP Web site (www.ISMP.org). The tool may be printed and questions evaluated, and the user may then return to the ISMP Web site for data entry. Each item in the self-assessment tool has a weighted response. The user receives a summarized numeric value for his or her hospital that can then be used to assign priorities and monitor progress. Unfortunately, ISMP has not reported individual answer weights with the potential maximum weight for each question. This makes it difficult to use the survey tool as a basis for ranking potential corrective actions in order of priority.

Many other tools are available for safety assessments. ASHP has published the Medication-Use System Safety Strategy (http://www.ashp.org/patient-safety/MS3-1.pdf) and the ASHP Best Practices Self-Assessment Tool (www.ashp.org/emplibrary/SAT-PrintableSurvey.pdf). Another tool is JCAHO's Periodic Performance Review. A demonstration of this tool, which includes standards and accreditation participation requirements, is available online (www.jcrinc.com/onlinebooks.asp?durki=5509&site=78&return=3105). The Wisconsin Patient Safety Institute has a publication entitled Maximizing Patient Safety in the Medication Use Process: Practice Guidelines and Best Demonstrated Practices (http://www.pswi.org/Patient_Safety_Booklet.pdf). These tools may be used as part of a rigorous self-assessment process or as checklists for routine medication-use system review.

EXTERNAL SELF-ASSESSMENTS

An external assessment uses knowledgeable outside specialists or consultants. Their experience and understanding of assessment methodology provide for a more efficient assessment, shorter project duration, and the possibility of performing comparative analyses. It also is less of a strain on the organization, since staff do not have to be pulled from their jobs to perform the assessment. (Some staff time will be required, even for an external assessment.) This efficiency is partially offset by the consulting fees, but using large amounts of staff time over a greater period of time to achieve a similar result will also incur costs.

External self-assessments are available from a number of sources. ISMP has been performing them for many years. In addition, many technology vendors have consulting services wrapped around, or incorporated into, their product lines. They are sometimes willing to perform limited assessments for no charge, or at a reduced fee, in return for product evaluation. Such an arrangement might make one question the objectivity of the analysis relating to that technology, and users should question the data and assumptions used in the analysis. In any case, staff participation is necessary to identify and evaluate the assumptions and potential biases in such an analysis.

Another advantage of external consultants becomes clear after the assessment is complete. An assessment produces a list of problem areas, but good consultants will also provide focused solutions and strategies to address each of the findings. These strategies are based on the literature and on the expertise they have garnered in multiple facilities.

The organization's leaders must develop a clear vision and then communicate it repeatedly and consistently to all stakeholders. Organizational leaders are also responsible for removing any obstacles to project success. These steps are necessary to create project buy-in and support both initially and throughout the project.

Key resources for external assessments include an American Hospital Association (AHA) toolkit focusing on leadership (www.aha.org). In addition, publications such as AHA Strategies for Leadership: An Organizational Approach to Patient Safety (www.aha.org/aha/key_issues/patient_safety/contents/VHAtool.pdf) and AHA Strategies for Leadership: Hospital Executives and Their Role in Patient Safety (http://www.aha.org/aha/key_issues/patient_safety/contents/conwaytool.pdf) may be of use.

Regardless of the reason for the assessment or the method to be used, it is essential to establish project goals and scope. Before the project is initiated, the organization's leaders should meet with key managers, clinicians, and line-level staff to determine the project goal, which segment of the medication-use system should be evaluated, key responsibilities, budget and staff allocations, anticipated time lines, and similar matters. Large projects require a substantial commitment at all organizational levels. If no additional resources are to be allocated, a frank negotiation of what current departmental and individual responsibilities will be suspended during the project will be necessary. The project goals and scope will be used throughout the project to keep the team focused on the primary objectives and to ensure that the team does not waste time.

Steps in the Self-Assessment Process

FORMING A PROJECT TEAM

Before the assessment gets under way, a primary project team should be established that includes representatives from the key stakeholders of the medication-use system. This group should remain relatively small in order to maintain functionality. It might include representatives from hospital administration, medical staff, nursing, pharmacy, the patient- or medication-safety officer, representatives from quality assurance or risk management and information systems, and a patient/consumer representative. Other members might include ward clerks, transport aids, or couriers, as well as representatives from departments such as respiratory therapy and clinical laboratories. The individuals with the most knowledge of the medication-use system are the line-level staff that interact with it directly and on a daily basis; consequently, team members should include both professional and technical staff.

The primary project team will likely need to create smaller action teams for focused initiatives or patient care areas related to the larger goal. These initiatives might include process mapping a specific portion of the medication-use system or performing a root-cause analysis (RCA).

SELECTING GOALS AND METRICS

During the early phase of the process, stakeholders should be asked to identify evaluation tools and interim goals that can be used to monitor progress and gauge project success. These interim goals may also form a focal point for celebrating project successes and provide an early indicator of the need to redirect project activities if interim results are not optimal.

As an example, if the goal is to evaluate the medication turn-around time (TAT), the definition of TAT needs to be established using easily measurable metrics. A metrics that might be used for evaluating processes might include the time that elapses between when a medication order is written and the time when the patient is administered the medication. A subprocess measurement might include the time between when the medication order is written and the time it is received in the pharmacy, or the time from receipt of the order in the pharmacy till the time it is entered into the pharmacy information system.

IDENTIFYING OPPORTUNITIES FOR PROJECTS OF LIMITED SCOPE

As the assessment gets under way, every organization should review medication-safety issues identified through outside sources. These sources include reference books, the professional literature, news reports, and publications from professional, government, and nonprofit organizations devoted to medication safety. As an example, the ISMP distributes the biweekly *ISMP Medication Safety Alert* and the *Quarterly Action Agenda*, each issue of which contains a series of actionable items relating to medication safety.

Staff interviews may be extremely useful sources of information on medication safety if the proper organizational culture exists and the interviewer is knowledgeable about medication safety and is a skilled interviewer. Various staff members may be asked about errors or potential errors that they have seen or in which they have been involved. They might also be asked to name those aspects of the medication-safety system that they believe pose a potential patient risk. Additional questions such as, "Do you believe that something bad would happen to you if you reported an error?" may provide clues as to whether the existing reporting culture is perceived as punitive or nonpunitive. Additionally, staff may be queried about what drugs, processes, or conditions (e.g., staffing, lighting, work space, lack of policies or protocols, training, education, communication) contribute to errors.

EXAMINING CURRENT DATA

Hospitals are a rich source of data that may be analyzed to identify latent and active error modes. Because of inconsistent reporting nomenclature, lack of communication between departments and members of different professions, and the absence of technical expertise, many of these sources often go unrecognized and untapped.

The volume and quality of the data that are available within a voluntary reporting system depend on a number of variables. For example, if the organizational error-reporting culture is perceived as punitive, many errors will likely not be reported, and the errors that are reported will be only significant events that would likely be identified through other means (e.g., patient death) or events that are relatively minor. The number and quality of reports will also suffer if the reporting system is too complex or if it does not provide feedback to reporters.

Spending time identifying what types of errors or error-related data might be available within the organization is highly recommended. Sources of such data include medication-error reports, adverse drug event or reaction reports, pharmacy clinical interventions, incident reports, intravenous (i.v.) therapy events, radiology reports, laboratory reports, medication administration record (MAR) reconciliation reports, automated-dispensing-device fill and variance reports, prescriber order clarifications, tracer drugs or tracer laboratory results, and e-code reports. (E-code reports are a specific group of diagnosis-related group codes relating to external causes of injury, such as falls, motor vehicle accidents, and adverse events, including adverse drug events.)

Components of an Organizational Safety Self-Assessment

There are eight areas in which problems are most commonly found during the course of hospital medication-safety assessment: organizational leadership and commitment to safety, organizational culture, medication-safety teams, technology, pharmacy and therapeutics (P&T) committees, communication, error reporting and analysis, and sentinel event preparation. Although other areas also bear investigation, each of the eight areas in this list is worth exploring in greater detail because it has often proved fruitful in identifying safety opportunities.

ORGANIZATIONAL LEADERSHIP AND COMMITMENT TO SAFETY

Any discussion about safety and organizational leadership should be anchored in an understanding of change management. Among the excellent references on this subject is a series of books by John P. Kotter of the Harvard Business School.[1] Kotter describes an eight-stage change process that is necessary for creating major transformation. These eight stages are establishing a sense of urgency, creating the guiding coalition, developing a vision and strategy, communicating the change vision, empowering broad-based action, generating short-term wins, consolidating gains and producing more change, and anchoring new approaches in the culture. One may review the list and easily determine why most organizational safety initiatives fail. They fail for the same reasons that most business initiatives fail—because they do not adequately address each of the eight stages.

Anchoring a safety program to these strategies is necessary for organizational success and requires the commitment of the hospital board of directors and hospital administration. For the individual pharmacist or medication-safety officer charged with implementing individual safety goals, the eight steps are also pertinent and should be reviewed before engaging in any new program or initiative.

If a medication-safety program is to be of value, everyone in the organization should have a knowledge and an awareness of, and a sensitivity to, patient and employee safety. However, even if the staff attend medication-safety educational programs and seminars and score high on all the subsequent competency tests, the organization will most likely not move forward if its leaders are not committed to safety. Moreover, if hospital staff do not hear and see their leaders actively involved in discussions and actions relating to safety ("Talk the talk, and walk the walk"), many will likely become frustrated and either surrender their well-meaning safety efforts or leave the organization altogether.

Patient safety should be clearly stated as an organizational goal. The hospital should have long-term strategic goals and plans related to patient safety, with accountability at the chief executive officer (CEO) level. Indeed, the CEO should have his or her own individual medication-safety objectives. Safety goals and objectives should be clearly communicated to all staff. Safety initiatives at the organizational level should be integrated into the departmental and individual yearly goals and objectives. Both organizational and individual performance should be evaluated in part on the basis of safety-related criteria.

Organizational leaders make safety a priority by being directly involved in it. Leaders should participate in committee meetings involving safety. Administrators should conduct routine patient-safety rounds during which they ask the staff about safety events, their potential causes, and how they could have been prevented.

A highly reliable organization (HRO) may be defined as one that has fewer-than-normal accidents through changes in culture. HROs operate correctly for the first time, every time, and honor the absolute avoidance of catastrophic failure. In HROs in fields other than health care, all staff members involved in potentially high-hazard activities have the ability to "push the red button," that is, to suspend operations that they perceive to be potentially hazardous. A similar policy, which allows suspension of the chain of command when a responsible staff member believes it is necessary, may be seen on aircraft carriers during takeoffs and landings. It is difficult to imagine this as a pervasive activity in the health care environment; however, the idea has enormous merit. For example, would it not be helpful if a staff pharmacist were able to stop or delay an order for chemotherapy if the appropriate staffing and expertise were unavailable for the appropriate order evaluation and safe preparation of the medication?

Organizational resources must be devoted to safety. If the self-assessment is organization-wide, one administrator should be assigned responsibility for the project and for addressing the findings. Key resources are necessary to maintain a viable safety program. A staff member should be assigned to serve as a medication-safety officer or coordinator, and a budget must be provided for safety-related education and training. Technology to improve patient safety should be routinely evaluated for potential implementation. Before large-scale facility or medication-use system changes are implemented, the leaders assess the potential impact of any planned changes on organizational resources (i.e., ensuring staff performing new technology tasks and activities are not pulled from tasks required for medication safety).

ORGANIZATIONAL CULTURE

Safety needs to be a visible initiative at all levels and across all disciplines of the organization. The organization should have a medication-safety plan and a medication-safety officer. Safety initiatives should be transparent to staff as well as to patients and the community. Publicizing and promoting safety initiatives makes a powerful statement about the level of organizational commitment.

There is a philosophical difference between risk management and risk avoidance. In other words, there is an inherent conflict between protecting the institution from liability related to the potential discoverability of released error data (*risk avoidance*) and the possible liability in not remediating system failures by disseminating institutional data to assist in identifying real and potential failure nodes through open, active dialogue (*risk management*). The practice of risk avoidance should never interfere with the management of potential risk.

Another potential source of conflict stems from use of the word *nonpunitive*. The error-reporting environment must be nonpunitive; however, the hospital environment should not necessarily be so. A hospital needs to be able to deal with matters of clear malevolence, such as directly and intentionally causing patient harm as well as engaging in illegal activities such as drug diversion. A broad nonpunitive environment may be a necessary interim step for organizations that have been perceived as taking a punitive approach to error reporters in the past. It is far more important for an organization to establish a nonpunitive reporting environment and to encourage the open and honest communication of errors than to "circle the wagons" against the far less common possibility of actual malevolent intent. Mature organizations create an environment that encourages reporting, rather than punishes reporters, and then accepts responsibility for dealing with clear ethical or practice violations. This environment might also be called a "just" environment.

In the past, health care tended to focus on the blaming and disciplining of individuals in response to an error. In more recent times, the focus has shifted to systems, to the exclusion of individuals. Now the pendulum has begun to swing back toward individual performance but from a different perspective. There are many reasons for human performance failure.[2] Table 20-2 presents cognitive system components.[3]

Table 20-2. Cognitive Systems Components[3]

Task	Intrapersonal	Organizational
• General job stress, hours worked • Interruptions, mental distractons • Number of breaks, scripts filled per hour • Task-specific tension, time counseling, time on 3rd-party paper-work, pharmacy volume, perceptions of task components	• Age, sex, job experience • Cognitive factors: cognitive capacity, focus on details, illusion/ error-prone, mental hardiness • Emotional: anxiety, depression, error worry, positive mood, tense arousal, impulsiveness, sensation seeking • Physical hardiness, resources for coping, Type A personality	• Norms: reporting error/ errors held against people • Supervisory style: encourages independence, encourages excellence, helps to establish goals • Teamwork climate
Environment • Perceptions of noise, disorderliness, lighting, equipment, and heating and A/C		**Extraorganizational** • Influences of 3rd party, BOP, manufacturers, physicians • Life changes
Interpersonal • Social life stress, other significant stress		

With respect to medication-use systems, the line between evaluating the system and the individual often becomes blurred. For example, what might be a department's course of action if a pharmacist clearly did not follow established procedures with respect to an important matter such as checking the final i.v. product against the label rather than against the original order? Would the department response be different if this pharmacist had made that error constantly, even though other staff did not? What if he or she made the error only one time—at the end of a double shift? Would pharmacy management review the procedures for double-checking and staffing guidelines, would they review the cognitive components list above for failure nodes, or would the investigation stop with the individual? Of additional importance would be the individual's response when made aware of his or her own role in a sequence of errors. Would the individual become defensive or unilaterally attempt to make changes in his or her practice to minimize the potential for future errors and then periodically reassess his or her performance? The responses to this question reflect the degree to which individual staff members have internalized the organizational culture of safety.

Interviews with staff should reveal that they see themselves as part of an environment where staff are actively encouraged to report and to discuss errors openly. Follow-up activities for medication errors are investigative in nature and are directed toward solving systems-related problems rather than assigning blame. Optimally, incentives such as rewards and recognition programs (e.g., occasions where hospital administrators publicly present gift cards or coupons to staff) are provided to those who consistently report errors, report important errors, or demonstrate the greatest improvement in the frequency of reporting. Some hospitals have minimal error-reporting requirements for staff as part of performance evaluations.

If a staff member is involved in an error that has caused significant patient harm, he or she may need to be removed, at least temporarily, from direct clinical responsibilities. The organization should find a place for such an individual to work within the hospital and ensure that he or she receives peer support. These staff could be assigned to work on the overall hospital medication-safety program with responsibilities for analyzing error- or event-related data. Who understands failure nodes within the medication-use system better than someone who has been victimized by it (i.e., the person who happened to be closest to an error and therefore is blamed for it, even though the error could have been prevented at any of several steps earlier in the medication-use process)? Supervisors should also ensure that such staff members receive emotional support from the facility's employee assistance program.

The organization needs to take an active interest in self-improvement related to safety. As an example, the hospital may have used the ISMP self-assessment tool as part of an organizational self-improvement program. Ideally, it will then continue to use the tool to benchmark its current position and perform a yearly self-assessment to determine areas of progress as well as areas requiring attention.

Safety initiatives are multidisciplinary by nature, with committees and project teams containing representatives from key departments and clinical areas. Pharmacy, nursing, and medical staff orientation and safety-education programs should also be multidisciplinary. During orientation, each discipline should spend time in the pharmacy department and on patient care areas, rounding with the other disciplines, or participating in mentoring programs. Ideally, each discipline will become more familiar with the interfaces among the disciplines as well as with their unique roles and responsibilities related to the medication-use system.

Safety activities and expectations should extend to patients, their families, and other hospital customers (e.g., vendors). Patients should be educated routinely upon admission to assist health care professionals with proper identification by showing staff their name bracelets or other form of identification and by stating their names clearly before medications are administered or treatments performed. Patients should be instructed on when and whom to call if they have questions about their drug therapy or any other issue after discharge.

Formal medication-error and safety education should occur not only at the time of orientation but also on a routine basis. Communications relating to errors and medication safety need to be a routine part of staff meetings. It is useful to discuss both internal and external error sources. External error reports may be especially important for organizations that are trying for the first time to create a nonpunitive environment and staff are still reluctant to discuss errors. External sources include newspaper reports, *ISMP Medication Safety Alerts*, JCAHO sentinel event reports, and other safety-related publications and news items. Posting these documents in break or lounge areas can be an effective way to initiate discussion.

Also important to communications is the manner in which the organization and staff deal with intimidation and conflict resolution. Incredibly, the March 11, 2004 issue of the *ISMP Medication Safety Alert* reported that 88 percent of survey respondents experienced intimidating behavior within the past year and 7 percent reported that they had been involved in an error in the past year in which intimidation had played a role.[4] Organizations can assist their hospital and medical staff by providing effective training in communication and decision making in dynamic environments. One example of such training is the aviation-based Crew Resource Management (CRM) training.[5] All health care providers should have a clear, easy, and effective path to follow to resolve conflicts when prescribers or supervisors do not agree with their concerns about the safety of an order.

MEDICATION-SAFETY TEAMS

Every institution, regardless of size, should have a multidisciplinary medication-safety team.

At a minimum, a pharmacist and nurse should review error reports and provide recommenda-tions to the reporting body, which may be the P&T committee, the medication-safety com-mittee, quality-assurance committee, or similar body. In larger institutions with greater re-sources, the ideal team components should include a risk manager, a representative from hospital administration, information systems, and a patient or consumer representative. Phy-sicians are a necessary component of the team, but may be used in an ad hoc capacity. Critical needs for the medication-safety team include adequate staffing and appropriate support from hospital administration.

TECHNOLOGY

New technologies, such as point-of-care, machine-readable coding for drug administration, computerized prescriber order entry (CPOE), and robotics, must be assessed with regard to their impact on medication safety.

As part of an overall self-assessment, the organization should make a formal effort to identify medication-use-system failure nodes and rank them in order of priority. Once it has done this, the organization can select technology and decide how best to use it. This entails the following six steps:

1. Process map the segment of the medication-use system to be evaluated.

2. Identify and evaluate medication-use system failure nodes that have been revealed by error reporting or other methods.

3. Prioritize the degree of risk (i.e., the frequency and severity of error or potential error) associated with each failure node.

4. Identify which type or types of technology or processes would best improve the failure node.

5. Gather baseline and postimplementation data around the failure node in order to measure the impact of the technology or process change.

6. Prioritize and allocate resources.

Technologies can produce, as well as prevent, error. The potential for a particular tech-nology to induce or propagate error, either directly or indirectly, should be assessed prior to their implementation. Failure mode and effects analysis (FMEA) is an effective means to ac-complish this task. Questions to ask include the following:

• Will new technologies require additional steps (e.g., processes, interfaces) to make them compatible?

• How will bedside bar-code verification affect the pharmacy order-entry process?

• Will the new CPOE system require staff to reenter orders because it is not compat-ible with the current pharmacy information system?

• Will computer software or hardware upgrades or changes be made during busy or-der-entry times?

• Will automated dispensing cabinets be filled during busy medication administration times?

• How would the medication-use system function during a catastrophic electrical or computer failure?

The possibility of competition for technology resources must be addressed. Several sites have attempted to introduce multiple technologies simultaneously, without regard to resource competition. They fail to recognize that technology implementation and operation often use unbudgeted staff and require that staff be pulled from patient care areas or other critical tasks. Facilities also need to determine how many staff will be needed and what levels of expertise they will require following implementation.

It is also important to determine whether existing technologies are being used to their optimal effect. For example, does the hospital maintain multiple i.v. drug delivery or patient-controlled analgesia (PCA) devices or automated drug-dispensing devices? Does the hospital attempt to maintain both unit dose carts and automated drug-delivery devices as primary drug-delivery systems? One common area of concern relates to order communication. Often, multiple technologies (e.g., phone, facsimile, hand-carried, courier, digital) are employed to communicate medication orders from the patient care area to the pharmacy.

ASHP has a number of guidelines that might assist in this evaluation. Available at www.ashp.org, they include the following:

- ASHP Technical Assistance Bulletin on Hospital Drug Distribution and Control
- ASHP Discussion Guide for Compounding Sterile Preparations
- ASHP Guidelines on Quality Assurance for Pharmacy-Prepared Sterile Products
- ASHP Guidelines on Preventing Medication Errors with Antineoplastic Agents
- ASHP Technical Assistance Bulletin on Handling Cytotoxic and Hazardous Drugs
- ASHP Technical Assistance Bulletin on Compounding Nonsterile Products in Pharmacies
- ASHP Technical Assistance Bulletin on Pharmacy-Prepared Ophthalmic Products
- ASHP Guidelines on the Safe Use of Automated Compounding Devices for the Preparation of Parenteral Nutrition Admixtures
- Safe Practices for Parenteral Nutrition Formulations

Another tool is the American Hospital Association publication AHA Strategies for Leadership: Assessing Bedside Bar-Coding Readiness (http://www.medpathways.info/medpathways/tools/content/Section_3.pdf). In addition, the California HealthCare Foundation (http://www.chcf.org/) has several publications on CPOE, including Computerized Physician Order Entry in Community Hospitals: Lessons from the Field, a CPOE fact sheet, and A Primer on Physician Order Entry.

Another critical part of the technology assessment is to determine whether employees have been adequately trained on the new technology. This includes not only current employees but also new staff, temporary staff, and on-call staff. Seemingly small oversights in training may produce a major impact on hospital services. For example, one hospital that had just implemented an electronic order-transfer system failed to train the staff of two critical-care units on its appropriate use. In particular, the use and exact placement of the "stat" sticker on order forms containing stat orders prior to scanning was not communicated. As a result, the scanned orders containing stat orders were put on the same list as routine orders were. Nurses were frustrated and blamed the pharmacy staff for their order delays. The pharmacists, who were not involved in the nursing training sessions, were angry at the nursing staff for repeatedly calling to check on the status of the scanned orders. The additional calls generated by nursing (averaging two or three per shift for about 200 nurses) cost each department more than eight hours daily in phone time. There is no telling the number of additional errors produced by the telephone interruptions and distractions to both departments. This incident also points out the need for postimplementation follow-up to ensure that new processes and systems work as expected.

PHARMACY AND THERAPEUTICS COMMITTEE AND FORMULARY FUNCTIONS

P&T committee functions are covered well elsewhere[6,7] and will not be outlined here. The formulary should be a strong and robust. Practitioners should be able to easily determine the formulary status of any agent. Though it is a good practice to limit the formulary for both safety and cost reasons, this is not always feasible, given the impact of local payer formularies and the limited staff available to address each nonformulary drug order.

All drugs that are on the formulary, or being considered for it, should be assessed for error potential and risk. This potential for errors and adverse events may be secondary to system failures due to look-alike or sound-alike, packaging, labeling, or dosing confusion. A literature and Internet search (e.g., www.ISMP.com) should be performed to identify and evaluate previous error reports relating to the product. Duplication of generic or therapeutically equivalent agents should be minimized or avoided.

An interdisciplinary committee (either the P&T committee or a subcommittee) should use FMEA to assess new drugs being considered for the formulary. A detailed health care FMEA (HFMEA™) approach may be found on the Department of Veterans Affairs Web site. Such a process[8-12] might include the following steps:

Step 1. The committee explores how the product would be procured and used, from acquisition through administration. Who would prescribe the drug, and for what type of patient? Where would the drug be stored? Who would prepare and dispense it? How would it be administered?

Step 2. Potential failure modes are identified. Could the drug be mistaken for another similarly packaged product? Does the label clearly express the strength or concentration? Does the name sound or look like that of a drug already on the formulary? Are dosing instructions complex? Is the administration process error-prone?

Step 3. The committee determines the likelihood of making a mistake and the potential consequences of an error. What would happen if the drug were given in the wrong dose, at the wrong time, to the wrong patient, by the wrong route, or at the wrong rate?

Step 4. Staff identify any processes already in place that could help detect the error before it reaches the patient and evaluate the effectiveness of these processes.

Step 5. If failure modes could cause errors with significant consequences, the committee outlines actions that would be taken to prevent the error, detect it before it reaches the patient, or minimize its consequences. Examples include using an alternative product; preparing the drug in the pharmacy; standardizing drug concentrations, order communication, and dosing methods; using auxiliary warning labels or computer alerts; and requiring entry of specific data into computer systems before processing orders.

Acceptance of formulary requests must be justified on the basis of specific criteria (e.g., "Patient stable on medication at home with no comparable existing formulary agent," "Failed therapy or adverse events with existing comparable formulary agent"). Nonformulary request forms should be in place and used effectively. The hospital and medical staff should understand both the safety and cost impact of a nonformulary request. Nonformulary requests should be summarized by practitioner and by drug and reported at each P&T committee meeting.

If such a medication is approved for inclusion on the formulary, the safety issues addressed should be the same as those reviewed before the use of any agent. Safety measures such as order forms, guidelines, check systems, reminders, limitations or restrictions on use, administration, and storage should be established before any drugs with potential safety problems are used. Questions to be asked include the following: Once a nonformulary agent is allowed into the pharmacy department, how will it be sequestered and controlled? How will staff be notified of potential safety concerns for nonformulary agents and new agents prior to release and of new safety concerns for existing agents?

The P&T committee should also play a role in evaluating drug-delivery devices for safety. Limiting the types of syringe pumps, infusion pumps, and PCA pumps, as well as ensuring that a FMEA has been performed, are important committee functions.

Product lines in a hospital pharmacy often change rapidly. This may be due to changes in availability resulting from product shortages or to shifting wholesaler product lines. Changes in contracts or in item availability may create an opening for a safety problem to enter the medication-use system. For instance, when a contract changes, a hospital's entire generic line may change. These generic items may all look similar as a means of gaining brand recognition and loyalty but may create inadvertent safety issues because of look-alike products with sound-alike names. A strategy to address potential safety issues that may arise during product shortages and changes is necessary. The strategy must include timely communication plans, reasonable evaluation of potential substitutes, and stocking and labeling procedures for new look-alike and sound-alike products. Product differences may also require changes in dosing, preparation, administration, and monitoring procedures that must be communicated to staff members.

Appropriate safety measures must be in place for any drugs with previously reported or perceived safety issues. Also needed is a procedure for unusual circumstances, such as the emergent admission of a patient on immunosuppressant transplant drugs in a hospital that does not perform transplants.

All drugs should undergo a routine evaluation period after being added to the formulary. If a physician requests a new product for the formulary, he or she should be involved with monitoring and subsequent reporting to the committee. If monitoring needs to be done, medication-use evaluation criteria should be in place before the drug is released for use.

Vendors need to understand their roles in medication safety, and the hospital can take a lead role in this educational process. This may be done, for example, by creating an introductory vendor packet that defines the safety responsibilities of vendors. Many hospitals provide vendors with written information regarding hospital security badges, floor plan, key contacts, formulary processes, visiting rules, general rules of conduct, and information on scheduling appointments. Vendor guidelines and controls, and the hospital's role in responding to those who violate them, should be clearly defined in such information packets. Vendor disciplinary actions should be handled by the P&T committee, which is a committee of the medical staff, rather than by the pharmacy alone.

Medication samples should be not be stored in an acute-care institution. If physician or clinic offices are located within the hospital and if medication samples are kept in these areas, they should be subject to the same assessments and actions of medication safety as are other nonformulary agents. Vendors should be instructed on the rules governing appointments, restricted areas of the hospital, and sample medications. They should be required to sign an agreement to abide by the rules, and disciplinary action should be taken against those who intentionally violate them.

Internal and external reports of medication-safety issues should be made routinely to the P&T committee. Once an issue has been reported to it, the committee must initiate procedures to improve patient safety by eliminating a drug or drug package, initiating or modifying protocols or guidelines, or initiating or changing the physician's privilege to prescribe specific agents.

COMMUNICATION

Two types of communication plans need to be developed in association with a self-assessment. The purpose of the first type of plan is to inform staff about the self-assessment project, medication-safety initiatives, potential high-hazard areas and potential solutions, and information gathered from the error-reporting program. Internal department communication plans should be developed and implemented for issues relevant to specific departments or areas. Part-time, on-call, and temporary or agency employees should be included in the communication plan, as should patients, families, vendors, and community members.

A second type of communication plan is required when serious events occur and a chain of communication is required to rapidly notify caregivers and managers so that they may continue to appropriately care for their patients, administrators and risk managers for public relations and liability purposes, and human resources staff. The plan should include detailed guidance on what information to disclose and when.

ERROR REPORTING AND ANALYSIS

Hospital leaders must directly and visibly encourage error reporting. They may do this through administrative walk-arounds, reward or recognition programs for error reporting, or other activities. The hospital board of directors should receive error and safety reports on an ongoing basis. The process flow for error reporting, ownership, investigation, analysis, and data reporting should be clearly defined.

In most hospitals, nursing and pharmacy personnel generate most of the event reports. All types of professional staff (e.g., physicians, pharmacists, nurses, radiology, physical therapy, laboratory, i.v. team) and nonprofessional staff involved in the medication-use system (e.g., pharmacy technicians, unit clerks, couriers) should participate in error reporting. Their various perspectives provide a rich source of information relative to error cause and prevention.

The policy and procedure for medication-error reporting should describe what type of event is to be reported, how reporting should be performed, follow-up steps (e.g., participation in an investigation and RCA), and appropriate notification when patient harm has occurred. Error reporting and analysis needs to be a robust system that ensures that problems are addressed with an action plan and monitored to ensure the problems have been addressed.

Multiple sources of safety-event data should be reviewed for potential common root causes and for latent system failures. Sources of such data include adverse drug event reports (including tracer drug or laboratory reports), e-code reports, medication-error reports, quality assurance or sentinel event reports, pharmacy clinical interventions, i.v. therapy reports, unit dose cart-fill errors, MAR reconciliation reports, and radiology, laboratory, and dietary reports. Table 20-3 summarizes data from one year's event reporting at a hospital. In this institution, each type of event was reported through a different reporting system, usually residing in a different department. The hospital administration knew of the rare sentinel events but was unaware of the larger body of data representing potential risks to the organization. The hospital did not centrally capture any data relative to errors in other areas, such as MAR reconciliation data, and cart-fill and automated-dispensing-device drawer-fill errors, that caused no patient harm.

Table 20-3. Summary of Events Reported at One Hospital during One Year

Number of Events	Type of Event
2–3	Sentinel event
112	Adverse drug event
3,595	Medication error
3,095	Clinical intervention
73,000–109,500	Phone call for missing doses

One matter of concern is that errors occurring in laboratory, dietary, or radiology that were secondary to patient identification would not be captured or analyzed in the error database. Events reported in just one department might not be perceived to be as serious as those revealed in multiple departments.

For the same reason, "minor errors," that is, those that do not propagate to the patient or do not cause patient harm, should be reported to the same database. Potential errors or "near misses" (National Coordinating Counsel for Medication Error Reporting and Prevention [NCC MERP] categories A through D) are often considered less important than those events that cause harm. Some committees choose not to review them and thus lose valuable opportunities to identify potential failures in the medication-use system before a significant patient event actually occurs. JCAHO standards state that the organization must identify and address these errors as "any process variation that did not affect the outcome but for which a recurrence carries a significant chance of a serious adverse outcome."

When an error or a potential error is discovered, it should be quickly reported. The reporter should have no fear of disciplinary action or reprisal. The reporting form or system should be easy to use; it must also capture the data required for analysis. It is useful if reporting can be done by multiple methods (e.g., computer, hard copy, phone transcription). Reported data should be entered into the system in a timely fashion. Ideally, the data are entered into a program with drop-down boxes to minimize data-entry errors. Data should be entered and reviewed by key personnel who are knowledgeable about medications and medication-error taxonomy.

The reporting system should be able to capture all error-related events, and all error data should reside in a single data system that can easily analyze the data for common system weaknesses. Communications systems should ensure that current events that have caused, or have a significant possibility of causing, patient harm can be quickly routed to clinical staff, the medication-safety team, risk management staff, and hospital administration.

A completed medication-error report should be accessible to unit managers so that they might (1) ensure proper patient management, (2) initiate support for the involved staff (e.g., referral to an employee assistance program), (3) investigate the event to determine its root cause, and (4) undertake unit-based changes to reduce future error risk, but not for disciplinary purposes. Ideally, the report should be electronically routed so that the unit manager, the medication-safety team and data-entry individual, and risk-management staff can see it immediately. Comments and edits can be added as an electronic appendage, but only a small group of people should have "write" access to the original data files.

If the hospital has not made the successful transition to a nonpunitive reporting culture, it might be best if the medication-error reporting system is not used in this type of notification process. If the reporting system is ever used to initiate disciplinary action, voluntary reporting will cease and the system will be of no value.

Another common problem with error-reporting systems is failure to use standardized nomenclature such as the NCC MERP medication-error taxonomy. From a process-improvement perspective, it is essential to have shared definitions for any processes that will be evaluated. As an example, different professionals have their own definitions of medication turn-around time. Pharmacy typically defines it as the time between the moment that the pharmacy receives the order and the time the medication is sent to the patient. Nursing might define it as the time between when the order is sent to pharmacy and the time the nurse receives the medication on the unit. Others might define it as the time between writing of the order and administering the medication to the patient. It is important to define the process and subprocesses being examined within the medication-use system. Some hospitals use process-flow mapping to enable staff to gain agreement on various process steps and key definitions. Information on this technique is readily available on the Internet.

A multidisciplinary committee should routinely review and analyze medication safety and error data from both internal and external sources (e.g., *ISMP Medication Safety Alert*, news stories, published reports), identify potential system-based causes of error, develop strategies to address these causes, and coordinate strategy implementation. The committee should also evaluate failure points identified by error reporting or other methods; prioritize by risk (frequency and severity of error or potential error), identify which type of technology or process would best correct the at-risk system failure point, and gather baseline and postimplementation data around the failure node being corrected in order to measure impact and success, with an eye toward the appropriate allocation of resources. In addition, the organization should appoint one individual who will be responsible for medication-safety activities.

Ideally, practitioners directly involved in significant medication errors should participate in the investigation, analysis, and development of recommendations.

Discussions of medication events should be a regular agenda item for P&T committees. The committee should see a variety of event-related data, such as medication-error and adverse drug reaction reports, accounts of clinical interventions, illegible order reports, and requests for nonformulary items.

RCA should be promptly performed on events that caused harm or that have the potential to cause harm. All failure points (primary, intermediate, and terminal) in the medication-use system that contributed to the error should be evaluated.

On an ongoing basis, hospital and medical staff should receive safety information feedback about the type and frequency of errors, high-alert drugs or situations, and recent initiatives. Patient care units or departments that have created medication-safety initiatives should be encouraged to share their experiences with other units. As an example, if one unit develops a poster designed to alert staff to certain look-alike products, it should be shared with other units and the issue should be addressed housewide.

PREPARATION OF SENTINEL EVENT POLICIES

A *sentinel event* is an unexpected occurrence involving death or serious physical or psychological injury, or the risk thereof. Serious injury specifically includes loss of limb or function. The phrase "or the risk thereof" includes any process variation for which a recurrence would carry a significant chance of a serious adverse outcome. Such events are called "sentinel" because they signal the need for immediate investigation and response (Sentinel Event Policy And Procedures. Revised July 2002. Available at: www.jcaho.org/accredited+organizations/sentinel+event/se_pp.htm).

There are various levels of sentinel events, each of which requires a clearly defined policy and procedure outlining responsibilities, actions, and follow-up. Every hospital should be prepared for these events. Early missteps may give the public the impression that the hospital is trying to cover up the event or may prevent the preservation of equipment or documentation that might later exonerate the facility.

A good sentinel event policy defines

- who is responsible for securing and sequestering all goods (e.g., labels, pumps, syringes, wraps), documents, and records in a timely manner;
- how equipment, labels, preparations, and documentation should be sequestered labeled and managed;
- the appropriate public relations response;
- notification of the hospital insurance carrier;
- guidelines for providing patient and family care, support, information (patient disclosure), and counseling;

- a plan describing how the involved employee(s) will be handled, including provision for counseling, placement on administrative leave, or assignment to nonclinical activities such as event investigation and RCA; and

- periodic practice runs and postpractice run evaluations in different hospital locations and for various scenarios (e.g., medication, pump failure, surgery, patient fall).

Developing an Action Plan and Time Line

At the end of an assessment, the institution finds itself faced with a list of newly identified problems. The project team must now develop an action plan and time line to begin to tackle these problems. At this point, Kotter's eight-stage change process should be reviewed.[1] As these eight stages are being addressed, the project team should begin to prioritize the identified problem areas.

The team may find it valuable to list the problem areas and potential strategies to address each problem. Individual team members may want to rank each problem in terms of its potential for harm and to evaluate proposed solutions in terms of ease of implementation. Problems that have little potential for harm and would cost a great deal in terms of money, staff time, or technology should be deferred. For maximum impact, it is often helpful to begin by focusing on solutions that promise early, short-term wins. The following is an example of how this process might be done.

The strategies are listed and then assigned two values: one for potential harm and another for difficulty in implementation. These assignments can be made by each member of the team or by the team as a whole. The product of these values may be used to loosely assign a rank order for prioritization. The prioritized list is then presented to the entire project team for validation.

The project team should also define criteria defining potential harm, frequency, and degree of difficulty of implementation. An example of some of the criteria that might be used to define potential harm might be similar to those used by the Veterans Administration (http://www.patientsafety.gov/HFMEA.html):

4—Catastrophic Event (FMEA rating 10). Failure could cause death or injury.

3—Major Event (FMEA rating 7). Failure causes a high degree of customer dissatisfaction.

2—Moderate Event (FMEA rating 4). Failure can be overcome with modifications to the process or product, but there is minor performance loss.

1—Minor Event (FMEA rating 1). Failure would not be noticeable to the customer and would not affect delivery of the service or product.

Error frequency may be defined using HFMEA criteria such as these:

4—Frequent. Likely to occur immediately or within a short period (may happen several times a year).

3—Occasional. Probably will occur (may happen several times in 1 to 2 years).

2—Uncommon. Possible to occur (may happen sometime in 2 to 5 years).

1—Remote. Unlikely to occur (may happen sometime in 5 to 30 years).

Finally, the team should determine how difficult or easy the criteria will be to implement. Criteria might include expense, staff resources, multiple departments, ability to establish buy-in from key constituents, and total time to completion. Examples of these criteria are as follows:

4—Easy to Implement. Low expense, internal to department, low staff resources.

3—Somewhat Difficult. Requires no or little funding, few people from one to two departments, or low level of staff resources.

2—Moderately Difficult. Requires budgeted funding, multiple departments, or moderate staff resource commitment.

1—Very Difficult. Requires substantial funding, multiple departments, or high staff resource commitment.

The completed list of strategies with accompanying scoring might look like **Table 20-4**, with a priority value calculated by the product of the severity, frequency, and implementation difficulty scores.

Table 20-4. Results of Analysis and Prioritization of Error-Reduction Strategies

Item #	Strategy	Severity	Frequency	Severity x Frequency	Difficulty	Priority Value
1	Remove concentrated potassium chloride from patient care units.	4	2	8	4	32
2	Establish periodic wakening as part of continuous sedation protocol.	3	4	12	3	36
4	Dose confusion. Place recommended maximum dose ranges on all order forms with high-alert medications.	2	3	6	2	12
5	Look-alike, sound-alike picking errors. Relabel pharmacy stock areas with boldface and "tall-man" lettering to identify look-alike and sound-alike medications.	1	4	4	3	12
3	Prescriber errors. Implement CPOE system.	1	4	4	1	4

Another way to encourage discussion about prioritization is to use graphic representations (see **Figure 20-1**). In this case, the product of the severity and frequency scores is graphed against the difficulty of implementing proposed solutions. Strategies falling in the upper-right quadrant should be among the first scheduled for implementation, because they have the highest potential risk to the organization and are the easiest to implement. Strategies with the lowest risk and the greatest difficulty in implementation appear in the lower-left quadrant and should be scheduled for later implementation.

As part of the communication plan, the list of strategies should be shared with other staff, and their input regarding prioritization should be sought. It is especially important to share these discussions with individuals who are in positions to be either critical obstacles or enablers. Gathering buy-in from key constituents at this phase can dramatically increase the probability for project success.

Once the team has created a prioritized list, it is time to establish a project time line. The time line should consist of key milestones or accomplishments. The action plan and time line should be widely shared, and key individuals on the project team should be held responsible for meeting the key milestones and interim goals.

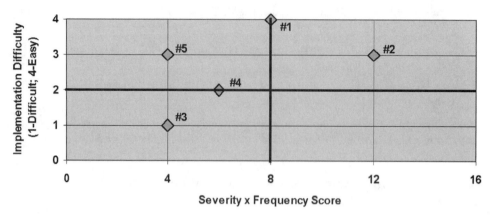

Figure 20-1. *Prioritization of Implementation Strategies*

Many organizations erroneously perceive that technology will solve all of their problems. Most safety technologies will take a substantial investment in terms of money, staff time, and political capital. If the project team leads its solution list with technology and the technology implementation goes poorly or does not cause a perceivable reduction in the errors that were trying to be prevented, its ability to implement further safety initiatives will be endangered. It is better to consider a prioritization strategy such as that described above, which will provide some short-term wins. This will build the political capital needed to implement those strategies that will weigh heavily on other departments, such as the medical staff with CPOE systems or the nursing staff with bedside bar-code systems.

Monitoring and Periodic Reassessment

Measurable and attainable goals are an important part of the action plan. The value of a measurable goal is that it enables one to determine when it has been achieved. Once met, goals should be celebrated.

Ongoing monitoring is also essential. Systems that are not monitored will rapidly return to their previous state. Measurable goals can ensure that the strategy put into place has (1) met the intended goal, (2) continues to meet the intended goal, and (3) does not produce new and unintended errors. This being said, it is essential to keep the measures simple and straightforward. One should measure only what is needed to determine compliance or success. Monitoring for the sake of monitoring is a waste of resources. Asking for too much data or too much detail will cause "paralysis by analysis," resulting in a team that can never meet project goals because it is always waiting for "just one more piece of data."

One valuable method of reassessment is repeating the original assessment. As an example, if the 2004 ISMP Medication Safety Self Assessment® for Hospitals was used for the initial assessment, the hospital could repeat the process using the same tool and compare the answers and scoring to determine where more action is required, where action has improved the scores, and where scores have fallen.

Summary

This chapter has presented a brief overview of how to perform a medication-safety self-assessment, an organized approach to identifying and addressing medication-safety issues. It has also reviewed several frequently identified problem areas within hospital medication-use systems. Many individuals and organizations that have long sought to make medication safety an integral part of professional practice are available to provide assistance in self-assessment and overall medication-safety efforts. As a hospital moves toward its safety goals, staff should be encouraged to seek information in a wide variety of areas, including the safety and change leadership literature outside of health care. They should also participate in the many seminars, workshops, and learning communities that are now available on the subject. Several schools of pharmacy now offer courses in medication safety, and Web-based programs will be available soon.

Finally, an action plan should be developed for addressing the identified initiatives. The plan should define the specific strategy, individual steps, prioritization, a time line and interim milestones, and champions.

In summary, the key steps in performing a medication-safety self-assessment would minimally include the following:

1. Determine project scope and objectives.

2. Engage administrators, managers, and other key stakeholders.

3. Form a multidisciplinary team.

4. Develop a communication plan to share information on the project and issue periodic updates.

5. Identify and define the nature of the problem or problems.

6. Perform an assessment and analysis.

7. Review findings.

8. Develop an action plan and time line.

9. Identify measurable metrics to gauge and sustain change.

10. Celebrate and communicate wins.

References

1. Kotter JP. *Leading Change*. Boston: Harvard Business School Press; 1996.

2. Institute for Safe Medication Practices. Insights into people will improve our safety system. *ISMP Safety Alert!* 2001;6(13):1-2.

3. Grasha A. A Cognitive Systems Perspective on Human Performance in the Pharmacy: Implications for Accuracy, Effectiveness and Job Satisfaction. Executive Summary Report. Report No. 062100. Alexandria, VA: National Association of Chain Drug Stores; October 2000.

4. Institute for Safe Medication Practices. Intimidation: practitioners speak up about this unresolved problem (part I). *ISMP Medication Safety Alert!* 2004;9(5):1-3.

5. Agency for Health Research and Quality. Making Health Care Safer: A Critical Analysis of Patient Safety Practice. Evidence Report/Technology Assessment No. 43. Publication No. 01-E059. Rockville, MD: AHRQ; July 2001. Available at: www.ahcpr.gov/clinic/tp/ptsaftp.htm. Accessed December 27, 2004.

6. American Society of Health-System Pharmacists. Principles of a Sound Drug Formulary System. Bethesda, MD: ASHP: 2000. Available at: www.ashp.org/bestpractices/formulary-mgmt/Form_End_Principles.pdf. Accessed December 27, 2004.

7. Quintiliani R, Quercia RA. How to create a therapeutics committee that is scientifically and economically sound. *Formulary* 2003;38:594–602.

8. Cohen MR, Davis NM, Senders J. Failure mode and effects analysis: a novel approach to avoiding dangerous medication errors and accidents. *Hosp Pharm.* 1994;29:319-324.

9. Williams E, Talley R. The use of failure mode effect and criticality analysis in a medication error subcommittee. *Hosp Pharm.* 1994;29:331-337.

10. Senders JW, Senders SJ. Failure mode and effects analysis in medicine. In: Cohen M, ed. *Medication Errors: Causes, Prevention and Risk Management.* Washington, DC: American Pharmacy Association; 1999.

11. Joint Commission on Accreditation of Healthcare Organizations. Sentinel Event Alert. No. 16. Oak Brook Terrace, IL: JCAHO; 2001. Available at: www.jcaho.org/about+us/news+letters/sentinel+event+alert/sea_16.htm. Accessed December 27, 2004.

12. National Council for Patient Safety. The Basics of Healthcare Failure Mode and Effect Analysis. Ann Arbor, MI: VHA National Center for Patient Safety; 2001. http://www.va.gov/ncps/HFMEAIntro.doc. Accessed December 20, 2004.

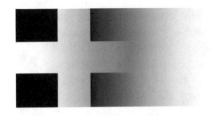

CHAPTER 21

Characteristics of High-Reliability Organizations

Henri R. Manasse, Jr., and
Kasey K. Thompson

Introduction

Elsewhere in this volume, Turnbull discusses several key characteristics of high-reliability organizations. The author highlights major cultural and practical paradigm shifts that will be essential if health care is to transform from its present, antiquated culture of hierarchy, fragmentation, blame, and opacity to a culture of flexible authority structures, integrative systems thinking, "justness," and transparent exchange of information. The purpose of this chapter is to elaborate on these principles, provide examples of how they have been applied in other industries, and demonstrate the feasibility and urgency of applying high-reliability theory to the medication-use process.

Intrinsic Hazard, Obsession with Safety, and Near-Errorfree Performance

Technology has now advanced to the point where the consequences of mechanical or human failure can be profoundly harmful, even lethal, to people, resources, and natural environments. This fact, reinforced by the hard lessons gained from numerous accidents, has engendered a commitment to safe systems design on the parts of such industries as the military, commercial aviation and air traffic control, space travel, petroleum refining and shipping, and nuclear energy production. In an environment where a defective sensor, a misread gauge, or a misinterpreted verbal instruction can result in a collision of aircraft or the release of dangerous chemicals into nature, it is incumbent on the organizations controlling these processes to adopt safeguards to avoid the disastrous consequences of errors.

These and other industries have applied learning about complexity and accident theory to a far greater degree than the health care services sector has done to date. The approaches and solutions developed so far in this relatively new branch of scientific and industrial inquiry cannot, of course, be imported wholesale into the medication-use process. We know that clinical practice is an art as well as a science, that hospitals are not factories, and that no two patients can be expected to have the same therapeutic needs or outcomes. However, we should candidly examine the way we do our work—and the way we view and interact with each other—to adapt whatever principles we can from our counterparts in other industries that have transformed their organizations into cultures that are just, trusting, preoccupied with safety, and committed to continual learning and operational refinement and have attained startlingly low error rates as a result.

319

A 2001 study by Singer et al.[1] helps demonstrate the gulf between health care and high reliability. Thousands of hospital workers (including physicians, nurses, and executives) and thousands of naval aviators responded to a survey asking for their perceptions of the presence, or absence, of a "safety culture" in their workplaces. Asked to agree or disagree with the statement, "Management provides adequate safety backups to catch possible human errors during high-risk activities," 23.7 percent of the hospital personnel disagreed while only 2.7 of the pilots disagreed. Similarly, the statement, "Management has a clear picture of the risks associated with [the organization's] operations," elicited a 21.9 percent disagreement rate from hospital personnel but only a 1.9 percent disagreement from aviators. The difference in error rates between the two disciplines is reflective of this disparity in cultures: While adverse medical events are estimated to happen in at least 3 percent to 4 percent of U.S hospitalizations, the rate of accidents among naval aviators is a staggeringly low 1.5 per 100,000 hours flown.

Pharmacists know that medications and the environments in which they are used are intrinsically unsafe. They know and appreciate that drug therapy is an invasive procedure, not simply the ingestion or injection of a "magic bullet" that cures disease and disappears without any residual effect. The number of medications on the market has increased, as have the potency and complexity of therapy, as evidenced by such innovations as biologicals and antineoplastic agents. The systems in which these potent medications are used have increased in complexity as well, with the introduction of new, and often un-integrated, technologies such as computerized prescriber order entry, bar coding, automated compounding devices, robots, and electronic decision support.

Intrinsic Complexity

High-reliability organizations are designed to accommodate highly complex operations, where the components of a system or process, or even the environments in which they operate, may interact in ways that are not intended or intuitive, to produce unexpected, undesirable outcomes. We have acknowledged that a number of factors contribute to the complexity of medication use (the nature of drugs and therapeutics, information technologies, etc.). However, we have not designed our systems to accommodate and compensate for those complexities. Instead, we have superimposed new layers of complexity onto existing systems. Moreover, we have not designed systems with a mindfulness of the effects of such seemingly trivial, but in fact quite essential, system elements as the physical environment and the competing personal and professional demands that affect human performance.

Consider this scenario: A new pharmacist is hired and scheduled to be trained in the room where intravenous (i.v.) products are prepared. On the day she is to be trained, the i.v. room supervisor, who also happens to coordinate staff training and competency assessment, has a family emergency that requires her to miss work. Coincidentally, that same morning, the most experienced i.v. technician is having car trouble and is delayed a few hours. So, at the last minute, less-experienced staff from other areas in the department are mobilized to cover the i.v. room. None of them recognizes that the newly hired pharmacist has not been adequately trained to work in that particular i.v. room; they assume that she is sufficiently competent and understands the organization's policies and procedures. Therefore, she is expected, without training, to "pitch in" as a member of the team. The new pharmacist has reservations about working untrained in the i.v. room, but she does not express them for fear that her new colleagues will perceive her as a complainer or someone who is not a team player. Inadvertently, an environment has been created where an error is apt to occur, through a cascade of unforeseen interactions among system elements whose interrelatedness is unrecognized.

Expecting the Unexpected

It is unlikely that the individual responsible for scheduling training for the new pharmacist would have anticipated any of the events just described. Nonetheless, a medication error and consequent adverse drug event could easily occur as a consequence of the above scenario— events that could have been prevented by better coordination between staff training and staff scheduling, by appropriate introductions of the new pharmacist to the other pharmacy personnel who were reassigned to the i.v. room that day, or by ensuring that more than one staff member was available to provide training in the i.v. room. These kinds of safeguards and redundancies are regularly built into high-reliability operations in an effort to "expect the unexpected" and to mitigate the effects of unintended system interactions.

Like any modern industry, health care is planned and provided in a "universe" where a vast number of systems and subsystems coexist and interact with each other and with their surroundings. We sometimes can and sometimes cannot anticipate their interactions in advance; sometimes, we cannot even comprehend them as we watch their consequences unfold. Electrical power supplies, water and air-sanitation systems, computers and computer networks, electronic and written communications systems, paper files, interpersonal and intraorganizational structures, pharmacy automation, drug inventory supply and management factors, weather conditions—all converge to determine the outcomes of our efforts to provide safe and effective therapies.

Anytime we superimpose one set of processes and resources upon another, we add complexity. As complexity increases within a system, so does the potential that things *will* go wrong, despite our efforts to anticipate every eventuality. If we think otherwise, we willfully depart from reality, and we fail to uphold our professional imperative to do our patients no harm.

The nuclear power industry has learned this reality the hard way, and transformed itself accordingly. The Diablo Canyon Power Plant in central California was plagued by design problems and regulatory violations during its first years of construction and operation. Since then, the facility has transformed its professional culture into one of active and diligent learning and a healthy respect for the unknown and unknowable potentials for danger associated with nuclear energy. The organization screens new employees on the basis of how creatively they can think and adapt to the reality that, in a complex system, the unexpected will occasionally occur.[3]

Communication

The medication-use process in a hospital can be viewed as one of many subsystems that function within the broader, organization-wide system of care delivery. Pharmacists play a vital role in ensuring safety and quality in all steps of the medication-use process, which is itself a set of subprocesses that can include between 80 and 200 steps, beginning with the placement of a drug product in the hospital's inventory and ending with its administration to the patient.[2] The subculture of the pharmacy department possesses some characteristics that are distinct from the cultures of other health professionals in the organization. The evolution of pharmacy education, practice, and workforce demographics has produced a curious "soup" of diverse educational and training backgrounds, gender- and culture-based worldviews and biases, types of institutional experience, and opinions on the nature and value of pharmacy services. These factors have an impact on the communication and collaboration between and among pharmacy directors, staff pharmacists, and pharmacy technicians—and therefore they affect the outcomes, quality, and safety of the work performed by pharmacy staff.

The fundamental requirement for establishing a high-reliability medication-use process is the establishment of a culture where an attitude of cooperation, communication, and openness across all levels of pharmacy personnel is the norm. This attitude must be embraced by all pharmacy staff, who must, in turn, radiate it to the other health professionals, services, and administrative components with whom they work. If a unity of purpose and spirit can be established, then when mistakes occur involving the medication-use process, communication channels are already in place to facilitate correction, learning, and improvement, not only within the department but also throughout the organization.

A common theme throughout this text is the concept of open and honest communication without fear of ridicule or blame. The Joint Commission on Accreditation of Healthcare Organizations recently adopted a patient-safety goal demanding better communication among health care providers.[5] Although it may be some time before all health care practitioners and administrators understand and embrace these concepts, it is possible for pharmacy leaders to nurture and support a team-based model, including open and honest communication within the pharmacy department, which can serve as an example for the entire organization.

Flexible Authority with Well-Defined Command Structures

The traditional, timeworn organizational model of hierarchical, or "top-down," authority is the nemesis of high reliability and of safety-centered operations. When a mistake, a near miss, or an impending emergency becomes apparent, frontline operators (frequently referred to as personnel at the "sharp end" of the system) may immediately know, or at least suspect, what solutions or interventions are needed (or worth trying) to correct it. However, in a traditional vertical organizational hierarchy, sharp-end personnel (who, ironically, will likely later be blamed for any accidents) find their hands tied by bureaucracy and protocol. They are powerless to step outside the constraints of their limited purview to halt or modify operations without consulting senior or supervisory personnel, who are likely inaccessible at the critical moment and in any event are not in a position to know the details of the situation.

Decisions that rest on reaction times of seconds or minutes cannot wait for communication to travel though bureaucratic channels: The people at the sharp end must be empowered to make those decisions. Authority must shift from those who normally possess executive power to those who possess clinical and technical expertise on, and who are in proximity to, high-risk operations. In health care, as on aircraft-carrier flight decks, any team member, regardless of rank, should have the right to stop the line at any time he or she observes a potential problem emerging.

Rochlin et al.[6] describe this phenomenon in naval aircraft operations: "Events on the flight deck . . . can happen too quickly to allow for appeals through a chain of command. Even the lowest rating on the deck has not only the authority but also the obligation to suspend flight operations immediately, under the proper circumstances, without first clearing it with superiors. Although his judgment may later be reviewed or even criticized, he will not be penalized for being wrong and will often be publicly congratulated if he is right."[4]

In health care as in the military, a high-reliability environment requires managing the tension between adherence to procedures, protocols, and best practices and an atmosphere of continuous learning and organizational responsiveness. Also required is a balance between a *vertical* command structure—where key individuals bear executive and operational responsibility for the overall outcomes of the enterprise and the integrity of the organization and its component divisions—and *horizontal* authority structures, where operators in or near the "trenches" are empowered to make decisions on the basis of their expertise, experience, and the facts and observations available to them as a situation presents itself. If such organizational flexibility is to occur, there must be an atmosphere of trust, respect, and openness among personnel at different levels of seniority, training, and expertise.

In health care, this means that the social and cultural barriers between physicians, pharmacists, nurses, technical specialists, and health administrators that impede the open sharing of information and accountability must be abolished. All too often we hear of pharmacists, technicians, and nurses who are chastised by physicians for questioning medication orders that are unclear because of handwriting or verbal transmission or because the pharmacist's or nurse's expertise or experience leads him or her to believe that the medication order is in some way inappropriate or unsafe for that patient.[5] This kind of interaction is completely counterproductive to fostering a culture of safety; it hampers communication and invites error.

If a flexible authority mechanism can be achieved in the military, where command and subordination are so entrenched and critical to success, then how much more feasible should it be in health care, where most authority is perceived rather than real and is simply the product of obsolete historical and cultural biases and assumptions? Health organizations should study and emulate the leadership of institutions such as Children's Hospitals and Clinics in Minneapolis, whose "stop-the-line" policy permits pharmacists and nurses to refuse medication orders that contain unsafe order-writing practices and that permits any physician, hospital worker, or patient to stop a procedure if there is a safety concern. Another example is Elizabeth's Hospital in Youngstown, Ohio, where nurses in the cardiac intensive-care unit are authorized to refuse a doctor's medication order if their knowledge of the patient's history indicates that the order is inappropriate.[6,7]

Repetitiveness of Key Tasks: A Double-Edged Sword

In most organizations, ensuring safe and consistent operations depends largely on the monitoring and preservation of the status quo—repeatedly performing various tasks that keep products, people, and information flowing through the system according to plan. However, when a task becomes routine, workers may not notice when something is wrong because they have become conditioned, over time and through repetition, to see what they expect to see.

Consider the acute-care pharmacist whose job is to verify the accuracy of thousands of similar repackaged unit dose medications per day. In the majority of cases, accuracy is perfect; no unusual action is necessary. However, in the rare event that a medication has been placed in the wrong container among many other correctly packaged medications, the probability that the pharmacist will catch the error is substantially decreased, because the pharmacist is unwittingly biased toward the belief that he or she is correctly executing the familiar task of inspecting and verifying the package contents. The high-reliability approach to this problem might be to rotate staff between tasks at periodic intervals, so that important tasks are approached with the renewed vigilance brought by a new set of eyes.

The numbing effect of repetition can extend beyond individuals to groups or organizations. An organization often becomes so entrenched in "the way we do things" that it misses the opportunity to learn alternative or innovative approaches. If pharmacy directors made a point of asking newly hired staff how their previous organizations would solve a particular problem, learning would increase dramatically and opportunities for improvement would not be so frequently missed.

Training and Learning as Priorities

The public expects health care workers to possess and exercise competency. A fundamental requirement for all health care organizations is the allocation of sufficient resources to train and assess the competency of their workers. It is often assumed that someone who has completed the educational requirements to work in a patient care environment is automatically qualified to do so. This assumption is false, and it is often damaging. Each organization is unique in terms of standard operating procedures and general operational approaches. An organization must provide new employees with enough time to become familiar with organizational policies and procedures, and the organization must have a reliable mechanism to assess the proficiency of all employees on an ongoing basis.

When budgets are cut, the first item to be jettisoned is often support for education and training. This is illogical. The competency of the workforce determines the effectiveness of the system. Support for ensuring continuing employee competency should be preserved when resource allocations are examined.

Individual competency is frequently brought into question when an error occurs. But rarely do we ask, Did the system fail the individual? A system can be a nebulous entity, often lacking clear definition and perspective on the part of its designers and participants. When we consider training and assessment as part of the fundamental criteria by which the system, its safety and effectiveness, and the performance of its personnel are judged, the concept of identifying and correcting problems from a systemic, rather than a personal, perspective becomes ever clearer.

Multidisciplinary Review and Response to Errors and Near Misses

A hallmark of a high-reliability organization is an extensive degree of cooperation across disciplines and specialties. In the event of an error, it is imperative that disciplines collaborate to seek answers to how and why the error occurred and to ensure that the event is not repeated. Highly reliable teams recognize that they are subject to the biases associated with knowing the outcome of the error. They recognize the challenges in seeing the "big picture" and think about the myriad ways the error might have occurred, rather than point to the most obvious solution, i.e., blaming the individual closest to the event at the time it occurred.

Multidisciplinary teams must also be cognizant of the biases associated with the subcultures within their professions. They must try to forget about which profession (pharmacist, nurse, physician) was closest to the error when it happened and to think instead about how things need to be changed to improve processes and systems in the future. This might result in ideas or practices that threaten some individuals' or groups' perceptions of their professional prerogatives. For example, a pattern of recurring medication administration errors might compel an organization to train certified pharmacy technicians to administer medications, freeing nurses' time for patient monitoring and assessment. This should not be viewed as a collective punishment of nurses but rather as recognition that their time and expertise would be better spent ensuring that patients are responding appropriately to therapy.

Anesthesiology: An Early Adopter of High Reliability in Health Care

Anesthesiology is a good example of a medical subspecialty that, faced with an increasing number of patient injuries and deaths associated with anesthesia and increasing malpractice premiums, began to apply principles of high reliability to its practice. The key causes of these incidents were identified as "heterogeneity of design in anesthesia devices; fatigue and sleep deprivation [among practitioners]; and competing institutional, professional, and patient care priorities."[8] Although anesthesiology is only a segment of the medication-use system, many of the principles it has adopted are applicable to broader organizational-improvement efforts. For example, anesthesiology educational and training programs have implemented electronic simulators that permit trainees to experience and react to crises using "dummy patients" that respond in lifelike ways to treatment.

Work in Teams . . . Train in Teams

It is feasible to consider designing scenarios that encompass the key segments of the medication-use process and applying those scenarios to simulations in a team-training model that includes pharmacists, nurses, physicians, patients, technical support personnel, and others. This concept, though time-intensive, would be a good step to transform the current "silo"-based training model to one that is consistent with the high-reliability concept that those who are expected to work in teams should also be trained in teams.

Team training does not alleviate the need for practitioners to be individually trained and skilled to be experts and leaders in specific aspects of the medication-use process. Distinct expertise in one area represents the need for organizations to establish defined areas of responsibility and accountability for component parts of the entire system, but it does not minimize the importance of team training. Every member of the team must know the role that he and his fellow team members play, and they must then work in concert to ensure the system is working to achieve the desired outcome.

Can High-Reliability Principles Be Applied in Blanket Fashion to Medication Use?

The decks of aircraft carriers and the control rooms of nuclear power plants differ significantly from hospitals. However, this does not mean that the concepts of high reliability developed in other areas and industries are not applicable to health care. Proven approaches, such as teamwork, open communication, defined responsibility, a nonpunitive culture that embraces learning and improvement, standardization, training and retraining, and the right of any member of the team to "stop the line" at any time because or to a safety concern are all transferable to patient care in hospitals.

Fundamental changes are necessary in health care as a whole. However, efforts to effect improvement in the cultures of individual services and departments, such as pharmacy, can serve as highly productive and potentially influential examples to the broader health care system to drive the fundamental changes that must occur over time. The medication-use process is consistently, and rightly, recognized as the low-hanging fruit. It is an obvious place to start. Pharmacists and hospital pharmacy departments should lead the charge of applying high-reliability theory to help ensure safe and effective medication use, spread the high-reliability "gospel" to other health disciplines through example and enthusiasm, advocate for adequate resources to make the needed changes in process and system design, and assume accountability for doing everything possible to ensure that no patient is ever harmed by a medication.

References

1. Singer S, Gaba D, Geppert J, et al. Safety climate survey results from12 hospitals, 2001 and 2002. Bay Area Health Care Quality and Outcomes Research Conference. (Abstract.)

2. Brennan TA, Leape LL, Laird NM, et al. Incidence of adverse events and negligence in hospitalized patients: results of the Harvard Medical Practice Study I. *N Engl J Med.* 1991;324:370-376.

3. Pool R. When failure is not an option. Technol Rev. 1997;100(5):38-45. Available through: www.technologyreview.com/articles/pool0797.asp?p=2, accessed 5/27/2003.

4. American Society of Health-System Pharmacists. Pharmacy-nursing shared vision for safe medication use in hospitals: executive session summary. *Am J Health-Syst Pharm.* 2003;60:1046-1052.

5. Joint Commission on Accreditation of Healthcare Organizations. 2005 Hospital National Patient Safety Goals. Available at: www.jcaho.org/accredited+organizations/patient+safety/05+npsg/05_npsg_hap.htm. Accessed July 21, 2004.

6. Rochlin GI, LaPorte TR, Roberts KH. The self-designing high-reliability organization: aircraft carrier flight operations at sea. Available at: http://www.Nwc.navy.mil/press/Review/1998/summer/art7su98htm. Accessed October 28, 2004.

7. Institute for Safe Medication Practices. Suggestions for resolving conflicts in drug therapy. *ISMP Medication Safety Alert.* 2001 (June 11). Available at: http://www.ismp.org/MSAarticles/resolve.html. Accessed July 21, 2004.

8. Runy LA. The American Hospital Association Quest for Quality prize. *Hosp Health Network.* 2002;76(8):49-56.

9. Weick KE, Sutcliffe KM. *Managing the Unexpected: Assuring High Performance in an Age of Complexity.* San Francisco: Jossey-Bass; 2001.

10. Kohn LT, Corrigan JM, Donaldson MD, eds. Committee on Quality of Health in America, Institute of Medicine. *To Err Is Human: Building a Safer Health System.* Washington, DC: National Academy Press; 1999.

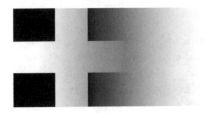

CHAPTER 22

International Perspectives on Patient Safety

David Cousins

Introduction

In a report entitled "Reducing Risks and Promoting Healthy Life," the World Health Organization (WHO) identified adverse events as a major risk to world health, alongside other major problems such as malnutrition, tobacco and alcohol consumption, high blood pressure, and unsafe sex.[1] The report states that there is a growing understanding that health care practices may be a source of disease and death, as well as of health. It also notes that health care comprises a complex combination of processes, technologies, and human interactions. It states that harm arises from human shortcomings, substandard or faulty products, side effects of drugs and drug combinations, and hazards caused by medical devices, procedures, and systems. There is a possibility of failure at every point of the caregiving process and in every setting in which care is delivered, including the patient's home.[1]

In 2002, the Fifty Fifth World Health Assembly, WHO passed Resolution A55/13 "Quality of care: patient safety," which recognizes the need to promote patient safety as a fundamental principle of all health care systems.[2] The resolution urged all WHO member states to pay the closest-possible attention to the patient safety and to establish and strengthen science-based systems necessary for improving patients' safety and the quality of health care, including the monitoring of drugs, medical equipment, and technology. The World Health Assembly (WHA), WHO's governing body, instructed the organization to develop and promote global standards to improve patient care, with particular emphasis on several topics, including the safe use of medicinal products.[2]

Also in 2002 the World Health Profession Alliance, or WHPA (comprising the International Council of Nurses, the International Pharmaceutical Federation [FIP], and WHO) published a fact sheet on patient safety.[3] This document defines an adverse event as "harm or injury caused by the management of a patient's disease or condition by health care professionals rather than by the underlying disease or condition itself." The alliance acknowledged the evidence of adverse incidents from research in hospitals but acknowledged that adverse events occurring in other health care settings, such as physicians' offices, nursing homes, pharmacies, and patients' homes, are not well documented. Identifying these errors, reducing their occurrence, and improving the safety and quality of health care have therefore been brought forward as a priority issue for health services around the world.[3]

This chapter examines international perspectives on patient safety and specifically focuses on medication errors.

Evidence of Adverse Events

A decade ago, researchers in Australia published an important early study on patient safety in health care. The Quality in Australian Health Care study drew attention to adverse events and iatrogenic injury in Australian hospitals. It reported that 16.6 percent of patients whose hospital charts were reviewed suffered an adverse event.[4] The Australian data demonstrated that morbidity stemming from adverse events was clearly a major public health problem.[5] Later studies revealed that more than 70 percent of identified adverse events were the result of failures in technical performance, failures to decide or act appropriately on the basis of available information, failures to investigate or consult, and a lack of care or failure to attend.[5,6]

A 2000 report issued by the Department of Health in England identified the impact of adverse events in that country.[7] Prepared by an expert committee chaired by the chief medical officer in England, the report focused on how the National Health Service (NHS) can more effectively learn from failures in clinical care. It concluded that the picture of error in the United Kingdom (U.K.), although admittedly incomplete, indicated that at least 400 patients died or were seriously injured in adverse events involving medical devices in 1999, and that nearly 10,000 people experienced serious adverse reactions to drugs (not all of which were preventable) in that same year. In 2001, Vincent and colleagues[8] published a pilot study of adverse events in two acute-care hospitals in London using methods similar to those used in the Australian study.[9] These researchers found that 10.8 percent of patients in these hospitals experienced an adverse event during their hospital stays. About one-half of these events were judged to be preventable. The authors conclude that adverse events are a serious source of harm to patients and a large drain on NHS resources.

Further analyses of the Vincent et al. study indicate that less than 20 percent of preventable adverse events were directly related to surgical operations or invasive procedures and that less than 10 percent were related to misdiagnoses. Fifty-three percent of preventable adverse events occurred in general ward care (including initial assessment and the use of drugs and i.v. fluids) and 18 percent occurred in care at the time of discharge. The authors suggest that probable contributory factors in these errors included dependence on diagnoses made by inexperienced clinicians, poor records, poor communication between professional caregivers, inadequate input by consultants into day-to-day care, and lack of detailed assessments of patients before discharge.[9]

Another study described the proportion of admissions to a medical ward in a U.K. hospital that were drug related and preventable. Of the 4093 admissions, 265 (6.5 percent) were judged to be drug related, and of these 67 percent were judged to be preventable.[10]

Studies of adverse events have been undertaken in other countries. Authors in Denmark reviewed medical charts sampled from 17 acute-care hospitals and reported that the prevalence of admissions to hospital as a result of adverse events was 9 percent.[11] In a French hospital, 9.9 percent of patients admitted had suffered an adverse drug event (ADE).[12] In a Spanish study, 2.25 percent of patients seen in an emergency department had experienced an ADE. More than half of these events were preventable.[13] In a meta-analysis of 22 studies from 12 countries, the reported drug-induced hospital admission rate range ranged between 1 percent and 28.2 percent, with an average of 7.2 percent.[14]

A worldwide review of the economic impact of ADEs has also been published recently.[15] Similar work has not been done in other countries, although two Canadian authors estimate a high likelihood of comparable levels of error in their own health care facilities.[16,17]

The incidence of adverse events in developing and transitional countries is not known but could be worse than in the industrialized nations, because of counterfeit and substandard drugs, and inappropriate or poor equipment or infrastructure.[1] The WHPA has reported that at least 50 percent of all medical equipment in most developing countries is unusable, or only partially usable, at any time.[3] In the newly independent states, about 40 percent of hospital beds are located in structures originally built for other purposes. As a result, the correct infrastructure for radiation protection and infection control is very difficult to install. Other problems include staff shortages, lack of technical skill, and low motivation among staff, as well as severe underfinancing of health services.[3]

Strategies for Reducing the Incidence of Adverse Events

Successfully tackling risks to health involves many stakeholders from different sections of society, a combination of scientific and political processes, many qualitative and quantitative judgments, a range of intersectional actions by different agencies, and open communication and dialogue. Risk management is not a linear process and involves iterative decision-making processes requiring actions in four main areas: risk surveillance, risk assessment, risk management, and risk communication (see **Figure** 22-1).[1]

Those who espouse a systems approach to safety, in health care and elsewhere, believe that risk is shaped and provoked by upstream systematic factors that include an organization's strategy, its culture, its approach toward quality management and risk prevention, and its capacity for learning from failures. WHO has identified system change as a potentially more effective means of potential error reduction than targeting of individual practice or products.[1] The WHPA[3] recommends that governments undertake the following actions:

- Establish national reporting systems to record, analyze, and learn from adverse incidents.

- Promote a culture of reporting.

- Emphasize safety as a prime concern in health-system performance and quality management.

- Implement mechanisms for ensuring that, where lessons are identified, the necessary changes are put into practice and progress is tracked.

- Develop evidence-based policies that will improve health care.

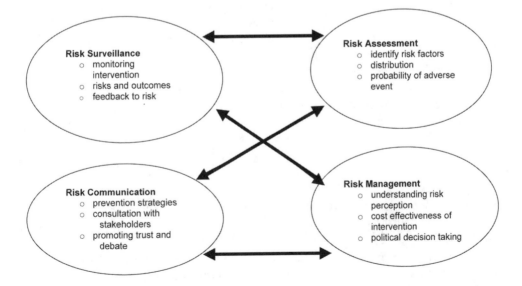

Figure 22-1. *Implementing Risk Prevention*[1]

- Develop mechanisms, for example, through accreditation, to recognize the characteristics of health care providers that offer a benchmark for excellence in patient safety.

Organizations Addressing Patient-Safety Issues

A National Expert Advisory Group on Safety and Quality in Australian Health Care was established in 1997, and its recommendations led to the formation of the Australian Council for Safety and Quality in Health Care. The Australia Patient Safety Foundation has responsibility for a national incident-monitoring system and has developed a classification system for coding and reporting of incidents and adverse events.[18]

The NHS in England and Wales has established a new agency and charged it with setting up a national patient-safety incident-reporting system to enable analysis and actions to reduce the risk and prevent the recurrence of adverse events.[19] The National Patient Safety Agency (NPSA) was established as a Special Health Authority of the NHS. The role of the NPSA is to

- collect and analyze information on adverse events from local NHS organizations, NHS staff, and patients and caregivers;

- assimilate other safety-related information from a variety of existing reporting systems and other sources in this country and abroad;

- learn lessons and ensure that they are fed back into practice, service organization, and delivery;

- where risks are identified, produce solutions to prevent harm, specify national goals, and establish mechanisms to track progress.

Reports from other countries have recommended setting up national organizations to promote patient safety.[20,21]

Medication Errors

In 1999, the FIP adopted the definition for medication error developed by the National Coordinating Committee for Medication Error Reporting Programs (NCC MERP) in the United States.[22] The definition is as follows:

> any preventable event that may cause or lead to inappropriate medication use or patient harm, while the medication is in the control of the health care professional, patient, or consumer. Such events may be related to professional practice, health care products, procedures, and systems including: prescribing; order communication; product labeling, packaging, and nomenclature; compounding; dispensing; distribution; administration; education; monitoring; and use.

Although there may be some degree of international agreement as to the overall definition of medication error, there is less agreement on other terms often used in discussions of patient safety. These terms include adverse drug event (preventable and nonpreventable), prescribing error, dispensing error, administration error, and others.

There is also no agreement on standardized methods to be used to measure and study medication errors. Some authors have started to make progress in standardizing the terminology and taxonomy[23] and methodology.[24] However, a good deal of work is still required. Details of international research studies that describe the incidence and types of medication errors will be presented later in the chapter, but the results from these studies are seldom comparable because of differences in definitions and methodologies.

Despite differences in definitions and study methods, health care organizations around the world have identified the prevention of medication errors as an important component of their patient-safety agendas and have developed action plans and targets to address this problem.

FIP published a statement on professional standards concerning medication errors associated with prescribed medicines in 1999.[25]

Participants in a European Expert Meeting on Medication Safety, held in The Hague in November 2002 and cosponsored by the Council of Europe and the Regional Office for Europe of the WHO, published a Consensus Document on Medication Safety.[26] This document recommends that medication errors be recognized as an important, system-based public health issue; that the approach to safe medication practices be multidisciplinary and include patients, professionals, and their organizations; that a recognized national focal point for safe medication practices be designated in each country; that there be active sharing and dissemination of data and strategies for risk reduction between countries; that a Europe-wide definition of medication error be developed; that there be Europe-wide standards for safe medication practices; that there be national systems for reporting medication errors, analyzing causes, and disseminating information on risk reduction; that a baseline assessment of the frequency, nature, and causes of medication errors is needed; and that local targets be considered valuable in implementing safe medication practices. An expert group has been established to network across Europe in order to help achieve these objectives.

The NHS has identified specific targets for action to improve safe medication practice in England. These targets include reducing to zero the number of patients being paralyzed by maladministered spinal injections by the end of 2001 and reducing by 40 percent the number of serious errors in the use of prescribed drugs by 2005.[19] In order to address these targets in England and Wales, national initiatives have been taken to improve safe medication practice with intrathecal chemotherapy,[27] the use of potassium chloride concentrate,[28] labeling and packaging of medicines by manufacturers,[29] and purchasing for safety.[30]

Fifteen case reports have been published in seven countries outside of the United States concerning the maladministration of potassium chloride concentrate.[31-45] These reports prompted the introduction of a national initiative in the U.K. Aronson[46] and Vandenbroucke[47] have described the benefits of publishing case reports concerning adverse drug reactions. They indicate that these reports provide important information concerning rare events, as these may be the only signals in the literature concerning these often-preventable events. At the same time, they caution that these reports may be susceptible to bias and that it would be beneficial to develop standardized guidelines for reporting patient harm from medicines. Case reports provide useful information concerning medication errors, and encouraging and standardizing this type of reporting internally would aid our understanding of medication errors and of methods to manage them.

Many national and local patient-safety programs include incident reports about medication errors. These programs emphasize that it is important that practitioners have a single system to use to report incidents of all types. A unified system offers the advantage of a single method for practitioners, and sometimes patients and family caregivers, to use to record, categorize, and report; perform analyses; receive feedback; and improve practice.

Industries other than health care have used incident reporting to reduce the number of serious incidents. **Figure 22-2** illustrates an increase in the number of air transport incident reports in the U.K. that provided opportunities for system improvements that have led to reductions in the percentage and in the actual number of serious incident reports.[48]

Government-sponsored organizations, as well as a number of other organizations, are undertaking initiatives to identify medication errors and develop methods to prevent them. These organizations are listed in **Table 22-1**.

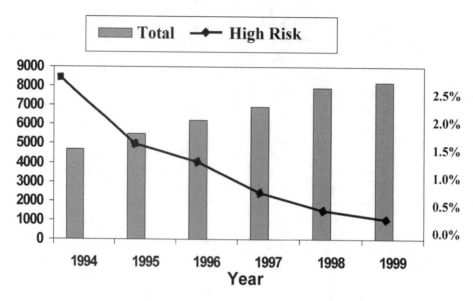

Figure 22-2. *Air Safety Reports (UK) Volume and Risk*

Interpreting Studies Internationally

Before reviewing international studies and initiatives concerning medication errors and their prevention, it is important to understand the context of the health care system and the drug products and medication-use processes that operate in that country. Products and processes that are used in one country may be very different from those used in another.

Following the European Directive (92/97), which came into force on January 1,1994, all prescribed tablets or capsules in European countries must be supplied in clearly labeled, original "patient packs" that contain a patient information leaflet.[49] The objective of the directive was to ensure that such a leaflet would be enclosed in the sealed manufacturer's pack. This initiative has minimized the dispensing of loose tablets in plain bottles. Medication errors associated with the dispensing, labeling, and packaging of medicines and the provision of patient information in countries that do not supply patient packs may differ from those in European countries.

Table 22-1. International Organizations Undertaking Actions to Identify and Prevent Medication Errors

Organization	Country/Region	Web Address
Australian Patient Safety Foundation	Australia	www.apsf.net.au.
Institute for Healthcare Improvement and British Medical Journal	International	www.qualityhealthcare.org.
Institute for Safe Medication Practice	Canada	www.ismp-canada.org
Institute for Safe Medication Practice	Spain	www3.usal.es/~ismp/marco.html
National Patient Safety Agency	England and Wales	www.npsa.nhs.uk

There are variations in the medicine-supply methods using patient packs within Europe. For example, in Germany, patient packs are dispensed from hospital and community pharmacies and do not require a pharmacy dispensing label. There is no requirement that the patient's name, date of dispensing, or dosage instruction be added to the patient pack.[50]

In the U.K., patients who are about to be admitted to the hospital are encouraged to bring in their own medicines, frequently in patient packs. The patient's own medicines are used during his or her inpatient stay, and the same pack is discharged with the patient. If new medicines or supplies are prescribed during the hospital stay, a patient pack is dispensed and used. If treatment is to be continued, the patient takes that pack with him or her at discharge from the hospital. This system of medicine distribution is intended to reduce patients' confusion over their medicines; to minimize unintended omissions, duplications, variations, and wastage of medicines; and to ensure that the patient has a patient information leaflet for each medicine that he or she is taking.[51,52]

Variations in medicine-processing operations in different countries can be illustrated by comparing hospital pharmacy survey data from European countries with data from the United States. In 2000, the European Association of Hospital Pharmacy conducted a survey and obtained responses from 748 hospitals from 16 countries.[53] The American Society of Health-System Pharmacists conducted a national survey on dispensing and administration in 2002 and received responses from 514 hospitals.[54] A 2001 survey of prescribing and transcribing resulted in responses from 535 hospitals.[55]

Hospital demographic data are presented in **Table 22-2**. On the average, European hospitals have higher numbers of inpatient beds, higher occupancy, and longer lengths of hospital stay than U.S. hospitals. The number of pharmacists and technicians per 100 beds is also significantly lower.

Table 22-2. Comparison of Demographic Data from Hospital Pharmacy Surveys in Europe[53] and the United States[54,55]

Data Field	Europe (n=748)	SD (SE)	U.S. (n=514)	SD (SE)
Number of beds	601	550	231	135
Average occupancy rate	74%	27%	51%	20%
Duration of stay	13 days	35 days	7 days	9 days
FTE pharmacists	4.0	7.0	8.6	0.3
FTE pharmacists per 100 beds	0.82	(0.04)	10.4	(0.54)
FTE pharmacy technicians per 100 beds	1.66	(0.06)	8.4	(0.28)

FTE = full-time equivalent.

Comparisons of pharmacy services are presented in **Table 22-3**. Hospital pharmacy services in the United States are available twice as many hours each week than in European hospitals. Only 9 percent of European hospitals provide oral unit dose systems or i.v admixture services outside of the preparation of total parenteral nutrition or cytotoxic medicines, whereas in only 19 percent of U.S. hospitals nurses have to prepare i.v. admixtures.

Table 22-3. Comparison of Hospital Pharmacy Services from Hospital Pharmacy Surveys in Europe[53] and the United States[54,55]

Data Field	Europe n=748	U.S. n=503
Hours of pharmacy inpatient activity	46	101
Pharmacist on call from home when pharmacy is closed	48%	
24-hour pharmacy service	6%	
Oral unit dose system	9%	81%
Centralized stock distribution from main pharmacy	83%	81%
Stock distribution from satellite pharmacies	22%	20%
Individually dispensed patient supplies	29%	
Medicine supplies on discharge	39%	
Days' supply on discharge	5	17
Pharmacist review and approve all medication orders before administration		79%
Robotic dispensing of inpatient packs	4%	8%
Automated point of use dispensing devices	4%	58%
Pharmacy preparation of cytotoxics	50%	
Pharmacy preparation of total parenteral nutrition	40%	
Pharmacy preparation of other i.v. doses	9%	
I.V. admixtures or solutions that require nurses to prepare from vials or ampoules		19%
Occasional pharmacist visits to ward	82%	
Daily pharmacist visits to ward	7%	
Decentralized clinical pharmacy services	4%	
Pharmacists attending medical rounds		30.4%

European hospitals have not implemented automated point-of-use dispensing cabinets to any significant extent; this is no doubt linked to the limited use of unit dose medicines. Implementation of robotic dispensing of inpatient packs is just beginning both in Europe and in the United States.

With the relatively small numbers of pharmacists and pharmacy staff and limited hours of pharmacy service, the provision of floor stock without required pharmacist review is the norm in European hospitals. Likewise, pharmacist approval of medications prior to administration is not common practice. Only 39 percent of European hospitals provide medications to patients at the time of discharge.

An understanding of the differences in drug products and systems from country to country can help health care professionals interpret medication-error data derived from another country and adapt it to their own practice settings. Such an understanding will also help them determine the appropriateness of proposed solutions to medication errors (e.g., new technology, policies and procedures, education and training). Solutions to medication errors identified in one country need to be validated, risk assessed, and evaluated in practice in another country before being accepted into mainstream practice.

International Comparison Studies

To overcome national differences, international comparison studies use the same definitions referred to in the previous section. These comparative studies can provide valuable benchmarking data concerning safe medication practices. They also help challenge paradigms and encourage innovative thinking concerning what constitutes safe medication practice.

One study compared medication errors in a hospital in the United States with those in a hospital in the U.K.[56] The U.S hospital had a unit dose drug distribution system, and the U.K. hospital had the ward-based system commonly used in that country, in which a pharmacist visits each ward several times daily and reviews each patient's medication chart. The physician uses the medication chart to order drugs, a process that obviates the need for transcription of orders. A disguised-observation technique was used to determine frequencies and types of medication errors. Medication errors were identified retrospectively in the U.S. hospital by comparing the observer's notes with the drug orders made in the patient's chart by the physician. In the U.K. hospital, identification of errors took place concurrently; as doses were administered, they were compared with the orders on the medication chart. A total of 919 and 2,756 opportunities for error were observed in U.S. and U.K. hospitals, respectively. The medication-error rate in the U.S. hospital was 6.9 percent; in the U.K. hospital, it was 3.0 percent. Omitted doses and incorrect doses were the most common types of errors in the U.K. hospital; incorrect doses and unordered doses were the most common errors in the U.S. hospital. This study challenged the established view in the United States that the unit dose system is always safer than alternative systems.

Some hospitals in Europe and elsewhere are introducing unit dose systems on the basis of research studies that took place in the United States in the 1960s and 1970s. It is important that unit dose system implementations in Europe and elsewhere be fully evaluated to help the health care community understand the benefits and new risks, as well as the resources required to operate these systems in health care settings other than those in the United States.

Taxis et al.[57] studied the rate of medication errors in hospital drug distribution systems in the U.K. and Germany. The aim of this study was to identify and compare the incidence of medication errors and the stages of the drug distribution system at which they occur in a U.K hospital using the ward pharmacy system, a German hospital using the unit dose system, and a German hospital using that country's traditional system. Medication errors were identified by observing the preparation and administration of regularly scheduled solid oral medications. In the U.K. hospital, the medication-error rate was 8.0 percent. The majority of these errors occurred at the stage of medication administration. In the hospital using the traditional German system, the error rate was 5.1 percent, and with the German unit dose system, the error rate was 2.4 percent. In both German systems, the errors occurred mainly at the time of transcription. In this study the patient turnover was much higher in the hospitals using the ward pharmacy system, and the study sites may, therefore, not have been comparable. Taxis and coworkers[57] made recommendations to reduce the error rate associated with each system. Errors associated with the ward pharmacy system may be reduced if medication is stored in individual patient medicine cabinets and if the patient's own drugs are used. Errors occurring with both the traditional system and the unit dose system may be reduced if the original prescription is used for medication administration.

This study provides some evidence of the benefits of operating a unit dose system in a European hospital. It does not provide information concerning how such a system would operate from a European hospital pharmacy department operating 50 hours a week or what would happen with new orders written when the pharmacy is closed. It is also important to note that unit dose systems in European hospitals are generally limited to solid medications and do not include i.v. additive services.

In 2003 Wirtz et al.[58] investigated the incidence and the severity of i.v. drug preparation and administration errors in the three hospitals in the United Kingdom and Germany. A disguised-observational method was used to record details of the preparation and administration of prescribed i.v. drugs on two wards in each of three teaching hospitals: one with a traditional British ward stock and daily visits to the wards by a pharmacists and two hospitals in Germany—one with a traditional ward stock supply and no pharmacist visits and one with a satellite pharmacy service that used a unit dose system. The preparation-error rates were 22 percent for the U.K. hospital, 23 percent for the German ward stock supply system, and 31 percent for the German hospital with the satellite and unit dose system. Administration-error rates were 27 percent in the U.K. hospital, 49 percent in the German hospital with ward stock, and 22 percent in the German hospital with the satellite and unit dose system. The percentage of administration errors in the German hospital with a traditional ward-stock system was higher than that in the other two services to a statistically significant degree. The most common errors in the U.K. hospital and in the German hospital with the satellite were omitted doses. Wrong rate of administration occurred most frequently in the German hospital with traditional ward-stock system. The outcomes of a majority of errors were considered to be moderate to severe.

This international study, alongside national studies to be described below, indicates that the rate of i.v. medicine errors in European hospitals is considerably higher than that involving oral medicines. Initiatives to improve practices with i.v. and parenteral medicines should be a priority for hospitals internationally.

Views concerning the severity and clinical outcome of medication errors vary significantly among practitioners in different countries. A study to assess the validity and reliability of a method used in the U.K. to score the severity of medication-administration errors was tested with 10 doctors, 10 nurses, and 10 pharmacists from German hospitals.[59] They were asked to score the potential clinical significance of 49 types of medication-administration errors on a visual analogue scale. Generalizability theory was used to determine the minimum number of judges required to obtain a reliable mean score. Validity was assessed by comparing the mean scores given by the judges with the known outcomes of the errors for a subset of the cases. German results were compared to original U.K. data. The mean scores were found to be valid indicators of the potential severity of the errors. German scores were significantly below U.K. scores for the same cases. The authors concluded that the fact that German health professionals see cases as less dangerous than their U.K. counterparts do is worthy of further investigation.[59]

Prescribing Errors

Dean et al.[60] in the U.K., working with groups of health professionals, developed a definition of prescribing error. The definition was "a prescribing decision or prescription-writing process that results in an unintentional, significant reduction in the probability of treatment being timely and effective or increase in the risk of harm when compared with generally accepted practice."[60] Prescribing without taking into account the patient's clinical status, failure to communicate essential information, and transcription errors were all considered prescribing errors. Failure to adhere to standards, such as national guidelines or the medicine's product license, were not considered an error if the prescribing reflected accepted practice.

Dean and coworkers[61] undertook a qualitative study to understand the causes of prescribing errors in hospital inpatients. Pharmacists in a U.K. teaching hospital prospectively identified 88 potentially serious prescribing errors. A research pharmacist interviewed prescribers who made 44 of these errors. The results suggest that the mistakes were made because of slips or inattention or because the prescriber did not apply relevant rules. The doctors identified many risk factors: work environment, heavy workload, whether or not they were prescribing for their own patients, communication with their team, physical and mental well-being, and lack of knowledge.

Many doctors did not seem to consider the task of prescribing medicines as important. The act of prescribing was often restricted to naming a product (e.g., "Put her on verapamil"); details concerning dosage, form, frequency, route, and duration were delegated to junior doctors. Mastering these matters supposedly occurs at some indeterminate moment between medical school (where, according to the sample of doctors interviewed, the subject is not taught) and employment. Junior doctors find themselves in a position where they are expected to prescribe without having been taught how to do so. The culture and power in medical teams led junior doctors and nurses to hesitate to question the decisions of senior doctors or to ask for clarification if they were unsure of how to prescribe a medicine. Pharmacists were seen as the main source of defense against prescribing errors. Some junior doctors suggested that they trusted pharmacists to such an extent that they would sometimes not bother to look up doses themselves. U.K. pharmacists not only supply the medications but also visit the wards each day to monitor prescriptions to detect errors. However, the less time that a pharmacist has to spend on each prescription, the less time he or she can spend checking for errors. Concerns have been raised over maintaining the quality of this service in times of pharmacist shortages.

Medical staff in the U.K. are responsible for writing new medicine charts on admission, rewriting full charts, and writing discharge prescriptions. Hospital medical staff saw these acts of transcription, or represcribing what other doctors had initiated, as a mechanical task that was not done with the same care as prescribing a new medicine is.

Details of quantitative studies of prescribing errors are presented in **Table 22-4**. Prescribing errors in hospital ranged between 0.56 percent and 9.9 percent. Results were partly dependent on the definition and study methods used. Prescribing errors in community practice ranged from 4.35 percent to 10.2 percent. The studies provide some evidence that electronic prescribing does reduce the number of prescribing errors. In community practice, Shah et al.[62] found the prescribing-error rate among general practitioners to be 10.2 percent for handwritten prescriptions and 7.9 percent for computer-generated prescriptions. Fowlie and coworkers[63] found the prescribing rate for handwritten prescriptions by hospital doctors to be 7.5 percent; this rate dropped to 4.7 percent following the introduction of a computer-prescribing system.

Nightingale[69] described the use of a computerized system in a 64-bed renal ward in a U.K. teaching hospital. The system had a software decision-support system that produced information concerning maximum recommended single and daily doses, interactions with other drug classes, contraindications, and side effects to the new prescription. During the study, 87,789 prescription items were generated. The system canceled 0.07 percent of the prescriptions on the grounds of clinical safety. In addition, 57 percent of attempted prescriptions that generated high-level warnings and 8 percent that generated low-level warnings were not completed. In a user survey 82 percent (31 of 38) of doctors and nurses considered the system to be an improvement on conventional procedures.

These findings confirm those of Steven et al.[70] in 1999 in Australia. These authors reviewed anonymous adverse incident reports from general practitioners and found that 50 percent of these incidents were associated with ADEs. The reviewers estimated that computer-based prescribing with decision support could eliminate at least a third of these problems in general practice.

Although results such as these support the inclusion of decision-support functions in electronic-prescribing systems, there is still much to learn on this topic. Magnus et al.[71] analyzed questionnaires returned from 220 U.K. general practitioners who routinely used elec-

Table 22-4. International Prescribing Error Studies

Type of Study	Reference	Country	Data Collection	Site	Study Design	Results
Chart review	Dean et al. 2002[60]	U.K.	4 weeks	Hospital	Prospective chart review by pharmacists visiting wards 36,200 prescription items	1.5% prescribing errors were identified 0.4% serious errors 1.1% as less serious.
Chart review	Van den Bemt et al. 2002[64]	Netherlands	5 days	Two hospitals	Prospective chart review by pharmacists visiting the wards 3,540 prescriptions items	9.9% prescribing errors
Chart review	Shah et al. 2001[62]	U.K.	2 months	Community practice/ ambulatory care. 23 doctors (from 3 general practice sites) 3 community pharmacies	Prospective chart review of prescriptions taken to community pharmacies 37,821 prescription items	7.46% 10.2% prescribing errors for hand written prescriptions 7.9% for computer generated prescriptions
Chart review	Buurma et al. 2001[65]	Netherlands	1 day	Community practice/ ambulatory care 141 community pharmacies	Prospective chart review of prescriptions taken to community pharmacies 4,595 prescriptions	4.3% prescribing errors 22.2% of prescribing errors could potentially have had clinical consequences
Chart review	Westein et al. 2001[66]	Netherlands	1 week	Community practice/ ambulatory care 23 community pharmacies	Prospective chart review of prescriptions taken to community pharmacies 39,357 prescription items	10% prescribing errors
Chart review	Fowlie et al. 2000[63]	U.K.	17 months	Hospital Orthopedic ward	Prospective chart review by pharmacists visiting wards 2,230 handwritten prescription items 2,030 computer-generated prescription items 826 handwritten discharge prescription items 1,658 computer-generated prescription items	7.5% prescribing errors of hand written inpatient prescriptions 4.7% prescribing errors of computerised inpatient prescriptions 7.5% prescribing errors of hand written discharge prescriptions 4.8% prescribing errors of computerised discharge prescriptions
Chart review	Ho L et al. 1992[67]	Canada	25 weeks	Hospital	Prospective chart review by pharmacists reviewing prescriptions in a central pharmacy Review of prescriptions sent to a central pharmacy 237,798 prescription items	0.56% prescribing errors. 11% of errors were defined as potentially fatal or severe

tronic-prescribing systems with decision-support functions. Twenty-two percent of the general practitioners responding to this survey admitted that they "frequently" or "very frequently" overrode the drug interaction alerts without properly checking them. One reason for overriding the alerts was the perception that they were frequently irrelevant. Nevertheless, 90 percent of the general practitioners agreed that it should be more difficult to override alerts for potentially lethal drug combinations.

Contributory factors have been identified for prescribing errors. Westein et al.[66] 2001 in the Netherlands found that the first prescription in a new treatment episode significantly increased the risk of a prescribing error in community practice (OR = 1.75). Buurma et al.[65] 2001 in the Netherlands confirmed that prescribing errors in the community were three times as frequent for handwritten prescriptions as for computer-generated prescriptions (OR = 3.30). Also, compared with prescriptions by the patient's own general practitioner, prescriptions of specialists (OR = 1.82), other general practitioners (OR = 1.49), and other prescribers, such as dentists and midwives (OR = 1.95), gave a higher probability of prescribing error.

Few computerized-prescribing systems are in use in hospitals worldwide. In the majority of hospitals, prescribing errors have been identified and corrected by pharmacists reviewing these prescriptions in the central pharmacy or on wards. Dale et al.[72] reported a U.K. study of pharmacist interventions to prevent prescribing errors after visiting ward areas to review prescription charts. Details of 740 interventions to correct prescribing errors were collected over a 12-week period. When these interventions were reviewed independently by a senior hospital doctor, more than 25 percent of them were considered to be major or life saving. Seventy-nine percent of the pharmacists' interventions were implemented by prescribers.

Barber, Batty, and Rideout[73] in 1997 developed and validated a model to predict the number of accepted pharmacists interventions on prescribed therapy in a U.K. hospital. The model was validated by comparing prospective pharmacist intervention data from several hospitals with the model-predicted number of interventions. The expected number of interventions in an intensive-care area was 3.17 times as great as that in a pediatric ward and 5.31 times as great as that in any other type of ward.

Although there is evidence that pharmacist review is an effective means to prevent prescribing errors, there are issues concerning the comprehensiveness and extent of this service. Farrar et al.[74] in 1997 examined all pharmacist-intervention data in a U.K. hospital over a five-month period. The interventions were analyzed to determine the time between the moment that the prescription was written and the moment when the pharmacist visited the ward to review the prescription and make any needed intervention. The analysis revealed that only 27.5 percent of interventions were made within 12 hours of the prescription being written. The number of interventions increased to 56.9 percent after 24 hours; however, it took 96 hours to make 88.8 percent of interventions. In some cases, even more time was needed for the pharmacists to make 100 percent of their interventions. The time delays were due to the lack of regular pharmacist visits to the wards during much of the weekends and at night, when the clinical pharmacy service was not open.

Scobie et al.[75] described a U.K. initiative to promote safe prescribing and administration of medicines. Medical students in their last year of training underwent a program of structured teaching and assessment. Teaching comprised five practical exercises covering seven skills. One month later, a random sample of taught and nontaught students participated in a nine-station objective structured clinical examination to assess the impact of the teaching. The taught group achieved higher scores in eight of the nine stations. At four stations, their scores were higher than those of the nontaught students to a statistically significant degree.

Preparation and Administration Errors

Studies reviewing drug administration errors in hospitals are presented in **Table 22-5**. Drug preparation and administration error rates ranged between 2.12 percent and 52.5 percent.

Table 22-5. International Drug Administration Error Studies

Type of Study	Reference	Country	Data Collection	Site	Study Design	Results
Observation	Angalakuditi, 2003[76]	India	n/a	Hospital pediatric ward	Observation of liquid medicine dose measurement and administration in 175 children; followed by an educational initiative and a second data collection in 162 children	52.4% administration error rate 2.3% administration error rate following education initiative
Observation	Pourrat et al., 2003[77]	France	1 month	Hospital: Medical ward Surgical intensive care Pediatric vascular ward	1,632 opportunities for error	13.4% administration error rate
Retrospective chart review	Fontan et al., 2003[78]	France	2 months	Hospital pediatric nephrology ward	4,532 prescribed drugs	29.3% administration error including wrong-time error with handwritten prescriptions or 24.3% excluding wrong-time errors 22.5% administration errors including wrong-time errors for computerized prescriptions or 9.7% excluding wrong-time errors
Incident reporting	Ito and Yamazumi, 2003[79]	Japan	2 months	44 psychiatric hospitals	221 incident reports	Administration to wrong patient 35.7% 24.9% of errors intercepted before being administered to patients Errors more frequent in units with no patient name on medicine pouches
Observation	Bruce and Wong, 2002[80]	U.K.	4 weeks	Hospital medical admissions ward	Observation of i.v. preparation and administration 107 opportunities for error observed	25.2% preparation and administration error rate including wrong-time errors 10.3% error rate excluding wrong-time errors
Observation	Taxis and Barber, 2002[69]	U.K.		Teaching and nonteaching hospitals (10 wards)	Observation of i.v. preparation and administration 430 opportunities for error	49% error rate 1% severe errors 29% moderate errors 19% minor errors Frequent errors administering bolus doses too quickly Incorrect preparation of doses that required multiple-step preparation

Method	Study	Country	Duration	Setting	Opportunities	Findings
Observation	Almond, 2002[81]	U.K.	6 months	Hospital medical/renal ward	1,169 opportunities for error	10% administration error with manual system; 5% administration error with computer system and bar-code reader
Incident reporting	McNally KM, et al., 1998[82]	Australia	23 days; 31 days	Hospital surgical ward	Self-reporting and baseline measurement, followed by FMEA to identify and improve systems and a further self-reporting period	3.3% administration error rate; 2.3% administration error rate
Observation	Hartley and Dhillon, 1998[83]	U.K.	39 days	Hospital 154 patients	Observation of preparation and administration of i.v. doses	26.9% i.v. preparation and administration error rate; 4.7% of errors classified as major; 17.3% of errors classified as moderate; 77.9% of errors classified minor
Observation	Ho CY, 1997[68]	U.K.	16 days	Hospital care of the elderly ward	2,170 opportunities for error observed by independent observer	5.5% administration error rate; Omission errors were the main type of error
Observation	Cavell and Hughes, 1997[84]	U.K.		Hospital 1: medical ward with computer prescribing and administration records; Hospital 2: medical ward with manual prescribing and computer records	1,295 opportunities for error; 1,206 opportunities for error	18% administration errors including wrong-time errors; 5.5% excluding wrong-time errors; 40% administration error including wrong time errors; 5.7% excluding wrong-time errors
Observation	Ridge and Jenkins, 1996[85]	U.K.	3 months	Hospital 2 medical wards 2 surgical wards 2 medicine for the elderly wards	Observation of oral dose administration; 3,312 opportunities for error	2.5% administration error rate; Errors of omission were the largest category; Wrong dose accounted for 155 of errors
Chart review and self-reporting	Kruse et al., 1992[86]	Australia	46 weeks	Hospital geriatric assessment and rehabilitation unit	129,234 opportunities for error	2.98% administration errors, excluding wrong-time errors, for a two-nurse system; 2.12% administration errors, excluding wrong-time errors, for a single-nurse system

Observational methods have been proved to be a valid and reliable method to detect preparation and administration errors.[24] Retrospective chart review and incident reporting are less robust methods to study drug-administration errors, and the validity of the results depends on the research method used. Error rates differ significantly, depending on whether wrong-time errors (i.e., whether the medicine was administered within an agreed time period of the time prescribed) are included in the count. The accepted window within which a drug may be administered is normally within 30 to 60 minutes of the prescribed time.

Studies by Bruce and Wong,[80] Taxis and Barber,[87] and Hartley and Dhillon[83] concerning the administration of i.v. doses are important. Error rates for these types of medicines are much higher than are those for oral medicines. Further studies are required to identify effective methods to minimize errors with these products.

Ho et al.[68] found that patients were at greatest risk of experiencing a medication-administration error in the first 48 hours of admission and in the first 48 hours after the drug is prescribed.

Methods to lower administration-error rates are included in some studies. An educational initiative that targeted for oral-medicine measurement was followed by significant improvement.[76] Two studies showed that computerized prescriptions and use of an administration record that included a bar-code reader helped reduce administration errors.[78,81] However, the time required for nursing staff to administer medicines may double when they use an electronic system.[81] Cavell and Hughes[84] did not find any reduction, indicating the significance of administration errors due to causes not affected by electronic prescribing, such as ambiguous strength designation on labels or in packaging, product nomenclature (look-alike or sound-alike names, use of lettered or numbered prefixes and suffixes), inaccurate dosage calculations, inadequately trained personnel, and lapses in individual performance.

Nurses' views concerning two-nurse versus single-nurse medicine administration systems have changed over the last 10 years. Under the former practice, used in many hospitals internationally, two nurses check and administer each medication dose. In recent years, in the wake of nursing shortages and in view of the lack of a research base to support this practice, hospitals have switched to single-nurse administration for most medicines. There are little data to determine the effect of this change on drug-administration error rates; however, two Australian studies have been published on this subject.

Kruse et al.[86] published a crossover study comparing error rates when medications were administered by two nurses and by a single nurse. Errors were detected by retrospective chart review and voluntary reporting. The error rate for single-nurse administration, 0.298 percent, was significantly higher than the 0.212 percent rate for two-nurse administration. The rates of drug-administration error were less than those reported in other studies. The authors acknowledge that more errors might have been recorded if an observational method had been used.

The authors concluded that the use of two nurses to administer medication does reduce the administration-error rate to a statistically significant degree. However, because the majority of errors were considered minor and had no serious adverse consequences, the manpower requirements for two nurses to administer all medicines on a routine basis could not be justified.

Jarman et al.[88] found that 74 percent of the hospitals in the State of Victoria in Australia operated a single-nurse medicine-administration system. A comprehensive literature review revealed no reliable evidence to support this practice. A research study was undertaken in the hospital to change the system of medicine administration from a two-nurse system to a single-nurse system for most medicines, but with a continuing requirement for double-checking in the following circumstances:

- medicines requiring calculations

- drugs of addiction
- cytotoxic agents
- new and unfamiliar drugs
- epidural and other nerve-blocking agents
- insulin according to sliding scale
- blood and blood products
- potassium chloride in excess of 2 grams

Data were collected concerning the number of reported medication-administration errors. Five administration errors were reported over seven months with the two-nurse administration system prior to the study, and four administration errors were reported in the hospital over seven months with the single-nurse system.

At the completion of the study, a convenience sample of 129 nurses completed a questionnaire concerning single checking and double checking systems for medicines administration. The nurses indicated that they were aware of the level of responsibility required for single-nurse administration of medicines. The majority of nurses appreciated the increased autonomy that the switch change to single-person checking provided. They also identified benefits to patients, including that nurses were able to be more responsive to patient needs with the time released from medication-administration duties.

In order to gain greater understanding of what constitutes safe practice for medication administration in hospitals, it would be helpful if a research study were carried out that used the observation method to compare single- and two-nurse drug preparation and administration of all medicines and routes, especially the i.v. route.

Few studies have explored drug-administration errors in the community (i.e., in patients' homes). Barat et al.[89] studied drug therapy in the elderly in Denmark. The results of the study indicated differences between medication orders in general practitioners' records and the medications that patients were actually taking; 22 percent of patients were taking different drugs, 71 percent were taking different doses, and 66 percent were using different regimens (frequency). Twenty-four percent of patients admitted they did not always follow their prescriptions, deviations from the prescription were toward lower doses and less-frequent drug intake. Only 60 percent of patients knew the purpose of their medicine. Persons living alone were more prone to medication errors than were those living with another person. Other studies have found similar results in the U.K.[90]

Other studies have found that many adverse reactions to medicines in older people could be prevented.[91,92] In addition, patients' medications often change at the time of discharge from hospital. This can cause particular confusion in elderly patients and lead to medication errors.[93]

National programs have been set up in Australia and England to ensure that elderly patients in the community have their medicines reviewed regularly. In Australia, the Domiciliary Medicines Management Review program, operated by doctors and pharmacists, has been available since October 2001. In England, as part of the National Service Framework for Older People, an initiative was taken to ensure that by April 2002 all patients aged over 75 years would have an annual review of their medications. Persons taking four or more medicines would be reviewed twice a year. By April 2004, all community health care authorities were to have schemes in place to ensure that older people get more help from their pharmacists in using their medicines.[94]

The implementation of medication reviews went ahead as planned. In a recent study in the UK, 872 patients aged over 80 were recruited during an emergency admission (any cause) if returning to their own home or warden (sheltered) accommodation and taking two or more drugs daily on hospital discharge. The intervention involved two home visits by a pharmacist within two weeks and eight weeks to educate patients and carers about their drugs and to remove out of date drugs, inform general practitioners of drug reactions and interactions, and inform the community pharmacist if a compliance aid was needed. Patients were randomly allocated into the implementation arm and the control arm (no pharmacist visits).

The outcome measures were the total emergency readmissions to hospital at six months and the death and quality of life measured with the EQ-5D method.

After six months 178 readmissions had occurred in the control group and 234 readmissions in the intervention group. In the control group there were 63 deaths and 49 deaths in the intervention group. The ED-5D quality of life scores decreased (worsened) by a mean 0.14 in the control group and 0.13 in the intervention group. The study concluded that patients who had their medicines reviewed by a pharmacist had a significantly higher rate of hospital admission and did not have a significantly improved quality of life or reduced death rate. More research is required to explain this counterintuitive finding and identify more effective methods of medication review.[95]

Dispensing Errors

There are fewer international studies examining pharmacy-dispensing errors than administration errors. This may indicate that there are fewer errors of this type, but the real reason for the discrepancy is not known.

In the U.K., pharmacy departments from 89 hospitals documented details concerning dispensing errors and sent this information to a single hospital pharmacy department, where it was entered into a database.[96] A dispensing error was defined as "an error which is detected and reported after the item has left the pharmacy department."

From 1991 to 2001, 7,158 error reports were received. Thirty-four percent of these reports were for medications prescribed for inpatient use, 28 percent were for discharge medicines, 20 percent were for outpatients, and 14 percent were for other uses. The errors were detected by nurses (45 percent), hospital pharmacists (17 percent), patients (17 percent), and other hospital staff (21 percent).

The most common errors were supplying the wrong medicine (23 percent), the wrong strength of medicine (23 percent), the wrong directions for use (10 percent), and the wrong quantity of medicine (10 percent). The remaining errors (44 percent) were categorized as "other."

Factors that contributed to the errors were recorded. The most common reasons were look-alike or sound-alike medicines (33 percent), high workload/low staffing (23 percent), inexperienced staff (20 percent), faulty transcriptions (14 percent), and other causes (10 percent).

Recorded outcomes of the errors included one fatality (0.02 percent), serious detrimental effects (0.08 percent), moderate detrimental effects (6.6 percent), and no or minor detrimental effects (92.5 percent).

The 10 drugs most commonly involved in dispensing errors accounted for 19 percent of the errors and 27 percent of the seriously detrimental or fatal outcomes. These drugs were prednisolone, morphine sulphate, isosorbide mononitrate, warfarin, aspirin, lisinopril, carbamazepine, diclofenac, co-codamol, and flucloxacillin. With this group of drugs, the most common error was dispensing the wrong strength. In an earlier report from the same group, the dispensing-error rate in U.K. hospital pharmacies was reported as 1.5 percent; of these, 0.4 percent were considered serious errors.[97]

Many hospitals in the U.K. are installing automation equipment to dispense original manufacturers' packs and patient packs. The main reason is to reduce the amount of time pharmacy staff spend dispensing. Other reasons include reducing the amount of shelf space required for dispensing stock and ensuring that physical stock level is the same as computerized stock level. Nevertheless, one U.K. study has reported that dispensing errors in a hospital pharmacy decreased by 50 percent following the introduction of automated dispensing equipment.[98]

The dispensing-error rate in U.K. community pharmacies is reported as 1 percent; of this total, serious errors account for 0.18 percent.[99] Chua et al.[100] found dispensing-error rates in community pharmacies to be 0.08 percent, with 0.48 percent near misses. Near misses occur six times as often as dispensing errors do, indicating the importance of a check from a second person. (This finding appears to be at odds with the trend toward single-nurse drug administration systems.) The most frequent types of errors in the community pharmacy studies were incorrect strength, followed, in decreasing order, by incorrect drug, incorrect quantity, incorrect dosage form, and inaccurate label. The study participants agreed that feedback from the reporting scheme was helpful and that the scheme was feasible and would continue to be used.

Summary

There is growing international awareness of the issue of adverse events in health care. World health care organizations, as well as national and local groups, are seeking to promote awareness of this problem, establish incident-reporting systems, and create a fair culture within health care so that these issues can be reported and discussed and action can be taken to manage these adverse events.

Adverse events involving medications are recognized as an important component of the overall problem. National targets and initiatives to reduce medication errors are under way in several countries.

The lack of standardization of terminology and methodology makes it difficult to study and compare information concerning medication errors internationally. The use of case studies to describe rare medication errors is likely to be helpful, but these reports should be developed using a standard methodology.

Research studies using the same terminology and methodology across more than one country provide important information about medication risks and how to manage them. Drug products and medication-use processes often differ significantly from country to country, and research results from one country cannot automatically be applied to another. It is necessary to understand the differences in the countries' health care systems and to perform validation studies in the local health care setting.

The types of risks and error rates associated with i.v. and parenteral medication process are much higher than those associated with oral medicines and require a high priority for the development and implementation of solutions.

Many safe-medication-practice recommendations and initiatives have been developed on the basis of expert opinion. The recommended solutions may not have been mistake-proof or risk assessed and in many cases are not evidence based. There is some evidence of the benefits of pharmacist prescription review, electronic prescribing, and automation as effective methods to help reduce medication errors. However, much more research is required to better understand the problem of medication errors and to develop solutions that are effective on a broad, even worldwide, scale.

References

1. World Health Organization. World Health Report 2002. Reducing Risks and Promoting Healthy Life. October 2002. WHO: Geneva, Switzerland. Available at www.who.int/whr/en/. Accessed November, 2004.

2. World Health Organization. Fifty-Fifth World Health Assembly Resolution 55.13. Quality of care: patient safety. 23 March 2002. WHO: Geneva, Switzerland. Available at www.wo.int/gb/ebwha/pdf_ files/WHA55/ea5513.pdf. Accessed November 2004.

3. World Health Professions Alliance. Fact Sheet on Patient Safety. 29 April 2002. Geneva, Switzerland. www.whpa.org/factptsafety.htm. Accessed November 2004.

4. Wilson, RM, Runciman WB, Gibberd RW, Harrison BT, Newby L, Hamilton JD. The Quality in Australia Health Care Study. Med J Austral. 1995;163:458-476.

5. Vincent C. The human element of adverse of adverse events. Med J Austral. 1999;170:404-405.

6. Wilson RM, Harrison BT, Gibberd RW, Hamilton JD. An analysis of the causes of adverse events from the Quality in Australian Health Care Study. Medical J Austral. 1999;170:411-415.

7. Department of Health [England]. An Organisation with a Memory. Report of the U.K. Department of Health. London: Department of Health; 13 June 2000. Available at www.doh.gov.uk/orgmemreport/index.htm. Accessed November 2004.

8. Vincent C, Neale G, Woloshynowych M. Adverse events in British hospitals: preliminary retrospective record review. Br Med J. 2001;322:517-519.

9. Neale G, Woloshynowych M, Vincent C. Exploring the causes of adverse events in NHS hospital practice. J Royal Soc Med. 2001;94:322-330.

10. Howard RL, Avery AJ, Howard PD, Partridge M. Qual Saf Health Care. 2003;12:280-285.

11. Schioler T, Lipczak H, Pedersen BL, et al. Incidence of adverse events in hospitals. A retrospective study of medical records. Ugeskr Laeger. 2001;163:4377-4379. Article in Danish.

12. Baune B, Kessler V, Patris S, et al. Medical iatrogenics. A survey on a given day. Presse Med. 2003;32:683-638. Article in French.

13. Otero-Lopez MJ, Bajo Bajo A, Maderuelo Fernandez JA, Dominguez-Gil Hurle A. Preventable drug effects in the emergency department. Rev Clin Esp. 1999;796-805. Article in Spanish.

14. Alonson-Hernandez P, Otero-Lopez MJ, Maderuelo Fernandez JA. Hospital admissions caused by medicines, incidence, characteristics, and cost. Farmacia Hospitalaria. 2002:26:77-79. Article in Spanish.

15. Rodriguez-Monguio R, Otero MJ, Rivora J. Assessment of the economic impact of adverse drug effects. Pharmaceconomics. 2003;21:623-650.

16. Millar J. System performance is the real problem. Health Care Papers. 2001:2:79-85.

17. Ohlhauser L, Schurman DP. National agenda: Local leadership. Health Care Papers. 2001;2:77-78.

18. Runciman WB, Helps SC, Sexton EJ, Malpass A. A classification for incidents and accidents in the health-care system. J Qual Clin Pract. 1998;18:199-211.

19. Department of Health (England). Building a Safer NHS for Patients: Implementing an Organisation with a Memory. London: Department of Health; 13 August 2001. Available at www.doh.gov.uk/buildsafenhs. Accessed November, 2004.

20. Swiss Expert Group on Patient Safety Improvement. Towards a safe health care system. A proposal for a national programme on patient safety improvements for Switzerland. 9 April 2001. Available at www.swiss-q.org/apr-2001/docs/Final_ReportE.pdf. Accessed November, 2004.

21. Baker GR, Norton P. Patient safety and health care error in the Canadian health care system. A systematic review and analysis of leading practices in Canada with reference to key initiatives elsewhere. A report for Health Canada. Ottawa, Ontario, Canada: 4 December 2002. Available at www.publications.doh.gov.uk/buildsafenhs. Accessed November, 2004.

22. National Coordinating Council for Medication Error Reporting Program. Council defines terms and sets goals for medication error reporting and preventing. 16 October 1995. United States Pharmacopoeia, Rockville, MD. Available at www.nccmerp.org/press/press1995-10-16.html. Accessed November, 2004.

23. Otero ML, Codina JC, Tames A, Perez EM. Medication errors: Standardising errors: Standardising the terminology and taxonomy. *Farm Hosp.* 2003;(3E)137-149. Article in Spanish.

24. Dean B, Barber N. Validity and reliability of observational methods for studying medication administration error. *Am J Health-Syst Pharm.* 2001;58:54-59.

25. International Pharmaceutical Federation (FIP). Statement on professional standards. Medication errors associated with prescribed medicines. 1999. FIP: The Hague, Netherlands. Available at www.fip.org/pdf/mrderror.pdf. Accessed November, 2004.

26. Council of Europe and World Health Organization Regional Office. Consensus document on medication safety adopted by experts. 2 December 2002. Strasbourg, France. Available at :www.coe.int/T/E/Social_Cohesion/soc-sp/Public_Health/Pharma_and_Medicine/consensusdocument_CoE_WHO_EnglishVersion.asp. Accessed November, 2004.

27. Department of Health (England). National guidance on the safe administration of intrathecal chemotherapy. London: Department of Health; 2001. Available at www.doh.gov.uk/intrathecalchemotherapy. Accessed

28. National Patient Safety Agency. Patient Safety Alert. Potassium Chloride Concentrate Solution 2002. Alert 01. Available at www.npsa.nhs.uk. Accessed

29. Medicines and Health Care Products Regulatory Agency (United Kingdom). Best Practice Guidance on the Labelling and Packaging of Medicines. Guidance Note 25. 2002. Available at www.mca.gov.uk/inforesources/publications/gn25.pdf. Accessed

30. National Health Service (England). Purchasing for safety 2003. Purchasing and Supplies Agency. London: Department of Health; 2003. Available at www.pasa.doh.gov.uk/pharma/purchasing_for_safety.stm. Accessed November, 2004.

31. Bermejo-Alvarez MA, Cosio F, Hevia A, Iglesias-Fernandez C. Accidental epidural administration of potassium chloride. *Rev Esp Anestesiol Reanim.* 2000;47(Aug-Sept):323-324. Article in Spanish.

32. Cousins DH, Upton DR. Medication errors: Is it time to make strong KCl a controlled drug? *Pharm Pract.* 2000;10:187.

33. Peduto VA, Mezzetti D, Gori F. A clinical diagnosis of an inadvertent epidural administration of potassium chloride. *Eur J Anaesthesiol.* 1999;16:410-412.

34. Cousins DH, Upton DR. Medication errors: Proceed with caution. *Pharm Pract.* 1999;9:132.

35. Cousins DH, Upton DR. Medication errors: Act now to prevent KCl deaths. *Pharm Pract.* 1996;6:307-310.

36. Liu K, Chia YY. Inadvertent epidural injection of potassium chloride. Report two cases. *Acta Anaesthesiol Scand.* 1995;39;1134-1137.

37. Cousins DH, Upton DR. Medication errors: Lethal drug ampoules still being issued to wards? *Pharm Pract.*1995;5:130.

38. Cousins DH, Upton DR. Medication errors: Stop these parenteral blunders. *Hosp Pharm Pract.* 1994;4:388-390.

39. Tessler MJ, White I, Naugler-Colville M, Biehl DR. Inadvertent epidural administration of potassium chloride. A case report. *Can J Anaesthesiol.* 1988;6:631-633.

40. Shanker KB, Palkar NV, Nishala R. Paraplegia following epidural potassium chloride. *Anaesthesia.* 1985;40:45-47.

41. Rendell-Baker L, Meyer JA. Hazards of potassium chloride solutions. *Lancet.* 1985; 2:329.

42. Pagani I, Carnevale L, Bonezzi C, Preseglio I. Description of a clinical case of inadvertent peridural administration of 15 percent potassium chloride. *Minerva Anestesiol.* 1984;50:407-410. Article in Italian.

43. Harsanyi L. Fatal errors in potassium therapy. *Morphol Igazsagugyi Orv.* 1983;2:150-152. Article in Hungarian.

44. Williams RHP. Potassium overdosage: a potential hazard of non-acid parenteral fluid containers. *Br Med J.* 1973;1:714-715.

45. Chambers DG. Dangers of rapid infusions of potassium (letter). *Med J Austral.* 1973; 20:945-946.

46. Aronson JK. Anecdotes as evidence. We need guidelines for reporting anecdotes of suspected adverse drug reactions (editorial). *Br Med J.* 2003;326:1346.

47. Vandenbroucke JP. In defense of case reports and case series. *Ann Intern Med.* 2001;134:330-334.

48. British Airways. Personal communication to the National Patient Safety Agency concerning the reporting of air transport safety incidents. 16 July 2002.

49. European Union. Council Directive 92/27/EEC of 31 March 1992 on the labelling of medicinal products for human use and on package leaflets. Brussels, Belgium. Available at www.ikev.org/docs/eu/392L0027.htm. Accessed November, 2004.

50. Lyftingsmo S. Improving the labelling of medicines internationally. 1 August 2002. Elverum, Norway. Available at www.lytingsmo.no. Accessed November, 2004.

51. Semple, JS, Morgan, JE, Garner ST, Sutherland K, Milligan, M. The effect of self-administration and reuse of patients' own drugs on a hospital pharmacy. *Pharm J.* 1995;255:124-126.

52. Audit Commission United Kingdom. A spoonful of sugar. Medicines management in NHS hospitals. London. December 2001. Available at www.audit-commission.gov.uk. Accessed November, 2004.

53. European Association of Hospital Pharmacists. EAHP Survey 2000. Paper presented at the EAHP Congress; 21<en>23 March 2001; Amsterdam, the Netherlands. Available at www.eahponline.org. Accessed November, 2004.

54. Pedersen CA, Schneider PJ, Scheckelhoff DJ. ASHP national survey of pharmacy practice in hospital settings: Dispensing and administration—2002. *Am J Health-Syst Pharm.* 2003;60:52-68.

55. Pedersen CA, Schneider PJ, Scheckelhoff DJ. ASHP national survey of pharmacy practice in hospital settings: Prescribing and transcribing—2001. *Am J Health-Syst Pharm.* 2001;58:2251-2266

56. Dean BS, Allan EL, Barber ND, Barker KN. Comparison of medication errors in an American and a British hospital. *Am J Health Syst Pharm.* 1995;52:2543-2549.

57. Taxis K, Dean B, Barber N. Hospital drug distribution systems in the U.K. and Germany—a study of medication errors. *Pharm World Sci.*1999;21:25-31.

58. Wirtz V, Taxis K, Barber ND. An observational study of intravenous medication errors in the United Kingdom and in Germany. *Pharm World Sci.* 2003;25:104-111.

59. Taxis K, Dean B, Barber N. The validation of an existing method of scoring the severity of medication administration errors for use in Germany. *Pharm World Sci.* 2002;24:236-239.

60. Dean B, Barber N, Schachter M. What is a prescribing error? *Qual Saf Health Care.* 2000;9:232-237.

61. Dean B, Schachter M, Vincent C, Barber N. Prescribing errors in hospital inpatients: Their incidence and clinical significance. *Qual Saf Health Care.* 2002;11:340-344.

62. Shah SN, Aslam M, Avery AJ. A survey of prescription errors in general practice. *Pharm J.* 2001;267:860-862.

63. Fowlie F, Bennie M, Jardine G, Bicknell S, Toner D, Caldwell M. Evaluation of an electronic prescribing system in a British hospital. *Pharm J.* 2000;265:R16.

64. Van den Bemt PM, Postma MJ, van Roon EN, Chow MC, Fijn R, Brouwers JR. Cost-benefit analysis of the detection of prescribing error by hospital pharmacy staff. *Drug Saf.* 2002;25:135-143.

65. Buurma H, de Smet PA, van den Hoff OP, Egberts AC. Nature, frequency and determinants of prescription modifications in Dutch community pharmacies. *Br J Clin Pharmacol.* 2001;52(July):85-91.

66. Westein MP, Herings RM, Leufkens HG. Determinants of pharmacists' intervention linked to prescription processing. *Pharm World Sci.* 2001;23(3):98-101.

67. Ho L, Brown GR, Millin B. Characterization of errors detected during central order review. *Can J Hosp Pharm.* 1992;45:193-197.

68. Ho CY, Dean BS, Barber ND. When do medication administration errors happen to hospital inpatients? *Int J Pharm Pract.* 1997;5:91-96.

69. Nightingale PG, Adu P, Richards NT, Peters M. Implementation of rules based computerised bedside prescribing and administration: intervention study. *Br Med J.* 2000;320:750-753.

70. Steven ID, Malpass A, Moller J, Runciman WB, Helps SC. Towards safer drug use in general practice. *J Qual Clin Pract.* 1999;(19):47-50.

71. Magnus D, Rodgers S, Avery AJ. GPs' views on computerised drug interactions alerts: questionnaire survey. *J Clin Pharm Therapy.* 2002;27:311-312.

72. Dale A, Copeland R, Barton R. Prescribing errors on medical wards and the impact of clinical pharmacists. *Int J Pharm Pract.* 2003;11:19-24.

73. Barber ND, Batty R, Rideout DA. Predicting the rate of physician-accepted interventions

by hospital pharmacists in the United Kingdom. *Am J Health-Syst Pharm.* 1997;4:397-405.

74. Farrar KT, Stoddart MJ, Slee AL. Clinical pharmacy and reactive prescription review—Time for a change. *Pharm J.* 1998;260:759-761.

75. Scobie SD, Lawson M, Cavell G, Taylor K, Jackson SH, Roberts TE. Meeting the challenge of prescribing and administering medicines safely: structured teaching and assessment of final year students. *Med Educ.* 2003;37:434-437.

76. Angalakuditi MV, Sunderland VB. Liquid medication dosing errors: A pre-post time series in India. *Int J Pharm Pract.* 2003;11:105-110.

77. Pourrat X, Antier D, Doucet O, et al. Identification and analysis of errors in prescription, preparation and administration of drugs in intensive care, medicine and surgery at the University Hospital Centre of Tours. Article in French. *Presse Med.* 2003;32:876-882.

78. Fontan JE, Maneglier V, Nguyen VX, Loirat C, Brion F. Medication errors in hospitals: computerized unit dose drug dispensing system versus ward stock distribution system. *Pharm World Sci.* 2003;25:112-117.

79. Ito, H, Yamazumi. Common types of medication errors in long-term psychiatric care units. *J Qual Health Care.*2003;15:207-212.

80. Bruce J, Wong I. Parenteral drug administration errors by nursing staff on an acute admissions ward during day duty. *Drug Saf.* 2001;24:855-862.

81. Almond M. The effect of the controlled entry of electronic prescribing and medicines administration on the quality of prescribing, safety and success of administration on an acute ward. *Br J Healthcare Comput Info Manage.* 2002;19:41-46.

82. McNally KM, Sunderland VB. Non blame medication administration error reporting by nursing staff at a teaching hospital in Australia. *Int J Pharm Pract.* 1998;6:67-71.

83. Hartley GM, Dhillon S. An observational study of the prescribing and administration of intravenous drugs in a general hospital. *Int J Pharm Pract.* 1998;6:38-45.

84. Cavell GF, Hughes DK. Does computerized prescribing improve the accuracy of drug administration? *Pharm J.* 1997;259:82-83.

85. Ridge KW, Jenkins DB, Noyce PR, Barber ND. Medication errors during hospital drug rounds. *Qual Health Care.* 1995:4:240-343.

86. Kruse H, Johnson A, O'Connell D, Clarke T. Administering non-restricted medication in hospital. The implications and cost of using two nurses. *Austral Clin Rev.* 1992;12:77-83.

87. Taxis K, Barber N. Ethnographic study of incidence and severity of intravenous drug errors. *Br Med J.* 2003;326:684-688.

88. Jarman H, Jacobs E, Zielinski V. Medication study supports registered nurses' competence for single checking. *Int J Nurs Pract* 2002;8:330-335.

89. Barat I, Andreasen F, Damsgaard EM. Drug therapy in the elderly: what doctors believe and patients actually do. *Br J Clin Pharm.* 2001;51:615-622.

90. Lowe CJ, Raynor DK. Intentional no-adherence in elderly patients: fact or fiction. *Pharm J.* 2000;265:R19-20.

91. Cunningham G, Dodd TRP, Grant DJ, McMurdo M, Richards RME. Drug-related problems in elderly patients admitted to Tayside hospitals, methods for prevention and subsequent reassessment. *Age Aging.* 1997;26:375-382.

92. Mannesse CK, Derkx FH, de Ridder MA, Man in't Veld AJ, van der Cammen TJ. Contribution of adverse drug reactions to hospital admission of older patients. *Age Aging.* 2000;29:35-39.

93. Duggan C, Feldman R, Hough J, Bates I. Reducing adverse prescribing discrepancies following hospital discharge. *Int J Pharm Pract.* 1998;6:77-82.

94. Department of Health (England). National Service Framework. Medicines and older people. Implementing medicines related aspects of the NSF for older people. London: Department of Health; 27 March 2001. Available at www.dh.gov.uk. Accessed November, 2004.

95. Holland R, Leneghan E, Harvey I, Smith R, Shepstone L, Lipp A, Christou M, Evans D and Hand C. Does home based medication review keep older people out of hospital? The HOMER randomized controlled trial. *Br Med J.* 2005;330:293-299.

96. Roberts DE, Spencer MG, Burfield R, Bowden S. An analysis of dispensing errors in U.K. hospitals. *Int J Pharm Pract.* 2002; 10(suppl):R6.

97. Spencer MG, Smith AP. A multicentre study of dispensing errors in UK hospitals. *Int J Pharm Pract.* 1993;2:142-146.

98. Slee A, Farrar K, Hughes D. Implementing an automated dispensing system. *Pharm J.* 2002;268:437-438.

99. Kaynes S. Negligence and the pharmacist: Dispensing errors and prescribing errors. *Pharm J.* 1996;257:32-35.

100. Chua SS, Wong I, Edmondson H, et al. A feasibility study for recording of dispensing errors and near misses in four UK primary care pharmacies. *Drug Safety.* 2003;26:803-813.

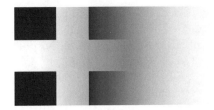

The Science of Patient-Safety Research

Richard J. Faris

Introduction

Health care professionals have been trained to "First, do no harm" when taking care of patients. This statement encompasses what we strive for caring for our patients—a safe medical care system. Yet despite our efforts to avoid harm and to do what is right for patients, evidence abounds that patients are injured from medical care.[1-12] Interest in improving the safety of medical care and of medication use has driven research efforts in hospitals and other organizations nationwide. The report *To Err Is Human*, released by the Institute of Medicine in 1999, called for an increase in funding for patient-safety research and for the creation of a national research agenda on the topic.[13] Other national groups have also called for better research into patient safety. A report from the National Patient Safety Foundation trumpeted the need for research into the underlying causes of errors and system failures that lead to safety lapses.[14]

Patient-safety research will require multidisciplinary efforts to better understand the medication-use system and the causes of safety problems. All health care professionals, including pharmacists, have the opportunity to participate in such research. To do so, they will require a set of basic research skills. These skills do not require a research-based degree, such as a Ph.D. However, for many practitioners it will take additional effort to gain the skills necessary to participate in the expanding science of patient-safety research.

This chapter reviews the impact that an unsafe medication-use system has on patient safety, describes the scientific method as a starting point for patient-safety research, and discusses some specific issues involved in understanding the science behind patient-safety research.

Impact of Patient Harm

Researchers have studied patient harm for many decades. It has been estimated that approximately 1.3 million persons are injured yearly as a result of the medical care they receive.[5] Research has implicated medications as the leading cause of injuries due to medical care.[3,9] Thus, despite advances in technology and in the education and training of health care practitioners, and the availability of newer, and presumably safer, drug entities, research suggests that patients are placed at risk when they seek medical care and are prescribed medications for therapeutic reasons. Adverse outcomes from medication use translate into drug-related morbidity and mortality, which is a huge financial burden for society. Johnson and Bootman[15] used a cost-of-illness model to estimate that drug-related morbidity and mortality cost U.S. society $76 billion a year (1995 dollars). Their model was updated by Ernst and Grizzle,[16] who determined that the figure was approximately $177 billion in 2000 dollars. This amount would place drug-related morbidity and mortality among the most expensive of all diseases.

The majority of research efforts on medication safety have centered on organized health care settings. Hospital costs account for the largest portion of health care spending in the United States.[17] Researchers have examined the impact of adverse drug events on hospital admissions. This work suggests that around 5 percent of all hospital admissions are drug related.[6,10,18-25] With hospital costs accounting for $511.2 billion in the year 2001, drug-related hospital admissions cost U.S. society $25.6 billion in unnecessary hospitalizations.[17] This amount translates into nearly $500 million for each of the 50 states and the District of Columbia, or nearly $100 for every man, woman, and child in the United States.

Drug-related deaths may be the most alarming quality issue in health care today. The 1999 IOM report estimated that approximately 98,000 patients die each year from preventable medical errors.[13] This report generated significant public debate, leading politicians to pledge additional funds to study and reduce these events. However, what is new to the politicians is not new to the health care system. Three decades ago, in 1974, Talley and Laventurier[26] estimated that up to 140,000 deaths each year were caused by adverse drug reactions. A 1998 meta-analysis concluded that 4.6 percent of recorded deaths in the United States were due to adverse drug reactions.[27] This result would place such events between the fourth and sixth leading causes of death in this country.[27] Thus, an unsafe medication-use system takes a tremendous toll on our society. Research directed at reducing the economic burden of drug-related morbidity and mortality would be highly beneficial for patients and society as a whole.

The Scientific Method

To engage in patient-safety research, a pharmacist or any other health professional must have a good understanding of research methods. Understanding and applying research has two purposes: (1) to add to the body of knowledge that is the discipline of patient safety; and (2) to increase one's own knowledge as a professional and consumer of patient-safety research.[28] Increasing knowledge within the patient-safety discipline can involve many mechanisms, including development of safety theory, practical applications of safety concepts, and development of tools to assess the medication-use system.[28] The two purposes are, moreover, not mutually exclusive.

One debate that often arises is that of theory versus practice. In truth, there is no clear line of demarcation between these two realms. Theory must be developed and refined in order to make practical application of the results. Likewise, practical applications should have theoretical underpinnings. Emphasizing one to the exclusion of the other can lead to ineffective research or to poorly designed interventions that introduce more harm than they alleviate.

What is research? *Merriam-Webster's Collegiate® Dictionary* defines research as "(1) a careful or diligent search, or (2) studious inquiry or examination; esp: investigation or experimentation aimed at the discovery and interpretation of facts, revision of accepted theories or laws in light of the new facts, or practical application of such new or revised theories or laws."[29] On the basis of this definition, we can deduce that research is a planned, organized activity that seeks to gather data to discover or apply new knowledge or to refine and apply existing knowledge. This process is often referred to as the *scientific method*. The scientific method is used to guide the research process in order to help ensure that the results are usable, reliable, and valid. As discussed below, this research process can be divided into six basic steps:

1. Identify the research question.
2. Develop a hypothesis.
3. Select a research method.
4. Collect and analyze the data.
5. Interpret the data
6. Acceptance or reject the hypothesis and conclusions.[30]

IDENTIFY THE RESEARCH QUESTION

The first step in the scientific process is to identify the research question. In other words, what are you trying to answer through research? Begin with a broad research question, then refine it until the data you need to answer the question are attainable. It is important to ask the question in a manner that will obtain an appropriate answer. For example, the question, "Can we reduce adverse drug events in our organization?" will yield simply a "yes" or "no" response. A more insightful question might be, "What is the current state of adverse drug events in our organization, and what can we do to reduce them?" Your research question will generate specific objectives that you wish to accomplish through your research.

DEVELOP A HYPOTHESIS

A *hypothesis* is a statement that contains two or more variables that are measurable or potentially measurable.[31] A *variable* is a characteristic of the people, process, or environment in a study that will have different values.[28] The hypothesis must be declarative and measurable. You must specify the relationship among the variables and be able to quantify each variable. For example, a research hypothesis could be, "Patients receiving heparin are at higher risk for bleeding than are those who are not on heparin." In this hypothesis, the variables are the use or nonuse of heparin and the presence or absence of bleeding. The hypothesis states the researcher's initial premise, namely, that bleeding will be higher in patients receiving heparin.

A study may have just one hypothesis or it may have several. The number of hypotheses depends on the research question and on objectives of the study. However, each hypothesis is under the same guidelines listed above, and each gathers evidence that leads to answering the research question.

SELECT A RESEARCH METHOD

The third step is to choose a research methodology that will allow you to test your hypothesis. A number of research designs are available; the choice should be based on the need to control for variables that influence the results. The level of control over the variables helps delineate the general type of research being conducted. This, in turn, requires that the investigator decide whether experimental or nonexperimental research is required. The distinction between experimental and nonexperimental research has to do with the control, or manipulation, of variables.

There are two types of variables. *Dependent* variables are the ones the researcher is looking at to see the impact of the experiment. These may often be referred to as the "outcomes" or "treatment effects."[32] *Independent* variables are not affected by the experiment, but rather are manipulated or controlled by it. An example of an independent variable is whether or not the patient received the intervention. This would be under the control of the researcher. Some independent variables are not under the control of the researcher and must be accounted for; examples in patient-safety research include age, gender, race, socioeconomic status, or nursing unit.

Experimental Research Designs

Experimental research is one of two types: *true experimentation* or *quasi-experimentation*.[32,33] The difference between them is the method in which patients or treatments are assigned to the study. In a true experiment, patients are randomly assigned so that each has an equal opportunity to receive the treatment or intervention. To achieve the highest level of evidence, random assignment is best.[32] When random assignment is not possible, the experiment is referred to as quasi-experimental. In patient-safety research, this is the method most often used.

Experimental designs may take several forms. In health care, the *randomized control trial* (RCT) is quite common. The randomization of a RCT makes it a true experiment. A RCT also uses two groups of patients: a control group and an intervention group. The intervention group receives the intervention or treatment, while the control group gets a placebo or, in the case of safety, "usual care." A control group is necessary for an experimental study design.[33]

Two additional types of studies that may be used in patient-safety research are the case-control study and the cohort study. A *case-control study* is done after the care or intervention has taken place. Patients who have the outcome of interest are identified (cases) and compared to similar patients who are absent of the disease or outcome of interest (controls). A case-control study identifies the risk of having the outcome of interest on the basis of the presence or absence of certain variables. A statistic similar to the odds ratio is calculated to obtain the relative risk of the outcome.

A *cohort study* is also referred to as a "prospective epidemiologic study." Cohort studies are prospective. Patients are followed after they are exposed to a treatment or an intervention to determine the outcome. These studies are difficult and expensive to conduct because it is generally necessary to follow patients for many years.[34]

Nonexperimental Study Designs

Nonexperimental study designs are very common in patient-safety research. They are termed "nonexperimental" because the researcher has no control over the variables or over the assignment of interventions to the patient. The most common nonexperimental research method is the *observational study* (also referred to as "correlational" or "associational" research). In such studies, the researcher merely observes the events and their outcomes, often retrospectively. He or she has no ability to control or manipulate the variables. For these reasons, observational research can determine whether a relationship exists but cannot assess causality.[28]

A second type of nonexperimental research design is *exploratory research*. In exploratory research, the investigator has no hypothesis but is merely trying to determine whether experimentation is warranted. Exploratory research often comes with descriptive research, where the variables of interest are described. This is also common in today's health environment. Most quality-assessment and quality-improvement activities fall under this category.

COLLECT AND ANALYZE THE DATA

Research into medication safety must involve some form of data collection. Many different mechanisms can be used to gather the information about which to make a decision. The researcher must know the strengths and weaknesses of each data-collection method. Using different methodologies may hinder comparison of results between studies.[35] There may also be differences in the scope of events monitored or in the intensity of data collection.[24,36] There is a need for consistency in both the terminology and methodology of studies investigating preventable drug-related morbidity (DRM).[37] Researchers must familiarize themselves with voluntary reporting systems, chart review, observational techniques, database research, and computerized surveillance.

Data must be collected in an unbiased and reliable manner, and the researcher must develop a data-collection tool that will meet these requirements. The tool must be clear and easy to understand, especially if more than one person will be responsible for data collection. The data-collection form should also flow in a logical format and be designed with data entry procedures in mind.

Reliability of data is very important. *Reliability* is defined as the consistency of measurement.[38] This means that if an investigator were to repeat a measure, or another person took the same measure, the results would be the same or very similar. If the reliability is low, the data are worthless for research purposes.

Continuous, Ordinal, and Nominal Variables

No discussion of research skills would be complete without some mention of statistics. Prior to performing any statistical analysis, one must define how the variables will be measured.

Measurement has been defined as the assignment of numbers to objects or events according to rules.[39] The objects or events of interest (that is, the variables) are measured on the basis of the rules set forth in the research plan.

There are three levels of measure for variables: continuous, ordinal, and nominal. It is critical that the variable be measured in the most appropriate level, depending on the characteristics of that variable.

A *continuous variable* is one that can take any value. Continuous values are often further segmented into ratio or interval numbers. *Ratio numbers* are those that have an absolute zero. A ratio value of zero indicates the absence of that characteristic. Examples of ratio numbers include weight, cholesterol level, and medication errors. *Interval numbers* are those that can take any value. The distance between any two consecutive interval numbers is the same, but there is no absolute zero. An example of an interval measurement is temperature as measured in degrees Fahrenheit. While you can have a temperature reading of 0°F, that does not mean an absence of temperature. An absolute zero makes it possible to calculate a ratio. For example, someone who weighs 100 pounds is half as heavy as someone who weighs 200 pounds. But for interval data, one cannot say that 30°F is twice as cold (or half as hot) as 60°F.

Ordinal data are used to measure characteristics of a variable where there is a specific order, but the relative distance between the measures is not known.[28] An example is the Likert scale, which may be used to measure preventability of adverse drug events. Using such a scale, one can rate how preventable an adverse drug event was on a 5-point scale, with 1 being definitely preventable, 2 possibly preventable, 3 neutral, 4 possibly not preventable, and 5 definitely not preventable. The assignment of numbers has a specific order. However, you cannot say that the distance between 1 and 2 is the same as that between 4 and 5. A common mistake is to use mean, or average, and standard deviation when analyzing ordinal data. This should not be done because the distance between the numbers is unknown. The median value is a better representation of the "average" response and frequency distributions. Ordinal values also limit the types of statistics used to analyze the data (see below).

Nominal values have meaning only in categorizing the variables. There is no order to the numbers, nor is there any representation of the distance between the values.[28] An example would be to assign the values 0 and 1 to male and female subjects, respectively. Other examples are categorizing drug-related problems and separating people by such factors as race, religion, or nursing unit. Once again, the type of statistical analysis is dictated by the level of measure. The chi-square test is one of the most common statistics used for nominal data.

When measuring a variable, one should try to measure it at the highest-possible level. This is because it is easier to collapse measurements into lower levels than to go the other way if the data were not properly collected. For example, you might collect data on patient income as a continuous value, which will allow you to later collapse the data into income categories for reporting data in a publication. If the data had been collected in income categories, you could not go back to continuous values.

Clinical versus Statistical Significance

There is a difference between statistical and clinical significance. Statistical significance depends on the effect size (i.e., the difference between the two study groups), the standard deviation, and the number of subjects in the sample. If a study had too low a power to detect true differences, you might not get statistical difference between the study group and the control group. However, the effect size might be large enough to make a subjective assessment that the difference was clinically significant. An example might be looking at two drugs that can have severe side effects. In a sample of the population, one drug might have a side effect rate of 10 percent while the second has a side effect rate of 5 percent; however, because of a small sample size, the results were not statistically significant. However, a 100% difference in the side effect rate (i.e., 5 percent versus 10 percent) would be considered clinically significant.

Inferential and Descriptive Statistics

Statistics can be descriptive or inferential. *Descriptive* statistics summarize the values. These statistics include the mean, median, and mode, as well as variance, standard deviation, and frequency distributions. *Inferential* statistics are used to determine the probability of a difference between the variables being measured. Statistical significance is determined on the basis of the chance that the results from the sample are truly different and are not due to drawing a sample that was outside a predetermined number of standard deviations from the population's mean.

Statistical significance is expressed in terms of a p-value. A p-value of 0.05 is the probability of obtaining a result as extreme as or more extreme than the actual result obtained given the null hypothesis of no difference if true. This level (i.e., 0.05) is often used as the cutoff point in research studies. The lower the p-value, the more confidence the researcher can be in the findings.

There are two broad classifications of inferential statistical methodologies: parametric and nonparametric. The test used depends on the measurement level, as discussed above, and on the distribution of the data. Data that are not normally distributed may require *nonparametric statistics*.[28] Data that are not normally distributed are usually skewed to the left or right, or may have more than one mode of distribution. The data may also exhibit a large variance relative to the mean. Nonparametric statistics include the chi-square analysis, Cochran's Q-test, Wilcoxon signed-rank test, Kruskal-Wallis statistic, Mann-Whitney U test, and the Spearman rank correlation test. Examples of *parametric statistics* include the student's t-test, analysis of variance (ANOVA), linear regression, and Pearson's product-moment correlation.

INTERPRET THE DATA

The fifth step is to make inferences from or to interpret the data. These inferences must be drawn from the hypothesis and based on the data analysis. At this point, the validity of the data and inferences are of prime importance. *Validity* is an integrated evaluative judgment of the degree to which empirical evidence and theoretical rationales support the appropriateness of inferences based on the data or measurement.[40] In terms of patient safety, validity is the degree to which the data indicating problems identify situations in which the quality of medical care is poor and can be improved.[41] Rigorous assessment of validity in evaluating medication safety has not received much attention in the literature.[35]

Determining Validity

The concept of validity has been evolving for several decades. Early in its development, validity was viewed as being three separate components: (1) content validity; (2) criterion-related validity; and (3) construct validity.

Content validity does not measure actual performance, but is based on professional judgment about the relevance of the content to a particular domain of interest and how well the items or tasks represent that domain. Content validity is evaluated by showing how well the content samples the class of situations about which conclusions are to be drawn.[40]

Criterion-related validity is evaluated by comparing the measurement results with one or more external variables, or criteria, that provide a direct measure of the characteristic in question.[40] The criterion is a gold standard by which the proposed measure is compared. Criterion-related validity is based on the degree of empirical relationship (correlation or regression) between the test scores and criterion scores. There are as many criterion-related validity measures as there are criteria.

Criterion-related validity can be divided into predictive and concurrent validity. *Predictive* validity indicates the extent to which future performance correlates with the current measure. *Concurrent* validity indicates the degree to which the measure estimates the present standing on the criterion.

Construct validity is evaluated by investigating the qualities that a test measures. It attempts to determine the degree to which certain explanatory concepts account for the measured results.[40] Construct validity may use any evidence that affects the interpretation or meaning of the measure. Almost any kind of information about a measure may contribute to an understanding of construct validity, but the analysis is stronger if the degree of fit of the information with the theoretical rationale underlying the interpretation is explicitly evaluated.

Today, validity has evolved into a unitary concept.[40] It is no longer neatly packaged into three categories that serve as independent indicators of validity. Many practitioners, especially those in health care, make the mistake of using expert judgment of content (i.e., content validity) as their sole assessment of validity and conclude that the measurement is valid for any use from that point forward. Validity must involve a measure and an intended use. Without a measure, there is no assessment of validity.[40] When validating a measure, what is being tested is not the measurement device, but the inferences about the meaning of the measure and the implications for actions taken based on that result.

Validity is not ensured after one, or even a few, observations. Rather, it is a matter of degree. It builds over time as evidence gathers either for or against the particular use or observation. Thus, validation is essentially a matter of making the most reasonable case to guide not only the current use of a measure but also research to advance understanding of what the score means.

One final issue to consider is that of *external validity*, which is also called generalizability. *Generalizability* is the ability to take the results from one study and apply them to another patient population or setting.[28] In its strictest sense, generalizability is a difficult concept to apply. For example, a study dealt with patients in a hospital in Memphis, Tennessee; there are no assurances that the results would be the same in Madison, Wisconsin. However, one can get a sense of the generalizability by looking at the study population and the study conditions (i.e., the organized health care setting) to determine whether the results are applicable.

ACCEPT OR REJECT THE HYPOTHESIS

The final step in the scientific method is to develop a statement as to whether the hypothesis is accepted or rejected. On the basis of this statement, the investigator then draws conclusions and develops a plan to intervene to effect the desired improvements. All conclusions must be supported by the data. Manipulating or falsifying the conclusions to fit a preconceived notion could cause readers to reject the entire study.

Issues in Medication-Safety Research

The scientific method is broad enough to be applied in virtually any research setting. There are other topics that are more specific to medication-safety research, and it is important that researchers understand them before proceeding with research efforts.

THE MEDICATION-USE SYSTEM

The medication-use system is a process that begins with the decision to prescribe a drug for a patient and ends with monitoring the effects of that drug. This complex process is commonly thought to include four major steps: prescribing, dispensing, administration and monitoring.[42] Physicians, pharmacists, nurses, and patients are the key players in the process. Quality-assessment and quality-improvement activities and research can have their greatest impact when medication use is viewed as a system. The outcomes by which success is judged will be better defined as research results on the medication-use system become more available.

TAXONOMY OF MEDICATION-SAFETY PROBLEMS

Research demands that words be defined and used in common, mutually understood ways. In the patient-safety arena, there is a lot of ambiguity surrounding the taxonomy of patient safety. This can hinder the validity of research and make comparisons of the results between studies difficult to impossible. Some of the taxonomy-related issues that researchers may confront are discussed in this section.

Medication Errors

Medication errors have been the target of safety research for some time.[43] A *medication error* has been defined as "an error in the process of ordering or delivering a medication."[44] In the ambulatory setting, errors would likely center on the prescribing or dispensing processes; in the institutional setting, errors would include the administration of the drug.

There is an important difference between a medication error and the other terms that are sometimes used interchangeably with it. A medication error deals with the *process* of medication use. Adverse drug reactions, adverse drug events, and drug-related morbidity, by contrast, all refer to the *outcomes* of drug use. There are many more "errors" in the system than there are adverse outcomes. Making this distinction is essential in any study and in data-collection methodology.

Many of the strategies employed to reduce medication errors involve targeting individual components of the process, such as order ordering, dispensing systems, or patient compliance, for improvement.[7,20,45,46] Component management operates in isolation from the system as a whole, and its intended impact is rarely realized. This is because one can rarely have an impact on one step in the process without affecting other steps downstream. These downstream effects may cancel the intended outcome. Thus, research efforts need to look across the medication-use system for improvement opportunities.

Researchers must be careful with how medication errors are measured and how causality is attributed. Labeling an event a "medication error" may lead to a misdirected search for causes. Efforts to assign or blame to specific individuals often follow.[47,48] Disciplinary action against the individual(s) identified is often the remedy. By blaming individuals as the cause for the adverse event, important system issues necessary for long-term improvement continue unabated.

Adverse Drug Reactions

The most widely recognized and studied adverse event involving drug therapy is an *adverse drug reaction* (ADR). In 1970, the World Health Organization defined an adverse drug reaction as "any response that is noxious, unintended, and undesired and that occurs at doses normally used in man for prophylaxis, diagnosis, or therapy."[49] Despite its wide use, this definition has limitations. For example, opinions differ as to whether the definition includes the failure to accomplish the intended purpose (drug therapy failure).[20,50] This definition would also call into question efforts to prevent occurrences, since the clinician could not have expected or anticipated them and the usual dose was given.[27]

Preventability received little, if any, attention in early research efforts to define and identify ADRs.[50] System solutions for ADRs are further hindered by the excessive focus on linking a specific drug entity to the adverse event. This is best illustrated by the algorithms developed to assist in identifying the causative agent.[51,52] Focusing on the drug, rather than on the use of the drug, hinders efforts to uncover problems in the medication-use system. The researcher must be open to any causes for the event.

Adverse Drug Events

The term *adverse drug event* (ADE) has been popularized in a series of articles by researchers from Harvard University.[1,2,9,44,53,54] These researchers have defined an ADE as "an injury resulting from the use of a drug."[44] An ADE differs from an ADR in that it relaxes the "normal dosage" requirement and allows for causes other than the drug entity. The definition does not cover patient risk stemming from the lack of drug use when medication therapy is clearly indicated. The definition of an ADE allows preventability to become a focal point for research. Research has suggested that ADEs are not random events but are system dependent.[9]

Drug-Related Morbidity

Drug-related morbidity is defined as the "clinical or biosocial manifestation of unresolved drug-related problems."[55] Drug-related problems are events or circumstances involving drug treatment that actually or potentially interfere with the patient achieving an optimal outcome of medical care.[56] Eight categories of drug-related problems have been defined: (1) untreated indications, (2) improper drug selection, (3) subtherapeutic doses, (4) failure to receive a drug, (5) overdoses, (6) adverse drug reactions, (7) drug interactions, and (8) drug use without indication.[57]

Drug-related problems signal a pattern of care that, if not changed, may lead to DRM. Drug-related problems may serve as the impetus for research to identify patterns in the misuse of medications. Thus, research directed at understanding and correcting drug-related problems may slow or eliminate DRM through changes in the medication-use system at the earliest sign. If research evidence identifies patterns of care indicative of a drug-related problem, prevention of DRM is theoretically possible. By viewing drug-related problems as the precursors to drug-related morbidity, the connection of preventability to a finding of human error is eliminated. This would allow practitioners to move beyond blaming simple causes, such as a person or a drug entity, toward a systematic approach to improving the entire medication-use system.[55]

PREVENTABILITY

For many decades, research on ADE prevention went largely unrecognized. In the 1950s, for example, one often heard adverse events described as "the price we pay" for using these chemical agents or as "a disease of medical progress."[58,59] The attitude was that patients and practitioners must accept the risk because the benefits outweigh any harm. Melmon[60] was one of the early authors to address preventability. He stated that 70 percent to 80 percent of ADRs were predictable.[60] And if such events were predictable, he continued, they should be preventable. His research further debunked the idea that adverse effects were a "disease of medical progress" by stating these events were preventable "without compromise of the therapeutic benefits of the drug."[60]

Approximately 50 percent of DRM is preventable.[1,2,10,15,19,22,23,36,61,62] What is important for the researcher to understand is how to assess preventability. Some may use a scale similar to the 5-point Likert scale and ask a health care professional to indicate whether a certain event was preventable or not on the basis of available information. One study of interest used the word avoidability, rather than preventability, to assess ADRs.[36] These authors classified events as definitely avoidable, possibly avoidable, not avoidable, or unevaluable.[36]

In 1990, Hepler and Strand[56] proposed a more consistent methodology to evaluate preventability of DRM. They used the framework and definition of DRM discussed previously and stated that an adverse outcome attributable to drug therapy could be deemed preventable if

- the adverse outcome was preceded by a recognizable drug therapy problem;
- the adverse outcome of the drug therapy problem had been reasonably foreseeable;
- the cause of the adverse outcome could have been identifiable with reasonable probability; and
- the cause of the adverse outcome could have been reasonably controllable within the context and objectives of therapy.[56]

This methodology may serve as a structured implicit evaluation tool for preventability. Health professionals can use such a tool to develop explicit criteria to assess preventability. Regardless of the methodology used, it is important to assess the preventability of ADEs. This will give the research team direction in designing system interventions to prevent their occurrence.

Implicit, Structured Implicit, and Explicit Review of Alleged Patient-Safety Events

Researchers need one final tool—a method to determine whether an alleged event occurred or not, the severity of patient harm, and whether it could have been prevented. The judgment mechanisms employed in the literature for this purpose can be classified into one of three categories: implicit, structured implicit, and explicit.[63]

IMPLICIT REVIEW

Implicit review in essence is peer review. To carry out such a review, experts compare the level of care provided with a standard that is consistent with their own knowledge, opinions, and beliefs.[63] The literature has many examples of studies where implicit judgment was used to determine the presence of DRM.[1,2,18,19,23] ADR studies have used implicit judgment for years. Kramer and colleagues[52] state that, "the diagnosis of an ADR has usually depended on unspecific clinical judgment, arising from the subjective impression and previous experience of individual clinicians." Thus, implicit review tends to be highly reviewer-dependent. It is often difficult to draw significant conclusions because of the broad responses received from reviewers.[63-65]

Some have suggested that implicit review is so subjective as to be invalid.[66,67] This may be especially true when an expert views a patient chart with the outcome known in advance.[68] This brings the results of the research into question.[65,69] Implicit review also suffers from being very expensive and time-consuming, limiting its usefulness for most health care organizations.[67]

STRUCTURED IMPLICIT REVIEW

A structured implicit review combines the expert's internalized standards with directions that lead reviewers to look at specific issues in care on which judgments are to be made.[63] A common use for structured implicit review has been in the area of ADRs. Algorithms to assess ADRs use a structured process to assist experts in judging their causality.[51,52] Each algorithm provides specific questions that direct practitioners to gather evidence to help them determine the probability of an ADR. A structured implicit review may increase the reliability of the measure because the reviewer can use the checklist to look for certain information in the patient's medical record. However, this method is still labor-intensive and costly.

EXPLICIT REVIEW

Explicit criteria compare the actual care process against a set of statements or criteria.[63] This method is highly reliable and has good predictive validity,[63,68] making it appropriate for use in examining the medication-use system. In addition to good measurement properties, practical support exists for the further development and testing of explicit criteria. Explicit criteria can be assembled into quality measures independent of the chart-review process.[70] This allows the criteria to serve as an ongoing and consistent measure that does not rely on chart review and abstraction. The IOM has recommended that the development of explicit criteria for assessing adverse medication events be a priority.[13]

Despite the potential value of explicit criteria, there are some pitfalls in using them as a research tool. Explicit criteria are only as good as the development process is. Some criteria are from leading experts and are grounded in evidence-based literature; at the other end of the spectrum are practice-based criteria that reflect only the opinions of local physicians.[67] The burden of accuracy falls on the researcher, and the biggest challenge is ensuring that standards to which criteria are compared are valid.[63]

Explicit criteria to evaluate patient safety have been used successfully; for example, to evaluate drug use in the elderly.[71,72] This work provides the opportunity to evaluate the prescribing of medications using explicit criteria developed by an expert panel. However, these criteria evaluated only whether the drug was appropriate or not on the basis of a global indicator. No attempt was made to incorporate clinical information or outcomes data.

Hanlon and colleagues[73] attempted to develop explicit criteria as an index of appropriate medication use in the elderly. They used a 10-item scale that judged the decision making on a broader scale than that of previous attempts.[71] However, they made no attempt to link to the patient outcome to determine the usefulness of the measure.

Recent research has developed definitions for preventable drug-related morbidity that links process and outcome.[74,75] These definitions were translated into explicit criteria and can be used to measure preventable drug-related morbidity using information system technology. The strength of this research is its ability to detect drug-related problems and adverse outcomes together.

Funding for Patient-Safety Research

Progress in patient-safety research field will require extramural funding. Thus, researchers must become familiar with funding sources and their requirements for grant submissions.

Grantsmanship is a skill that all successful researchers must acquire and polish. Persistence is essential: Successful grant writers have a history of failures and have learned from experience. Successful grant writing requires than the researcher clearly and accurately communicate his or her research idea. The request for proposals issued by the granting body must be reviewed carefully before the proposal is submitted to ensure that all necessary components are included. Funding organizations have widely diverse requirements; however, virtually all expect that grantees be able to express their research plan in a manner consistent with the scientific method as described above.

In the patient-safety arena, the biggest single funding source is the federal government. The Agency for Healthcare Research and Quality (AHRQ) is the branch of the government that distributes most patient-safety research grants. This agency has supported a number of patient-safety projects, including the Centers of Excellence for Patient Research and Practice. The funds enable grantees to explore best practices for improving patient safety in multiple care settings, to improve the scientific basis of patient safety research, to improve practitioner education in the patient safety arena, and to evaluate technology that may improve patient safety. AHRQ has also issued grant requests for demonstration projects that would study the use of medical-error data, the use of computers and information technology to prevent medical errors, understanding the health care working environment and its impact on patient safety, and the development of innovative approaches to improving safety.

Private foundations make money available to study patient safety. Chief among these are private foundations such as the Commonwealth Fund, the Robert Wood Johnson Foundation, the Kellogg Foundation, the Kaiser Family Foundation, the Aetna Quality Care Research Fund, the National Patient Safety Foundation, the ASHP Foundation, the Society of Critical Care Medicine, and the Anesthesia Patient Safety Foundation. Each foundation has different requirements for grant proposals. Researchers should monitor these groups' recent grants to determine any areas of common interest between the foundations' priorities and their own.

Other funding sources include the pharmaceutical industry. These grants may often be garnered through contacts with people inside the industry and through limited grant requests.

For any project, multidisciplinary research teams are more appealing to funders than single-discipline projects are. With respect to federal funding, this is particularly true for pharmacists. Few pharmacists have been successful in gaining federal research dollars as principal investigators. However, the doors to this opportunity have never been open wider than they currently are. Increasing the involvement of pharmacists in research will be critical to improving the medication-use system.

A number of Web sites provide up-to-date information on patient-safety research grants. Chief among these is the Community of Science (www.cos.com). This site allows users to search for grant opportunities that match their profiles. At the user's request, the site will e-mail information on patient-safety grants to the researcher on a regular basis.

Other Web sites of interest include the following:

- National Patient Safety Foundation (www.npsf.org)
- AHRQ Center on Patient Safety (www.ahrq.org/patient_safety)
- Leapfrog Group (www.leapfroggroup.org)
- Institute of Medicine (www.iom.edu)
- Veterans Affairs National Center for Patient Safety (www.patientsafety.gov)
- Patient Safety Institute (www.ptsafety.org)
- American Society of Health-System Pharmacists (www.ashp.org)
- Institute for Safe Medication Practices (www.ismp.org)

Conclusion

Being actively engaged in patient-safety research requires that pharmacists become knowledgeable about the scientific process. Knowledge of grant writing, research methods, and statistics is crucial. It is also important that patient-safety researchers continue to refine the taxonomy in the area to improve the consistency of results. By providing research information that can change and improve the medication-use system and save lives, such studies will more than justify their economic costs.

References

1. Bates DW, Cullen DJ, Laird N, Petersen LA, Small SD, Servi D, et al. Incidence of adverse drug events and potential adverse drug events. *JAMA.* 1995;274:29-34.

2. Bates DW, Leape L, Petrycki S. Incidence and preventability of adverse drug events in hospitalized adults. *J Gen Intern Med.* 1993;8:289-294.

3. Brennan TA, Leape L, Laird N, Hebert L, Localio AR, Lawthers AG, et al. Incidence of adverse events and negligence in hospitalized patients. *N Eng J Med.* 1991;324:370-376.

4. Classen DC, Pestotnik SL, Evans RS, Lloyd JF, Burke JP. Adverse drug events in hospitalized patients. *JAMA.* 1999;277:301-306.

5. Cullen DJ, Sweitzer BJ, Bates DW, Burdick E, Edmondson A, Leape L. Preventable adverse drug events in hospitalized patients: a comprehensive study of intensive care and general care units. *Crit Care Med.* 1997; 25:1289-1297.

6. Cunningham G, Dodd TR, Grant DJ, McMurdo MET, Richards RME. Drug-related problems in elderly patients admitted to Tayside hospitals, methods for prevention and subsequent reassessment. *Age Ageing.* 1997;26:375-382.

7. Dartnell JGA, Anderson RP, Chohan V, Galbraith KJ, Lyon MEH, Nestor PJ, et al. Hospitalisation for adverse events related to drug therapy: incidence, avoidability and cost. *Med J Austral.* 1996;164:659-662.

8. Holdsworth MT, Fichtl RE, Behta M, Raisch DW, Mendez-Rico E, Adams A, et al. Incidence and impact of adverse drug events in pediatric patients. *Arch Pediatr.* 2003;157:60-85.

9. Leape L, Brennan TA, Laird N, Lawthers AG, Localio AR, Barnes BA, et al. The nature of adverse events in hospitalized patients. *N Engl J Med.* 1991;324:377-384.

10. Nelson KM, Talbert RL. Drug-related hospital admissions. *Pharmacotherapy.* 1996; 16:701-707.

11. Rothschild JM, Bates DW, Leape LL. Preventable medical injuries in older adults. *Arch Intern Med.* 2000;160:2717-2728.

12. Tafreshi MJ, Melby MJ, Kaback KR, Nord TC. Medication-related visits to the emergency department: a prospective study. *Ann Pharmacother.* 1999;33:1252-1257.

13. Kohn LT, Corrigan JM, Donaldson MD, eds. Committee on Quality of Health in America, Institute of Medicine. *To Err Is Human: Building a Safer Health System.* Washington, DC: National Academy Press; 1999.

14. National Patient Safety Foundation. Agenda for Research and Development in Patient Safety. Arlington, VA: National Patient Safety Foundation. 1999; 1-12.

15. Johnson JA, Bootman JL. Drug-related morbidity and mortality: a cost-of-illness model. *Arch Intern Med.* 1995;155:1949-1956.

16. Ernst FR, Grizzle AJ. Drug-related morbidity and mortality: updating the cost-of-illness model. *J Am Pharm Assoc.* 2001;41:192-199.

17. Heffler S, Smith S, Keehan S, Clemens MK, Won G, Zezza M. Health spending projections for 2002-2012: spending on hospital services and prescription drugs continues to drive health care's share of the economy upward. *Health Aff (Millwood).* 2003;W3:54-65.

18. Bero LA, Lipton HL, Adair Bird J. Characterization of geriatric drug-related hospital admissions. *Med Care.* 1991;29:989-1003.

19. Bigby J, Dunn J, Goldman L, Adams JB, Jen P, Landefeld CS, et al. Assessing the preventability of emergency hospital admissions: a method for evaluating the quality of medical care in a primary care facility. *Am J Med.* 1987;83:1031-1046.

20. Bergman U, Wiholm BE. Drug-related problems causing admission to a medical clinic. *Eur J Clin Pharmacol.* 1981;20:193-200.

21. Lindley CM, Tully MP, Paramsothy V, Tallis RC. Inappropriate medication is a major cause of adverse drug reactions in elderly patients. *Age Ageing.* 1992;21:294-300.

22. Lakshmanan MC, Hershey CO, Breslau D. Hospital admissions caused by iatrogenic disease. *Arch Intern Med.* 1986;146:1931-1934.

23. Hallas J, Gram LF, Grodum E, Damsbo N, Brosen K, Haghfelt T, et al. Drug related admissions to medical wards: a population-based survey. *Br J Clin Pharmacol.* 1992;33:61-68.

24. Caranasos GJ, Stewart RB, Cluff LE. Drug-induced illness leading to hospitalization. *JAMA.* 1974;228:713-717.

25. Winterstein AG, Sauer BC, Hepler CD, Poole C. Preventable drug-related hospital admissions. *Ann Pharmacother.* 2002;36:1238-1248.

26. Talley RB, Laventurier MF. Drug-induced illness. *JAMA.* 1974;229:1043.

27. Lazarou J, Pomeranz BH, Corey PN. Incidence of adverse drug reactions in hospitalized patients. *JAMA.* 1998;279:1200-1205.

28. Gliner JA, Morgan GA. *Research Methods in Applied Settings: An Integrated Approach to Design and Analysis.* Mahwah, NJ: Lawrence Erlbaum Assoc; 2000.

29. *Merriam-Webster's Collegiate Dictionary.* 11th ed. Springfield, MA: Merriam-Webster, Inc; 2003.

30. Drew CJ. *Introduction to Designing and Conducting Research.* St. Louis, MO: CV Mosby Co; 1980.

31. Kerlingea F. *Foundations of Behavioral Research.* 3rd ed. New York: Holt Rinehart & Winston; 1986.

32. Cook TD, Campbell DT. *Quasi-Experimentation: Design & Analysis Issues for Field Settings.* Boston: Houghton Mifflin Company; 1979.

33. Campbell DT, Stanley JC. *Experimental and Quasi-Experimental Design for Research.* Boston: Houghton Mifflin Co; 1963.

34. Glantz SA. *Primer of Biostatistics.* 5th ed. New York: McGraw-Hill; 2002.

35. Ross SD. Drug-related adverse events: A reader's guide to assessing literature reviews and meta-analyses. *Arch Intern Med.* 2001;161:1041-1046.

36. Hallas J, Harvald B, Grodum E, Brosen K, Haghfelt T, Damsbo N. Drug-related hospital admissions: The role of definitions and intensity of data collection, and the possibility of prevention. *J Intern Med.* 1990;228:83-90.

37. Weingart SN, Wilson RM, Gibberd RW, Harrison B. Epidemiology of medical error. *Br Med J.* 2000;320:774-777.

38. Cronbach LJ. *Essentials of Psychological Testing.* 3rd ed. New York: Harper & Row; 1970.

39. Stevens SS. Measurement, statistics, and the schemapiric view. *Science.* 1968;161:849-856.

40. Messick S. Validity. In: Linn ER, ed. *Educational Measurement.* New York: American Council on Education; 1989:13-113.

41. Nadzam DM. Development of medication-use indicators by the Joint Commission on Accreditation of Healthcare Organizations. *Am J Hosp Pharm.* 1991;48:1925-1930.

42. Nadzam DM. A systems approach to medication use. In: Cousins DD, ed. *Medication Use: A Systems Approach to Reducing Errors.* Oak Brook Terrace, IL: Joint Commission on Accreditation of Healthcare Organizations; 1998:5-18.

43. Cohen MR, ed. *Medication Errors.* Washington, DC: American Pharmaceutical Association; 1999.

44. Cullen DJ, Bates DW, Small SD, Cooper JB, Nemeskal R, Leape L. The incident reporting system does not detect adverse drug events. *Jt Comm J Qual Improve.* 1995;21:541-548.

45. Aparasu R, Fliginger SE. Inappropriate medication prescribing for the elderly by office-based physicians. *Ann Pharmacother.* 1997; 31:821-829.

46. Nightingale PG, Adu D, Richards NT, Peters M. Implementation of rules based computerised bedside prescribing and administration: intervention study. *Br Med J.* 2000;320:750-753.

47. Reinersten JL. Let's talk about error. *Br Med J.* 2000;320:730.

48. Berwick DM, Leape L. Reducing errors in medicine. *Br Med J.* 1999;319:136-137.

49. World Health Organization. International drug monitoring: the role of the hospital—a WHO report. *Drug Intell Clin Pharm.* 1970;4:101-110.

50. Karch FE, Lasagna L. Adverse drug reactions: a critical review. *JAMA.* 1975;234:1236-1241.

51. Naranjo CA, Busto U, Sellers EM, Sandor P, Ruiz I, Roberts EA, et al. A method for estimating the probability of adverse drug reactions. *Clin Pharmacol Ther.* 1981;30:239-245.

52. Kramer MS, Leventhal JM, Hutchinson TA, Feinstein AR. An algorithm for the operational assessment of adverse drug reactions. *JAMA.* 1979;242:623-632.

53. Bates DW, Boyle BA, Vander Vliet MB, Schneider J, Leape L. Relationships between medication errors and adverse drug events. *J Gen Intern Med.* 1995;10:199-205.

54. Bates DW, Spell N, Cullen DJ, Burdick E, Laird N, Petersen LA, et al. The cost of adverse drug events in hospitalized patients. *JAMA.* 1997;277:307-311.

55. Hepler CD, Grainger-Rousseau TJ. Pharmaceutical care versus traditional drug treatment: Is there a difference? *Drugs.* 1995;49:1-10.

56. Hepler CD, Strand LM. Opportunities and responsibilities in pharmaceutical care. *Am J Hosp Pharm.* 1990;47:533-543.

57. Strand LM, Morley PC, Cipolle RJ, Ramsey R, Lamsam GD. Drug-related problems: their

structure and function. *DICP.* 1990;24:1093-1097.

58. Barr DP. Hazards of modern diagnosis and therapy—the price we pay. *JAMA.* 1955; 159:1452-1456.

59. Moser RH. Diseases of medical progress. *N Engl J Med.* 1956;255:606-614.

60. Melmon KL. Preventable drug reactions—causes and cures. *N Engl J Med.* 1971; 284:1361-1368.

61. Culler SD, Parchman ML, Przybylski M. Factors related to potentially preventable hospitalizations among the elderly. *Med Care.* 1998;36:804-817.

62. Dubois RW, Brook RH. Preventable deaths: who, how often and why? *Ann Intern Med.* 1988;109:582-589.

63. Ashton CM, Kuykendall DH, Johnson ML, Wray NP. An empirical assessment of the validity of explicit and implicit process-of-care criteria for quality assessment. *Med Care.* 1999;37:798-808.

64. Karch FE, Smith CL, Kerzner MB, Mazzullo JM, Weintraub M, Lasagna L. Commentary: Adverse drug reactions—a matter of opinion. *Clin Pharmacol Ther.* 1976;19:489-492.

65. Thomas EJ, Brennan TA. Incidence and types of preventable adverse events in elderly patients: population based review of medical records. *Br Med J.* 2000;320:741-744.

66. Lipton HL, Bird JA. Drug utilization review in ambulatory settings: state of the art science and directions for outcomes research. *Med Care.* 1993;31:1069-1082.

67. Donabedian A. The quality of medical care: methods for assessing and monitoring the quality of care for research and for quality assurance programs. *Science.* 1978;200:856-864.

68. Caplan RA, Posner KL, Cheney FW. Effect of outcome on physician judgments of appropriateness of care. *JAMA.* 1991;265:1957-1960.

69. Brennan TA. The Institute of Medicine report on medical errors—Could it do harm? *N Engl J Med.* 2000;342:1123-1125.

70. Geraci JM, Ashton CM, Kuykendall DH, Johnson ML, Souchek J, Junco DD, et al. The association of quality of care and occurrence of in-hospital, treatment-related complications. *Med Care.* 1999;37:140-148.

71. Beers MH, Ouslander JG, Rollingher I, Reuben DB, Brooks J, Beck JC. Explicit criteria for determining inappropriate medication use in nursing home residents. *Arch Intern Med.* 1991;151:1825-1832.

72. Beers MH. Explicit criteria for determining potentially inappropriate medication use by the elderly. *Arch Intern Med.* 1997;157:1531-1536.

73. Hanlon JT, Schmader KE, Samsa GP, Weinberger M, Uttech KM, Lewis IK, et al. A method for assessing drug therapy appropriateness. *J Clin Epidemiol.* 1992;45:1045-1051.

74. MacKinnon NJ, Hepler CD. Preventable drug-related morbidity in older adults: 1. Indicator development. *J Managed Care Pharm.* 2002;8:365-371.

75. Faris, RJ. Explicit definitions to identify preventable drug-related morbidity in an elderly population and their use as an indicator of quality in the medication use system. [unpublished dissertation]. University of Florida; 2001.

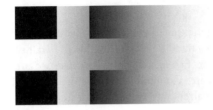

The Role of the Patient and Family in Preventing Medication Errors

Roxanne J. Goeltz

Introduction

The stories in this chapter are based on my own experiences and on experiences related to me by friends and family. In each story is a lesson to be learned—sometimes for the patient, sometimes for the health care worker, but most often for both. This chapter is from my heart as well as from my head.

I am an air traffic controller by trade. Teamwork and systems thinking are embedded in our work ethic. Ensuring safety is the core value of our culture. The errors that occur in our industry are examined from a systems view in order to determine whether or not that system supported the individuals involved in the error. This is not an easy task; the initial human reaction to error is to find someone to blame or take responsibility. In the world of air traffic, we have discovered that it is safer, more effective, and more efficient to work as a team and to be accountable to each other than to place blame on individuals.

I was drawn to the patient-safety movement for personal reasons; most importantly, the death of my brother Mike as the result of a health care system failure. I have also been treated for cancer in recent years and have had several opportunities to witness firsthand how health care workers interact with each other and with patients and their lay caregivers. From my reference point, the Institute of Medicine's recommendation that health care be culturally transformed into an activity that is patient centered and systems based is right on the money.[1] We have much to accomplish to make this vision a reality.

Key Role of Communication

Communication breakdowns among caregivers and between caregivers and patients are a major cause of errors. The lack of open and full disclosure surrounding even some of the smallest incidents has created distrust between the people providing care and those receiving it.

My brother's death was the result of numerous communication errors that ended in a fatal misdiagnosis. His death was my first experience of health care's "wall of silence" when an error occurs. The disbelief and betrayal I felt following that incident fueled my desire to make positive change. I have learned that as a patient I have a responsibility to help my health care team make my experience as safe as possible. I was not aware of this responsibility or, to be more accurate, did not want to accept it, until my brother's death.

Health care workers, especially physicians, are taught that they are responsible. Their model is perfection. When an error occurs, it is this misguided belief that builds the wall of distrust between those caring and those being cared for. Errors will occur because we are human: what makes the difference is how we communicate. Communicating before an error occurs is a step toward error prevention. Communication after an error occurs is a step toward healing and learning how to prevent a similar error from happening to someone else.

Why do we have to be more responsible patients? Why can't health care workers just do better jobs? More than one physician has told me that it is a sad state of affairs when patients and family members have to remind providers to wash their hands before touching them to prevent the spread of infection. This may be an unfortunate situation, but it is a reality, and we must deal in reality if we are going to make health care safer. We must acknowledge that it's a good sign when patients ask health care workers to wash their hands before touching them. It means that patients are trying to be partners; they are doing what they can to take responsible roles in their care. It is not an easy role to assume. Many patients have been taught not to question; now, they are being asked to do it for their own safety.

Patients today need not only to ask questions but also to become actively involved in decision making. Decisions can no longer be made for us; the ultimate decision maker is the patient or his or her appointed representative. Patients want to trust that health care workers know what they are doing and will do their best to care for them, but the culture in which health professionals work does not always provide the support that they need to make patients' expectations a reality. We enter a system that has failed to learn from mistakes and therefore continues to make them.

When my brother died, I found out how unsafe our health care system is. When I began to learn how complex the health system is, I became overwhelmed. I wanted to be involved in improving health care, but did not know what to do or how to do it. I began sharing my story with others, and others began sharing their stories with me. It is through stories that I have learned to be a partnering patient. It has not been easy, because I did not always know what I was trying to do, and it was hard to find someone in health care who was willing to help me figure it out.

Medication use is a key part of safe care. The stories that follow focus on barriers to safe medication use and how they can be overcome. In each story, good communication could have been the link that prevented a break in the chain of events leading to an error. Some of these stories had tragic consequences, but if we learn from them then the families' losses will have not been in vain.

Stories

STORY 1

Nine months after my brother Mike died, I developed a tumor in my chest cavity. Having learned a great deal from his experience, I was determined to be an active patient and do my part to make my experience safe. I called together my own team—a group of family and friends who would stay with me around the clock while I was in the hospital. They worked with the nurses and doctors, reviewing my medications and asking questions when I could not.

Despite these precautions, the day after my surgery, I developed a pulmonary embolism. In hindsight, there were things that could have been done better to prevent this complication, including my own education on the need for movement after surgery. Because of the embolism, I was put on anticoagulation therapy for a year.

During that year, I had to undergo a second surgery for suspected ovarian cancer. I met with the doctor who had prescribed my anticoagulation therapy to discuss what needed to be done before I could have my second surgery. He told me I was at high risk for this surgery and that I would have to stop taking my anticoagulation tablets four days before surgery. At that time, I would receive twice-daily injections of Lovenox®. Twenty-four hours before surgery, I would stop the injections. The anticoagulant could be resumed immediately after surgery. I asked a couple questions that I had written down. He said a nurse would call me to set up training for giving myself the shots.

I came in for my training. All went well until the nurse started to go over the orders for taking my medicine. What she told me was different from what I thought my doctor had said. I knew that this medicine, as well as the consequences of not using it properly, could be deadly. I also knew my surgery could be delayed if I did not stop receiving it prior to surgery. I did not relish questioning this woman, and her demeanor was not the most inviting, but I had learned that I needed to speak up, and so I did. Her response was defensive; she stated she was reading what the doctor had written in my chart. She read it to me. I realized there was indeed a discrepancy between my understanding and what the doctor had written in the chart. I told her again something was not right, and she offered to verify the orders with the doctor. Later that day, she called me and said that I should do what the doctor and I had discussed during my appointment. She had misunderstood his written instructions.

What lesson do we learn from this story? Communication, whether verbal or written, has the potential for error. The patient who listens, and who is listened to, can be a stopgap for error.

STORY 2

This story is also based on my own experience and likewise concerns my anticoagulation therapy. Following my second surgery, my dosage was lowered to 2.5 mg daily, 6 days a week, and 10 mg on the seventh day. My original prescription was for 5-mg tablets. This meant that I had to slice the tablets in half. This became a hassle; moreover, I knew that if I lost some of the medication, my dose could be inaccurate. I asked for prescriptions for 10- and 2.5-mg tablets. When my supply of 5-mg pills ran out, I took these new prescriptions to the pharmacy. It was the same pharmacy I always used.

I returned later in the day to pick them up. The clerk asked me how many packages there should be, and I said two. When she handed me just one package, I knew something was wrong. I looked at the label and noted the physician's name was not correct. The name listed was the surgeon from my first surgery, and it should have been the discharging physician from my second surgery. I started to understand what I thought had happened. I had refills left on the original prescription, and the pharmacist had filled the original prescription, rather than the two new ones.

The pharmacist stepped up and started giving me instructions on how to use the 5-mg tablets. I said, "This is not the prescription I turned in," and he said, "It is the same medicine; you just have to cut the pill in half." I said, "I realize that, but again, this is not the prescription I just turned in. Why was this one filled, and not the two I turned in?" He said, "I assumed you would prefer this one because there are two copayments involved with the prescriptions you turned in." When I heard the word "assumed," my antennae went up. One of the first things that an air traffic controller learns is never to assume anything. Always communicate until you *know*. The same applies for health care, which is also a high-risk industry.

What is the lesson in this example? Communication prevents assumptions from becoming errors. Pay attention to what you pick up at the pharmacy. When getting a prescription from your physician, write down the name of the medication. Ask how to spell it. Confirm the strength and dosage. Ask whether there are generic brands that may be substituted and what are they (your insurer may pay only for generic products). When you pick up the prescription, look at the label. Are the doctor's name, your name, and the name of the medication correct? Does the dosage match what you wrote down in the office? Even if you have gotten this medication before, take a look at it and make sure it is correct. If it is not, ask the pharmacist.

STORY 3

One of my friends takes two medications, one for allergies and one for a thyroid condition. Both tablets are yellow, but they look quite different. She has been a registered nurse for 30 years and knows to check the information on the prescription label. She did this when she picked up the two refills from her pharmacy. The labels were correct.

A few days later, her allergies were bothering her. She took an allergy tablet; later, she took two more on schedule. By this time she was feeling worse, and was wondering why her medications were not working. She then noted that her toes had started twitching (which indicated something was wrong, although she was not sure what). She looked at her medications and realized the pills she thought were allergy pills were actually her thyroid medication. When the prescriptions were filled, the tablets had been put into the wrong bottles! She was feeling so ill because of her allergies that she did not notice that she was taking the thyroid pills.

She was an educated, able-bodied person, and a health professional to boot. But because she was not feeling well, she did not see something that normally would be obvious. If my friend could have such a problem, think of what might happen to a person who is elderly or not versed in paying attention to these kinds of things.

What is the lesson in this case? Know how your medications work. What are signs that you have taken an overdose? How long should they take to work?

STORY 4

A woman took her mother to the hospital for admission. She brought along the three medications her mother was taking. She gave the medications to the health care workers and was assured that her mother would receive them while in the hospital.

The next day, the mother collapsed. She went through a series of tests. The health team told the family that they did not know what was wrong. On the third day, the woman discovered her mother had not been receiving two of the medications she had brought with her. She had collapsed because she was not receiving her seizure medication and her blood pressure medication. When the medications were resumed, the patient recovered.

The daughter came to me with her story and said, "What more could we have done but bring in the bottles of medications? Do we have to count the pills each time we visit to ensure she is being given her medications? We trusted them to care for her. The anxiety to our family, the unnecessary poking and prodding of my mother, not to mention the cost of the tests, could have been avoided if they had simply listened to us."

What lesson is learned here? Communication again comes to mind. When patients and families give input, health care providers appear to be listening, but they may not really be hearing what is said. We talk about the cost of error. What was the cost in this situation? There was certainly a cost for unneeded tests. A far greater cost was the suffering of the patient and family and the loss of trust between her family and the care team.

STORY 5

An elderly patient had liver, lung, and bone cancer, but the lung and bone cancer were in remission. She was hospitalized for a bladder infection. Her physician prescribed sublingual morphine, to be administered hourly, for pain relief. Instead, she was given a long-term, time-release morphine tablet (a form that is less time-consuming for staff to administer).

The patient became comatose. Three days later, she came out of the coma but was depressed and could not drink or talk. The family was told about the morphine substitution. They asked the nurse not to give her the time-release tablet. The nurse said she would inform the doctor, but the original order was never removed from the patient's chart. The patient was given another time-release tablet that evening. She went into a coma again and died two weeks later. The nurse who administered the tablet apologized for overmedicating their mother.

The lesson from this tragic experience is that we cannot leave our loved ones alone. If, because of staff shortages, treatment is based on the availability of staff rather than on patient need, we need to step in to help. We need to do whatever we can to keep patients safe. Family members are part of the health care team.

STORY 6

One of my coworkers had been taking medication for hypertension for quite some time. He developed side effects. He discussed the problem with his physician, who changed the medication.

A month or so later, his wife asked him what was wrong. He did not seem to be his lively, chatty self lately. My friend said, "I'm fine." A couple of people at work made the same observation. Finally, the wife convinced her husband to go to the doctor. She went along. The wife described her husband's personality change and some other things she has noticed. The doctor then said the word "depression."

Up to this point, my coworker did not think he had a problem, even though everyone around him did. It was not until the doctor mentioned the possibility of depression did my coworker become seriously concerned. He knew that his doctor's comment put his job at risk, because anyone in our profession who is suspected of being depressed cannot continue to have a medical clearance to work. The depression must be treated before medical clearance is reinstated. My colleague started thinking about how poorly he'd been feeling and realized that it began at about the same time that he started taking the new medication.

The doctor, who was not the same one who had prescribed the new antihypertensive agent, checked the patient's chart. He noted the dosage in the chart was not the dosage listed on the prescription bottle and indicated that my coworker had been taking twice the normal dose of this agent. The doctor who ordered the medication had used a computerized physician order entry (CPOE) device. The pharmacy received this order with the larger dose. The use of a CPOE was new to the doctor and this particular health clinic. Review of the situation would be vital to ensure there is not a problem with the software or hardware that make up the CPOE system for this health care group.

My coworker shared his story with me and asked what he should do. He wanted to make sure this did not happen to someone else. Since he and I are in a profession that looks at its errors and then figures out what to do, he wanted to do that in this situation. I advised him to call his health care provider and to explain that he wanted to talk about the experience.

This story illustrates the dangerous consequences of not taking an active role in your health care, especially when it has to do with medication use. If my coworker had done the things suggested in the other stories presented above, namely, reviewed names and dosages of medication, this error would have been caught before it affected him physically. He was lucky to have had a persistent wife and observant coworkers.

This story is also a good example of how systems thinking can be used to review the error. The health care professional's normal course of action is to blame the individuals involved—for example, to say that the doctor typed it wrong or that the pharmacist did not catch the dosage error. With systems evaluation of an error in air traffic, the assumption is that the individuals involved did their jobs; the purpose of the evaluation is to focus on how the system supported or failed them. A systems evaluation provides a broad picture, rather than a narrow view of individual behavior. It also takes a team-centered approach. Instead of singling out an individual, it looks at the total process and the parts played by all, including the patient, who had an opportunity to catch this error as well.

STORY 7

A friend was hospitalized, gravely ill with *Escherichia coli* infection. She was being desensitized to a drug to which she was allergic because it was needed to save her life. The immunologist spent eight hours in her room getting her through the desensitization process.

The doctor then turned to my friend and said, "Now, I'm going to tell you something very important and ask you to make me a promise. This drug must remain in your system until we beat the bacteria. The fluid in this i.v. bag lasts for 12 hours. This means that it must be replaced at 1:00 a.m. and 1:00 p.m., exactly. You cannot let a bag become empty before replacing it with another. You must promise to make sure this happens because if you do not, it will not get done! Medications are often administered late—by minutes or even by hours. Normally, it is not a big deal. For you, it is. At the least, we would have to do the desensitizing all over. At the worst, you could die. Promise me." My friend, along with her family members who were present in the room, promised to do what the doctor asked.

As 1:00 p.m. approached, her son went to the nursing station to inquire about the medication. The nurse said that the medication would be coming from the pharmacy soon. He said, "I would like you to call and get the medications here so they are in my mother's room and ready to be changed at 1:00 p.m." The nurse replied, "Don't worry, they will be here soon. We will take care of it." He said, "No, that will not do. My mother needs her medication bag changed out at 1:00 p.m., and not any later. I would like to see it in her room and ready before then." The nurse continued to try and placate the son, until he finally threatened to call the doctor.

This man was able to make such a statement because the doctor had given him and his family permission to do so by asking them to promise. This empowered the patient and family to become partners in care. Had they not been empowered, they more than likely would have fallen into the role so many of us do when we enter the health care system. We tell ourselves that our gut instincts are wrong. We think, "They know what they are doing; they are taking care of us." None of us wants to be the "difficult" patient or family member, but as partners in our health care we do have the right to be listened to.

If you are a health provider, the next time you encounter a difficult patient or a demanding family member, stop and listen to what they are saying. You may be surprised at what you learn. Many of us who have experienced error in health care remember hearing words such as, "Don't worry" or "We'll will take good care of her," and realize that if we had pushed, our loved one might still be alive or costly complications might have been avoided.

The immunologist in this story was aware of problems associated with late delivery of medications. But why was it necessary to make the patient promise to take responsibility? Why didn't the immunologist just did write it on the medication order? I am sure she did, but that might not necessarily have made a difference. The doctor knew that the one thing that would ensure the medication was delivered in a timely manner would be the active involvement of the patient or a family member.

The nurse in this case reacted in a predictable way. She was responsible for administering medications to many patients and for other duties as well. The unit may have been understaffed, a situation that, as I learned with my pulmonary embolism experience, can be even more challenging. It is important to use all members of the team to ensure that care is the safest it can be. The sooner we take advantage of and encourage the use of all members of the team, the better.

Conclusion

We need to educate patients and families in the roles they can play in error prevention, encourage them gently, and praise them for their input. Look at communications among caregivers and between caregivers and patients. Open your hearts to the fact we are all human and that we need the support of everyone to make sure that health care becomes safer for everyone.

Reference

1. Kohn LT, Corrigan JM, Donaldson MD, eds. Committee on Quality of Health in America, Institute of Medicine. *To Err Is Human: Building a Safer Health System.* Washington, DC: National Academy Press; 1999.